Renal Cell Carcinoma

Renal Cell Carcinoma

Immunotherapy and
Cellular Biology

edited by

Eric A. Klein
Ronald M. Bukowski
James H. Finke

The Cleveland Clinic Foundation
Cleveland, Ohio

Marcel Dekker, Inc.   **New York • Basel • Hong Kong**

Library of Congress Cataloging-in-Publication Data

Renal cell carcinoma: immunotherapy and cellular biology / edited by
    Eric A. Klein, Ronald M. Bukowski, James H. Finke.
        p.   cm.
    Includes bibliographical references and index.
    ISBN 0-8247-9033-2
    1. Kidneys--Cancer--Immunotherapy--Congresses. 2. Cytokines-
-Therapeutic use--Congresses. I. Klein, Eric A.
II. Bukowski, Ronald M. III. Finke, James H.
    [DNLM: 1. Carcinoma, Renal Cell--therapy--congresses.
    2. Immunotherapy--congresses. 3. Combined Modality Therapy-
-congresses. 4. Immunity, Cellular--congresses. WJ 358 R393 1993]
    RC280.K5R46 1993
    616.99'46106--dc20   93-20036
    DNLM/DLC   CIP

MARCEL DEKKER, INC.
270 Madison Avenue, New York, New York 10016

Current printing (last digit):
10 9 8 7 6 5 4 3 2 1

PRINTED IN THE UNITED STATES OF AMERICA

In memory of Milton Klein

Foreword

This book is a compilation of current scientific knowledge of the immunology and molecular biology of renal cell carcinoma. In the 100 years since the first case of spontaneous regression of renal cell carcinoma was reported, clinicians and researchers have been perplexed and fascinated by the peculiarities of this disease. Only in the last decade, however, have investigative tools become available, through the use of monoclonal antibodies and molecular and cytogenetic probes, to help us understand the complexities of this system. It is unlikely that a spectacular breakthrough will be forthcoming to eliminate the previously unsolvable problems of therapy for the patient with metastatic renal cell carcinoma. More likely, small pieces of the enormously complex puzzle of renal cell carcinoma will be painstakingly pieced together by many different laboratories.

It is in this context that the Second International Symposium on the Immunobiology of Renal Cell Carcinoma assumes its vital role. Instant communication among researchers worldwide is now feasible with electronic data transfer, but that communication will not happen unless a forum is established to initiate the dialog of common interest. Sharing information will minimize unnecessary duplication, stimulate alternative approaches, and verify areas of uncertainty. The First International Symposium on the Immunobiology of Renal Cell Carcinoma, in 1989, sponsored by The Cleveland Clinic Foundation and partially supported by the National Cancer Institute and private grants, was a pioneering effort to bring together the best scientists in this field. That symposium was an immense success and a second symposium was held in 1991.

This is a field with rapid improvements in technological methods and brisk expansion of clinical trials. The information presented herein will hopefully provide a stimulus for research efforts by those who have long been frustrated by dilemmas of understanding and treating renal cell carcinoma.

James E. Montie, M.D.
J. Edson Pontes, M.D.
Department of Urology
Wayne State University
School of Medicine
Detroit, Michigan

Preface

The treatment of advanced renal cell carcinoma is one of the most challenging problems facing oncologists today. More than half of the patients with newly diagnosed renal cancers present with tumors that are not curable by surgery alone. The relative ineffectiveness of standard chemotherapeutic regimens and the lack of adjuvant therapies for patients at high risk of relapse make treatment of these patients difficult at best.

Conceptual and technological advances in the fields of immunology and molecular biology have recently allowed progress in our understanding of the genetic origin of human tumors and their interaction with the immune system. Renal cell carcinoma became a prime target for study within these fields because of the relatively easy availability of normal kidney and tumor tissue, the existence of renal cancer in a familial form (von Hippel-Lindau disease), and long-standing observations suggesting that renal cell carcinoma is an immunologically active tumor.

The burgeoning knowledge in those fields and the development of immune-based therapies led us to organize the First International Symposium on the Immunobiology of Renal Cell Carcinoma in October 1989, sponsored by The Cleveland Clinic Foundation. For the first time in the era of molecular genetics, a range of scientists that included medical oncologists, urologists, and members of biotechnology corporations gathered to share their knowledge. The major themes of that symposium included the detailed characterization of lymphokine-activated killer cells and tumor-infiltrating lymphocytes, clinical and laboratory efforts designed to understand and improve cell-based immune therapy, reports on early trials of cytokine-based therapies, initial efforts in gene transfection of tumor-infiltrating lymphocytes and tumor cells, and the role of monoclonal antibodies in antigen characterization and therapy. A session on molecular biology also included descriptions of efforts to isolate a putative tumor suppressor gene on chromosome 3, the role of oncogenes in the progression of renal cell carcinoma, and molecular characterization of the multidrug resistance phenotype in renal tumors.

These reports laid the groundwork for continued investigations, and based on a very enthusiastic response from symposium participants, we held the Second International Symposium on the Immunobiology of Renal Cell Carcinoma in October 1991. The general themes of this symposium paralleled those of the first, although some changes in emphasis become apparent. Significant progress has been made in the last few years in identifying the gene associated with von Hippel-Lindau disease. The focus of cell-based immunity and therapy has shifted away from peripheral blood cells to tumor-infiltrating lymphocytes. Less toxic and outpatient cytokine-based treatments have emerged, with much anticipation regarding new cytokines alone or in combination with standard chemotherapeutic regimens. Reports of antitumor efficacy of cytokine-gene transfected tumor cells in the animal model are most exciting. This work has formed the basis for gene therapy of renal cell carcinoma, and this therapy is just beginning initial clinical trials.

This volume chronicles the proceedings of the 1991 symposium. We are grateful to the participants for their earnest presentations and contributions to this book. We hope that this volume will serve as a compendium of the basic and clinical immunobiologic aspects of renal cell carcinoma, a snapshot of knowledge in this field. Moreover, we hope that it will serve as a springboard for further advances in our understanding of renal cell carcinoma. In conclusion, we wish to thank Cynthia Jarrell of The Cleveland Clinic Cancer Center and Robin Fayman of Marcel Dekker, Inc., for their help in the preparation of this volume.

Eric A. Klein
Ronald M. Bukowski
James H. Finke

Contents

III The Molecular Biology of Renal Cell Carcinoma

IV Cell-Mediated Immune Responses and Adoptive Immunotherapy

I

The Challenge of Advanced Renal Cell Carcinoma

1

Overview

Eric A. Klein

The Cleveland Clinic Foundation, Cleveland, Ohio

Renal cell carcinoma accounts for about 3% of adult malignancies and is the third most common type of urologic tumor after cancers of the prostate and bladder. Its peak incidence occurs in the sixth and seventh decades. Males are more commonly affected than females by a 2:1 ratio. In 1989 there were approximately 23,000 new cases of renal cancer in the United States and more than 10,000 deaths (1). Most patients with localized tumors can be cured by surgical resection, and the incidence of incidentally discovered low-stage tumors that are amenable to partial or total nephrectomy appears to be increasing (2). Still, more than half of the new cases each year present with regionally advanced or metastatic disease, and these patients face a collective median survival of 7 months and a 1–2% chance of surviving 5 years or more (3).

The management of advanced renal tumors is problematic. Neither chemotherapy nor radiotherapy has proven efficacy in the management of bulky locoregional, metastatic, or locally recurrent disease. Surgery is the primary therapy for locally advanced or large tumors that have not invaded adjacent organs or metastasized. Recent reports have suggested a survival advantage in those patients undergoing extended regional lymphadenectomy concurrently with radical nephrectomy, documenting 5 and 10 year survival rates of 50 and 25%, respectively, in patients with resected microscopically positive lymph nodes (4). Patients with tumors that penetrate the perirenal fat, with positive surgical margins, or with unsuspected regional nodal metastases are at higher risk for local and distant recurrence. Although the need for additional treatment in these patients is manifest, there are no currently available adjuvant therapies with documented efficacy in lowering the incidence of tumor recurrence.

Locally advanced tumors as defined by extension of tumor thrombi into the renal vein or inferior vena cava do not carry a diminished prognosis in the absence of extension into perirenal fat or nodal metastases (5). En bloc excision of primary tumors with thrombi extending above the hepatic veins may require the use of carciac bypass or hypothermic circulatory arrest for complete removal (6,7). Although survival rates in these patients are similar to those without thrombi on a stage-for-stage basis, there is a higher risk of operative complication with the use of these specialized surgical techniques.

Surgery is also appropriate in selected patients with apparently solitary metastatic lesions. These are patients with pulmonary or bony metastases with a good performance status in whom resection of the metastasis does not result in a significant deficit in the patient's ability to function on a day-to-day basis. One series documented a 5 year survival of 33% in 40 patients undergoing radical nephrectomy and resection of metastasis from the lung, bones, brain, or retroperitoneum (8). Like patients with disseminated tumors, however, most patients with synchronous or metachronous solitary metastases are not cured surgically and would also be well-served by the development of effective adjuvant therapy.

The role of adjuvant nephrectomy in the face of more widely metastatic cancer is controversial. Significant local or systemic symptoms, such as pain, anemia secondary to hematuria, Budd-Chiari syndrome, uncontrollable hypercalcemia, or cardiac failure secondary to arteriovenous shunting, can be effectively palliated by nephrectomy. Spontaneous regressions following nephrectomy have been reported in patients with minimal pulmonary metastases, but most have not been documented histologically (9). Early reports of renal angioinfarction and delayed nephrectomy in conjunction with systemic progestins documented a 15% objective response rate but few long-term cures (10). Early evidence on the potential beneficial effect on response rates to immunotherapy by pretreatment nephrectomy is inconclusive, and decisions on nephrectomy in this setting must be individualized until the results of randomized trails are known. One disadvantage of pretreatment nephrectomy is that a significant proportion of patients (19% in the Cleveland Clinic experience) may be prevented from receiving therapy because of intercurrent tumor progression, operative complications, or insufficient renal function (unpublished observation).

Traditional chemotherapeutic approaches to the treatment of locally advanced and disseminated renal cancer have been ineffective, with overall objective response rates of the order of 10% (11). This resistance reflects the general insensitivity of adenocarcinomas to most chemotherapeutic agents, as well as the biologic heterogeneity of primary tumors and their metastases. Patient selection factors are also important in predicting response to chemotherapy. Those with good performance status and minimal pulmonary or nodal metastases generally respond better than those with more extensive disease (11). Approximately 70% of renal tumors retain the ability to express the multidrug resistance gene (MDR1), which confers resistance to such agents as Adriamycin (doxorubicin) and vinblastine (12). The earliest clinical trials using agents that reverse multidrug resistance in vitro failed to show an increase in response rates in nonrenal tumors (12). At present it is unclear whether this phenotype is a clinically important mediator of resistance in renal cancer, and it remains to be seen if currently available agents are capable of circumventing this phenomenon. Several trials designed to assess this in renal cancer are currently underway. It is likely that further advances in the chemotherapy of renal cell carcinoma will depend upon improved understanding of this and other specific mechanisms of drug resistance at the cellular level.

Poor clinical responses have also been seen with hormonal agents known to exhibit antitumor activity in animal models of renal cancer. Yagoda summarized results from 58 clinical trials, including more than 1400 patients treated with progestins, androgens, antiandrogens, or combination therapy, and found a 9–17% overall response rate (11). Recent experimental evidence on hormone receptor levels in renal tumors do not support a role for these agents in the treatment of renal cancer (13).

The poor results obtained with conventional therapies has led to attempts to modulate the immune system in patients with advanced renal tumors. Renal cancer has long been an object of interest in this regard because of circumstantial evidence that renal tumors are immunologically active. This evidence includes (1) the preponderance of renal cell carcinoma among cases of spontaneously regressing tumors, with more than 50 such cases on record (14); (2) experimental demonstrations of specific immune cell-mediated tumor lysis (15–17); and (3) occasional reports of responses to such agents as immune xenogeneic RNA, bacillus Calmette-Guérin (BCG), *Corynebacterium parvum*, and tumor vaccines that presumably work by modulation of immune effectors (18).

In the early 1980s, Rosenberg reported on the efficacy of a subset of lymphocytes that when appropriately stimulated could selectively lyse a variety of fresh tumor cells in vitro. When isolated from peripheral blood, stimulated in tissue culture with the lymphocyte growth factor interleukin-2 (IL-2), and reinfused into patients with additional IL-2, these lymphocytes (lymphokine-activated killer, LAK, cells) also demonstrated the ability to cause regression of human tumors in vivo. These observations served as the foundation for what is now known as adoptive immunotherapy and spawned further efforts to understand and improve this mode of therapy.

Of particular interest is the identification of the cells within the population of LAK cells that are most active against tumors and the development of ways of improving their tumoricidal activity. An initial approach was the isolation of the lymphocytes contained within excised tumors rather than from peripheral blood. The hypothesis was that lympocytes within a tumor, known as tumor-infiltrating lymphocytes (TIL), have a higher specificity for tumor cell lysis than those in the peripheral blood (19). A limited number of clinical trials have demonstrated that infusion of TIL is roughly equivalent in efficacy to LAK cells against renal tumors.

In parallel with trials of adoptive immunotherapy have been other efforts using relatively nonspecific immune modulators, such as interferon-α, interferon-γ, and tumor necrosis factor, as well as specific cytokine T cell growth factors. The overall response rate seen with these forms of biologic therapy has ranged from 10 to 35%, suggesting a modest improvement in responses over conventional chemotherapy. Although the optimum agents, routes of administration, and patient selection factors for this therapy have not been established, several general principals have emerged from experimental trials. Like chemotherapy, patients treated with immunotherapy who have isolated pulmonary metastases and small tumor burdens respond best. The combination of interleukin-2 and LAK cells appears to be no more effective than IL-2 alone, although there may be a slightly higher incidence of complete response when combined therapy is used (20). IL-2 appears to be more toxic than interferon alone, although responses to IL-2 are probably more durable. A combination of IL-2 and interferon produces response rates similar to those seen with either agent alone, without a resultant decrease in toxicity (20). Limited clinical experience with other agents, including novel combined chemoimmunotherapy approaches, preclude generalizations about their activity at present. Current trials with many of these agents are described in this volume.

A great deal of current research effort is being devoted to understanding the mechanisms by which modulation of the immune system might eradicate renal tumors. One exciting advance has been the recognition of specific cytolytic T cell clones derived from tumors, which exhibit marked specificity for autologous tumor (16,17). There is also mounting evidence that suggests that a subpopulation of TIL may respond to autologous tumor by cytokine secretion without displaying lytic activity (16). New evidence also suggests that although TIL isolated from renal cell carcinoma have the capacity to secrete cytoklines, many display a low proliferative response to a variety of stimuli (21). These and other factors in the T cell-tumor cell interaction remain to be elucidated.

Current state of the art immunotherapy appears to represent a modest advance over conventional therapy in the treatment of renal cell carcinoma. In addition to understanding the specifics of cell–cell interaction in the immune response, further understanding and reduction of immune-related toxicities must be achieved. Additional clinical trials are necessary to optimize patient selection factors and to select the best agents with optimal treatment schedules. Other molecular and technologically based therapies have yet to fully mature as clinical agents. These include monoclonal antibodies, agents, which inhibit the action of oncogene products, and genetically tailored tumor-infiltrating lymphocytes and/or tumor cells, which secrete high local concentrations of cytokines within the tumor bed and may be capable of generating immunologic memory. Whether these advances in immunotherapy will be effective enough to become the new standard for the treatment of disseminated renal cancer must await further clinical experience.

REFERENCES

1. Linehan M. Introduction. Immunotherapy of renal cell carcinoma. Heidelberg: Springer-Verlag, 1991; 1.
2. Konnak JW, Grossman HB. Renal cell carcinoma as an incidental finding. J Urol 1985; 134:1094.
3. deKernion JB, Ramming KP, Smith RB. The natural history of metastatic renal cell carcinoma: a computer analysis. J Urol 1978; 120:148.
4. Giuliani L, Giberti C, Martorana G, Rovida S. Radical extensive surgery for renal cell carcinoma: long-term results and prognostic factors. J Urol 1990; 143:468.
5. Cherrie RJ, Goldman DG, Lindner A, deKernion JB. Prognostic implications of vena caval extension of renal cell carcinoma. J Urol 1982; 128:910.
6. Klein EA, Kay MC, Novick AC. Management of renal cell carcinoma with vena caval thrombi via cardiopulmonary bypass and deep hypothermic circulatory arrest. Urol Clin North Amer 1991; 18:445.
7. Novick AC, Kaye MC, Cosgrove DM, et al. Experience with cardiopulmonary bypass and deep hypothermic circulatory arrest in the management of retroperitoneal tumors with large vena caval thrombi. Ann Surg 1990; 212:472.
8. Richie JP, Skinner DG. Renal neoplasia. In: Brenner BB, Rector FC, eds. *The Kidney*. Philadelphia: W.B. Saunders, 1991; 2126.

9. Bloom HJG. Hormone-induced and spontaneous regression of metastatic renal cancer. J Urol 1971; 74:42.
10. Swanson DA, Johnson DG, von Eschenbach A, et al. Angio-infarction plus nephrectomy for metastatic renal cell carcinoma—an update. J Urol 1983; 130:449.
11. Yagoda A. New cytotoxic single-agent therapy for renal cell carcinoma. In: Johnson DE, Logothetis C, von Eschenbach AC, eds. *Systemic therapy for genitourinary cancers.* Chicago: Year Book Medical Publishers, 1989; 112.
12. Klein EA. The multidrug resistance gene in renal cell carcinoma. Semin Urol 1989; 7:207.
13. Ahmed T, Benedetto P, Yagoda A, et al. Estrogen, progesterone and androgen-binding sites in renal cell carcinoma. Observations obtained in phase II trial of flutamide. Cancer 1984; 54:477.
14. Holland JM. Cancer of the kidney—natural history and staging. Cancer 1973; 32:1030.
15. Golumbek PT, Lazenby AJ, Levitsky JH, Jaffee LM, Karusuyamah H, Baker Pardoll M. Treatment of renal cancer by tumor cells engineered to secrete interleukin 4. Science 1991; 254:719.
16. Finke JH, Rayman P, Edinger M, et al. Characterization of a human renal cell carcinoma specific cytotoxic CD8[+] T cell line. J Immunother 1992; 11:1.
17. Koo AS, Tso C-L, Shimabukuro T, Peyret C, deKernion JB, Balldegrun A. Autologous tumor-specific cytotoxicity of tumor infiltrating lymphocytes derived from human renal cell carcinoma. J Immunother 1991; 10:347–54.
18. Crusinberry R, Williams RD. Immunotherapy of renal cell cancer. Semin Surg Oncol 1991; 7:221.
19. Rosenberg S, Spiess P, LaFreniere R. A new approach to adoptive immunotherapy of cancer with tumor-infiltrating lymphocytes. Science 1986; 233:1318.
20. Klein EA. The immunotherapy and cellular biology of renal cell carcinoma. Cancer Cells 1990; 2:58.
21. Alexander JP, Melsop KA, Hamilton TA, et al. T cells infiltrating renal cell carcinoma are unable to proliferate but exhibit normal interferon-gamma production. 1992; (in press).

II

Clinical Features of Renal Cell Carcinoma

2

Prognostic Factors in Metastatic Renal Cell Carcinoma

Jean-Pierre Droz, Annie Rey, Monder Mahjoubi, Isabelle Philippot, Carole Bouleuc, and Andrew Kramar

Institut Gustave-Roussy, Villejuif, France

I. INTRODUCTION

The median survival of patients with metastatic renal cell cancer is rather short, between 6 and 12 months (1–7). In the past no systemic treatment was available (2,8), but promising results are obtained by immunotherapy. Only few studies have addressed the question of whether prognostic factors may influence the survival of these patients (9–12). We published the first multivariate analysis of prognostic factors in a large series of patients (10,11) but decided to perform a new analysis with the objective of selecting more reliable and easily measurable prognostic factors.

II. MATERIALS AND METHODS

We reviewed retrospectively the charts of 207 patients with metastatic renal cancer treated at the Institut Gustave-Roussy between January 1976 and June 1990. Some of these 207 patients were included in a previous study of prognostic factors (10,11).

The histologic type of the tumor was classified according to the World Health Organization (WHO) classification (13) and was available in all but 36 patients, in whom the diagnosis was established by the presence of a renal tumor with metastatic sites and positive fine-needle aspiration of the tumor.

Patients with either relapse or primary metastatic disease were included in this retrospective study. All patients were classified at initial diagnosis according to Robson's anatomoclinical classification (14). The initial workup of patients included medical history, clinical examination, body weight, WHO performance status (PS), standard biochemical profile, complete blood count (CBC), erythrocyte sedimentation rate (ESR), chest x-ray, and liver morphologic examination (scintigraphy before 1980; echography or computed tomography, CT scan afterward). Bone x-ray, bone scintigraphy, and brain CT scan were performed only in patients with clinical suspicion of bone or brain metastases. Weight loss was considered significant when it was more than 10% of body weight within 3 months before entry on study. Fever was considered present if more than 38°C was registered for more than 8 days.

Patients were treated by surgery (of local tumor or metastases) and/or radiotherapy and/or systemic treatment (e.g., chemotherapy, hormonal therapy, or immunotherapy) and/or supportive care. None of these 207 patients had either solitary metastasis completely removed or first-line immunotherapy (either interferon or interleukin-2). In detail, 38 patients had metastasis surgery, 74 patients had radiotherapy on metastatic sites, and 192 patients had at least one systemic treatment. Chemotherapeutic regimens included nitrosourea in 90 patients (15), 9-methylhydroxyelliptinium in 40 patients (16,17), ifosfamide in 20 patients (18), a combination of dacarbazine, cyclophosphamide, cisplatin, doxorubicin, and vindesine in 14 patients (19), a combination of methyl-gag and melphalan in 14 patients (20), and miscellaneous agents in 44 patients. Of the 192 patients, 16 and 16 received interferon-α and interleukin-2, respectively. A total of 15 patients did not receive any treatment. The response to treatment was assessed according to WHO criteria (21).

The initial characteristics of the patients, the treatments, and the follow-up data were registered on a specific form. Data were analyzed using a general data base management system (22). Survival was the end point of the study. The origin of survival was the date of referral to the Institut Gustave-Roussy, and the end point was the date of last follow-up or death of the patient. Survival curves were estimated by the Kaplan-Meier method (23). The log-rank test (24) was used to select variables to be included in the Cox regression analysis (25). All variables that were significant at the 5% level in the univariate analysis were included in the multivariate analysis. Model selection for identifying the variables that have an important effect on survival was based on a forward stepwise procedure. The variables were entered on the basis of significance calculated from a large-sample partial likelihood ratio test. The threshold to enter a variable was 0.05 and was 0.15 to remove a variable.

III. RESULTS

A. Patient Characteristics

There were 154 males and 53 females, the median age of the patients was 54 years (extremes 17 and 75), histologic types were clear cells in 159 patients, granular cells in 2 patients, sarcomatoid cells in 3 patients, miscellaneous pattern in 7 patients, and unknown in 36 patients. Time between the diagnosis of primary and the diagnosis of first metastasis was less than 1 month in 98 patients (47%), 1–12 months in 60 patients (29%), 13–18 in 10 patients (5%), and >18 months in 39 patients (19%). A nephrectomy was performed in 55 of 98 patients (56%) with asynchronous metastases. Patient characteristics are shown in Table 1. An objective effect of medical treatment was observed in 8 patients with chemotherapy: 3 complete remissions (CR) and 5 partial responses (PR). No objective effect was observed in 32 patients treated by second-line immunotherapy.

B. Survival

The survival curve of the overall population is shown in Figure 1. At the time of analysis (March 1991), 137 patients were alive and 170 patients died (154 of evolution, 2 of toxicity, and 4 of other cause). Median survival was 10 months. The 1, 2, and 3 year survival rates were 48% (95% confidence interval, CI, 38–52%), 20% (CI = 14–26%), and 11% (CI = 6–16%), respectively.

C. Univariate Analysis

Table 2 shows the 35 variables selected for univariate analysis: 8 variables failed to achieve prognostic value: sex, histology, time between diagnosis of primary and metastases, lung metastasis, bone metastasis, brain metastasis, lymph node involvement, and treatment (either radiotherapy or systemic treatment); 7 variables attained significance. Unfavorable prognosis was associated with PS > 1, no nephrectomy, weight loss > 10%, elevated ESR, presence of liver metastases, increased number of involved sites, and shorter time between diagnosis of primary and metastases if the cutoff point of 12 months is considered. There was a significant interaction between weight loss and sedimentation rate, with a similar relative risk for a weight loss of more than 10%, for a sedimentation rate greater than 100, or for both. Thus a new variable was created, SRWL. It is coded 1 if the ESR ≥ 100 and/or weight loss is present and coded 0 if ESR < 100 *and* weight loss is absent. This new

Table 1 Patient Characteristics

	Number	%
Total number of patients	207	
Age, years		
Mean	54	
Range	17–75	
Gender (male/female)	154/53	
Time from diagnosis, months		
0	98	47
>12	49	24
≤12	148	76
>18	39	19
≥18	158	81
Weight loss		
No	105	51
Yes	102	49
ESR		
<50	104	56
50–99	51	27
≥100	31	17
Performance status		
0	34	16
1	103	50
2	62	30
3	8	4
Fever		
No	172	83
Yes	35	17
Lung metastases		
None	75	36
≤5/lung, ≤2 cm	28	
>5/lung, ≤2 cm	41	
≤5/lung, >2 cm	19	
>5/lung, >2 cm	43	
Lymph nodes		
Mediastinum	31	
Lumboaortic	31	
Bone metastases	53	
Skin metastases	12	
Brain metastases	12	
Liver metastases	42	
Number of involved sites		
1	108	52
2	65	32
3	25	12
4	9	4

Note: ESR = erythrocyte sedimentation rate.

% SURVIVAL

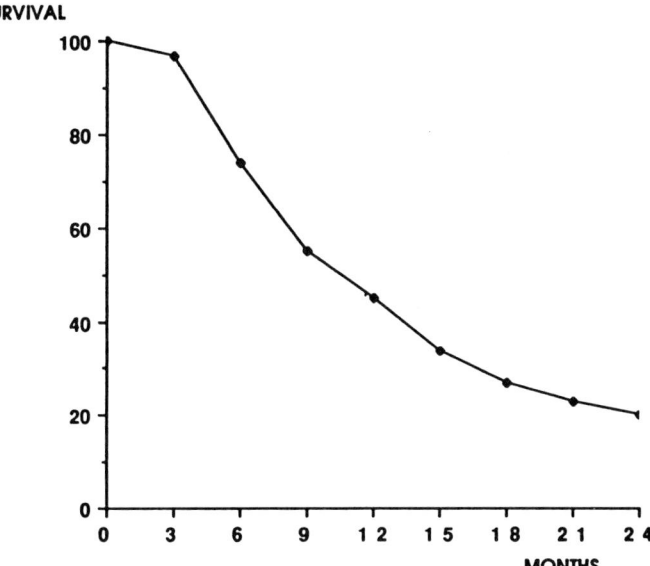

Figure 1 Survival of 207 patients with metastatic renal cell cancer.

variable retained prognostic value. The results of the univariate analysis are shown in Table 3.

D. Multivariate Analysis

The following variables retained prognostic value in the multivariate analysis: SRWL, PS, liver metastasis, nephrectomy, lung metastasis, and number of sites (Table 4). We considered that the conditions of selecting variables to be included in the prognostic model were (1) statistically significant variables in univariate and multivariate analysis; (2) variables for which the measure is easily reproducible; (3) the combination of variables that had clinical significance; and (4) the combination of variables that gave rise to prognostic groups with statistically different survivals. We chose the first three variables of Table 4, which seemed to fulfill all these conditions.

The predictive survival rate for each group of patients at time t was calculated from the Cox model according to $Sx(t) = Sp(t)^w$, where $Sp(t)$ was the predictive survival rate for the whole population at time t and $w = ea + iPFi$, where i was the estimated coefficient given by the model for each selected prognostic factor (PFi).

Table 2   Definition of the 35 Selected Variables

ETAT	=	status (dead, alive)
SURV	=	survival (months)
SEXE	=	sex
AGE4	=	age in four classes (<40, 40–50, 51–60, >60)
AGE60	=	age (<60, ≥60 years)
STAGE	=	initial stage of disease (Robson's classification) (14)
DELAI	=	time between diagnosis of renal cancer and metastases (>1, ≤1 year)
POUM	=	lung metastases (yes, no)
GG	=	lymph nodes (yes, no)
OS	=	bone metastases (yes, no)
FOIE	=	liver metastases (yes, no)
PEAU	=	skin metastases (yes, no)
SNC	=	central nervous system (CNS) metastases (yes, no)
AUTRM	=	other metastases (yes, no)
NBSIT	=	absolute number of metastases
OMS	=	WHO performance status (0, 1, 2, 3)
FIEVRE	=	fever > 38°C > 8 days (yes, no)
PDS	=	weight loss > 10% body weight in 3 months (yes, no)
VSED	=	erythrocyte sedimentation rate (<50, 50–99, ≥100)
CHIRR	=	nephrectomy (yes, no)
RTL	=	radiotherapy of the lumbar area (yes, no)
CHIRM	=	surgical removal of metastases (yes, no)
RTM	=	radiotherapy of metastatic sites (yes, no)
CHAMP	=	site of irradiated site (lung, bone, CNS, mediastinum, skin)
CT	=	chemotherapy (yes, no)
REPCT	=	response to chemotherapy (yes, no)
DEL1	=	time between diagnosis of renal cancer and metastases (>0, 0 month)
SRWL	=	sedimentation rate and weight loss (see text)
ZPM	=	lung metastases in five classes
PM2	=	lung metastases in two classes (>2 cm and >5/lung, other)
SITE	=	number of metastatic sites (1, ≥2)
ELSON	=	prognostic group in Elson classification (12)
CHIR2	=	nephrectomy in patients with synchronous metastases (yes, no)
PS	=	WHO performance status (0–1, 2–3)
GG1	=	mediastinal lymph nodes (yes, no)

Note: WHO = World Health Organization; CNS = central nervous system.

Table 3 Univariate Analysis (Log-Rank Test)

	Variables	p Value
1	OMS	10^{-5}
2	VSED	10^{-5}
3	SRWL	10^{-5}
4	CHIRR	10^{-5}
5	PDS	10^{-4}
6	SITE	0.0007
7	FOIE	0.0014
8	NBSITE	0.004
9	DELAI	0.01
10	DEL1	0.07
11	AGE4	0.09
12	PM2	0.10
13	ZPM	0.17
14	SNC	0.18
15	GG1	0.19
16	GG	0.29
17	AUTRM	0.45
18	OS	0.64
19	POUM	0.80
20	SEXE	0.81

Note: For legend, see Table 2.

Table 4 Multivariate Analysis (Cox Model)

Step	Variables	Improvement χ^2	p Value	Coefficient
0				
1	SRWL	20.03	10^{-4}	0.589
2	OMS	11.93	0.001	0.367
3	FOIE	7.48	0.006	0.552
4	CHIR2	5.13	0.023	
5	PM2	5.82	0.016	
6	SITE	4.45	0.035	

Note: For legend, see Table 2.

Table 5   Combinations of Factors, Proportions of Patients, and 1 and 2 Year Survival of Prognostic Groups

Groups	PS[a]	Liver metastases	SRWL[b]	No. patients (%)		Survival (%) 1 year	2 years
Good risk	0–1	0	0	69	85 (41)	70	34
	2–3	0–1	0	13 + 3			
Intermediate risk	0–1	0	1	45	68 (33)	35	15
	0–1	1	0	11			
	0–1	1	1	12			
Poor risk	2–3	0–1	1	38	54 (26)	15	0
				16			

[a] Performance status.
[b] Sedimentation rate + weight loss.

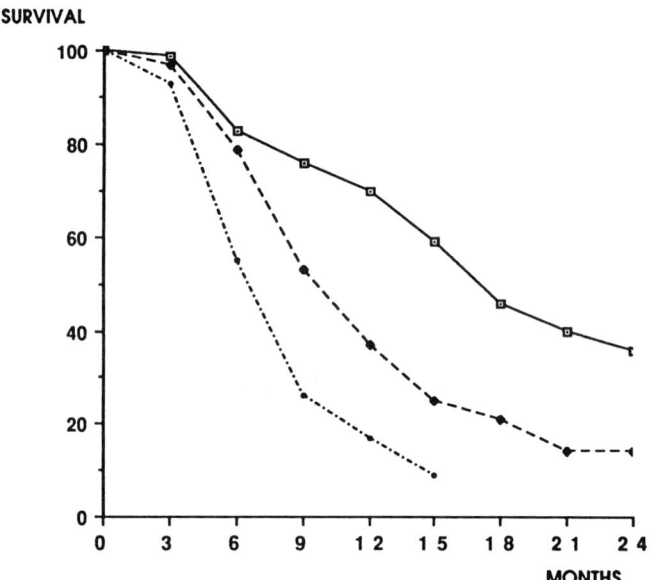

Figure 2   Survival of the three prognostic groups (good, intermediate, and poor) as defined by the mathematical model: good risk (solid line); intermediate risk (dashed line); poor risk (dot-dash line).

There were eight possible combinations of the three selected prognostic factors. These were combined into three subgroups with a clear difference in survival: good risk, intermediate risk, and poor risk groups.

The combinations of factors, the proportion of patients, and the 1 and 2 year survival rates in these three subgroups are shown in Table 5.

The survival curves of these three subgroups are shown in Figure 2.

IV. DISCUSSION

The survival of patients with metastatic renal cell cancer is poor: the median survival time of 10 months we observed is in agreement with other reports, where it is 6–12 months (1–7). It is interesting to note that authors reported the occurrence of unexplained spontaneous regression of metastases (26). A prospective trial of observation in patients with metastatic renal cancer confirmed this observation: 3 spontaneous CR and 2 PR were observed in 73 patients (27). However, 75% of the patients progressed by 3 months. This observation shows the need for an observation time before entering patients in a prospective trial of systemic treatments. The role of nephrectomy in such regressions has been advocated by some authors (1,5,12,28,29), but others failed to find any improvement in survival in nephrectomized patients (30). Elson et al. (12) found nephrectomy as a prognostic factor in an univariate analysis, as we did, but this factor did not retain prognostic significance in a multivariate analysis. It is, on the other hand, one of the prognostic factors in our multivariate analysis. The impact of nephrectomy in patients with synchronous metastases is shown in Figure 3. However, we decided not to include this factor in the final model because, even if it has an independent prognostic value, it is mainly influenced by the medical decision.

Univariate analyses of prognostic factors were reported in many papers. However, only three multivariate analyses have been reported until now. The first was published in 1983 and concerned 26 patients (9). Two factors retained prognostic value: initial albumin level and liver metastasis. We reported the first multivariate analysis on a large series of 134 patients (10,11). We found four independent prognostic factors: hepatic metastasis, lung metastasis, interval between primary and metastasis diagnosis, and SRWL (11). Six prognostic groups were defined. Elson et al. (12) later published a multivariate analysis of 610 patients. They found very similar variables and separated five prognostic subgroups defined by a score of the prognostic factors: performance status, interval between primary and metastasis diagnosis, weight loss, prior chemotherapy, and number of metastatic sites. Two major points led us to perform a new study of prognostic factors: (1) the need

% SURVIVAL

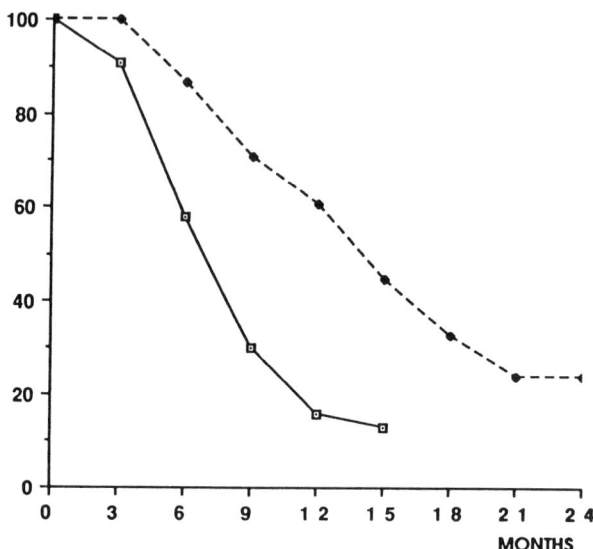

Figure 3 Survival of patients with synchronous metastases according to the performance of a nephrectomy (dashed line) or not (solid line).

to select easily measurable prognostic factors, and (2) the need to define a small number of prognostic subgroups that have clinical signification, as opposed to the use of a scoring system.

Many prognostic factors were recognized in univariate analysis. The time between diagnosis of primary and diagnosis of metastases is one of the factors most often mentioned (1,5,12,31). Katzenstein et al. did not find this factor important (32); this may be because of the selection of the patients in this study. One problem with this variable is that it depends widely on the frequence of follow-up visits and of the nature of the follow-up workup. The presence, number, and size of lung metastases were found significant in our first multivariate analysis (11), as they did in other papers (1,12). Because the majority of our patients had only chest x-ray and patients who are now proposed to participate in prospective trials have CT scan of the chest, this variable no longer has a significant value. One other reason not to select lung metastases as prognostic factors may be its high frequency (70%) (1,11,12) and the fact that the absence of lung metastases seems to be related to a different pattern of metastatic disease, which could have a different evolution

(33,34). The observation about workup techniques also concerns the number of involved sites, which is widely dependent on the initial workup procedure. It is nevertheless an important factor. In fact, some metastatic sites have no clear prognostic value, such as central nervous system involvement (12,35) and bone metastases (36), but liver involvement is found significant in many studies (9,12). This is easily explored by liver echography, which was available at the time when the different studies were done. This investigation gives quick results and is painless, noninvasive, and inexpensive. The results of liver echography are very satisfactory.

Constitutional factors are very important: performance status, weight loss, fever, and ESR. Performance status was found significant in most studies (1,11,12,35). We looked at the significance of separating patients in four or only two categories (PS 0 and 1 versus 2 and 3). The use of two categories was more significant, and in fact this assessment is more confident (37): there is a clear-cut difference between PS 0–1 and 2–3. Weight loss was found significant by Elson et al. in multivariate analysis and is easily assessable. Conversely, there is no information on ESR, which was found significant in both our analyses. In fact, this is very reliable information and has proved of strong prognostic value in Hodgkin's disease (38). Initial elevated ESR is not only predictive of poor risk in early-stage Hodgkin's disease, but elevated ESR after radiotherapy is predictive of early relapse and poor prognosis and justifies early aggressive therapy (38). We then observed that, combined with weight loss, ESR is a more powerful prognostic factor in metastatic renal cell cancer.

The three selected prognostic subgroups of our study have clearly different survival patterns: patients with poor risk have either poor performance status and elevated ESR or weight loss, or both; patients with good risk always have no elevated ESR and no weight loss and may have good or poor performance status with or without liver metastasis; patients with intermediate risk have good performance status but different combinations of SRWL and liver involvement. It should be kept in mind that other unknown prognostic factors may influence survival. For example, patients with diploid or nearly diploid deoxyribonucleic acid content in the primary tumor or in the metastasis have better survival than patients with an aneuploid deoxyribonucleic acid content (39).

The analysis of prognostic factors in metastatic renal cell cancer has shown that survival may vary widely from one patient to another. This may influence the interpretation of clinical trials. Because the complete response rate with either interferon or interleukin-2 with or without cells is rather low, the evaluation of survival is of importance in reporting trial results. Few trials clearly define the characteristics of patients entered in the studies, and few provide information about prognostic factors. This is important since randomized trials between immunotherapy and no treatment seem unethical. Thus an approach studying the impact of immunotherapy on survival may be obtained by the study of prognostic factors. We recommend that the major prognostic factors and their combinations be reported in the results of clinical trials in metastatic renal cell cancer.

ACKNOWLEDGMENT

The authors thank Mrs. M. Moussé for her excellent secretarial help in the preparation of the manuscript.

REFERENCES

1. Maldazys JD, deKernion JB. Prognostic factors in metastatic renal cell carcinoma. J Urol 1986; 136:376.
2. Talley RW, Moorhead EL, Tucker WG, San Diego EL, Brennan MJ. Treatment of metastatic hypernephroma. JAMA 1969; 207:322.
3. DeKernion JB. Treatment of advanced renal cell carcinoma. Traditional methods and innovative approaches. J Urol 1983; 130:2.
4. Thompson IM, Shannon H, Ross G Jr, Montie J. An analysis of factors affecting survival in 150 patients with renal carcinoma. J Urol 1975; 114:694.
5. DeKernion JB, Ramming KP, Smith RB. The natural history of metastatic renal carcinoma: a computer analysis. J Urol 1978; 120:148.
6. McNichols DW, Segura JW, De Weed JH. Renal cell carcinoma: long-term survival and late recurrence. J Urol 1981; 126:17.
7. Golimbu M, Joshi P, Sperber A, Tessler A, Al-Askari J, Morales P. Renal cell carcinoma: survival and prognostic factors. Urology 1986; 27:291.
8. Droz JP, Theodore C, Ghosn M, et al. Twelve years experience with chemotherapy in adult metastatic renal cell carcinoma at the Institut Gustave-Roussy. Semin Surg Oncol 1988; 4:97.
9. Brubaker LH, Troner MB, Birch R. Advanced adenocarcinoma of the kidney: therapy with lomustine, vinblastine, hydroxyurea and medroxyprogesterone acetate and regression analysis of factors relating to survival. Cancer Treat Rep 1983; 67:741.
10. Ghosn M, De Forges A, Rey A, Klink M, Kramar A, Droz JP. Prognostic factors of adult metastatic renal carcinoma: predictive survival rate studied by Cox regression analysis. Proc Am Soc Clin Oncol 1987; 6:103.
11. De Forges A, Rey A, Klink, M, Ghosn M, Kramar A, Droz JP. Prognostic factors of adult metastatic renal carcinoma: a multivariate analysis. Semin Surg Oncol 1988; 4:149.

12. Elson PJ, Witte RS, Trump DL. Prognostic factors for survival in patients with recurrent or metastatic renal cell carcinoma. Cancer Res 1988; 48:7310.
13. WHO. Histological typing of kidney tumors, No. 25. Geneva: World Health Organization, 1981.
14. Robson CJ, Churchill MB, Anderson W. The results of radical nephrectomy for renal cell carcinoma. J Urol 1969; 101:297.
15. Amiel JL, Cukier J, Droz JP, Ben Ayed F. Cancer du rein, essai de chimiothérapie. Nouv Presse Med 1979; 8:2235.
16. Caille P, Mondesir JM, Droz JP, et al. Phase II trial of elliptinium in advanced renal cell carcinoma. Cancer Treat Rep 1985; 69:901.
17. Piot G, Droz JP, Theodore C, Ghosn M, Rouesse J, Amiel JL. Phase II trial with high dose elliptinium acetate in metastatic renal cell carcinoma. Oncology 1988; 45:371.
18. De Forges A, Droz JP, Ghosn M, Theodore C. Phase II trial with ifosfamide/mesna in metastatic renal carcinoma. Cancer Treat Rep 1987; 71:1103.
19. Lupera H, Theodore C, Ghosn M, Court BH, Wibault P, Droz JP. Phase II trial of combination chemotherapy with dacarbazine, cyclophosphamide, cisplatin, doxorubicin, and vindesine (DECAV) in advanced renal cell cancer. Urology 1989; 34:281.
20. Guimaraes JL, Ghosn M, Ostronoff M, Azab M, Theodore C, Droz JP. Phase II trial of methyl-gag and melphalan in metastatic adult renal cell carcinoma. Cancer Invest 1990; 8:621.
21. WHO. Handbook for reporting results of cancer treatment. WHO offset publication No. 48. Geneva: World Health Organization, 1979.
22. Wartelle M, Kramar A, Jan P, Kruger D. PIGAS: an interactive statistical database management system. In: Proceedings of the international workshop on statistical database management, Los Altos, CA. Springfield, IL: National Technical Information Service, U.S. Department of Commerce, 1983; 124–32.
23. Kaplan EL, Meier P. Nonparametric estimation from incomplete observations. J Am Stat Assoc 1958; 53:457.
24. Mantel N, Haenszel W. Statistical aspects of the analysis of data from retrospective studies of disease. J Natl Cancer Inst 1959; 22:719.
25. Cox DR. Regressions models and life tables (with discussion). J R Stat Soc [B] 1972; 34:187.
26. Fairlamb DJ. Spontaneous regression of metastases of renal cancer. Cancer 1981; 47:2102.
27. Oliver RTD, Miller RM, Mehta A, Barnett MJ. A phase 2 study of surveillance in patients with metastatic renal cell carcinoma and assessment of response of such patients to therapy on progression. Mol Biother 1988; 1:14.
28. Klugo RC, Detmers M, Stiles RE, Talley RW, Cerny JC. Aggressive versus conservative management of stage IV renal cell carcinoma. J Urol 1977; 118:244.
29. Montie JE, Stewart BH, Straffon RA, et al. The role of adjunctive nephrectomy in patients with metastatic renal cell carcinoma. J Urol 1977; 117:272.

30. Johnson DE, Kaesler KE, Samuels ML. Is nephrectomy justified in patients with metastatic renal carcinoma? J Urol 1975; 114:27.

31. O'Dea MJ, Zincke H, Utz DC, Bernatz PE. The treatment of renal cell carcinoma with solitary metastasis. J Urol 1978; 120:540.

32. Katzenstein AL, Purvis R, Gmelich J, Askin F. Pulmonary resection for metastatic renal adenocarcinoma: pathologic findings and therapeutic value. Cancer 1978; 41:712.

33. Saitoh H, Hida M, Nakamura K, Shimbo T, Shiramizu T, Satoh T. Metastatic processes and a potential indication of treatment for metastatic lesions of renal adenocarcinoma. J Urol 1982; 128:916.

34. Weiss L, Harlos JP, Torhost J, et al. Metastatic pattern of renal carcinoma: an analysis of 687 necropsies. J Cancer Res Clin Oncol 1988; 114:605.

35. Decker DA, Decker VL, Herskovic A, Cummings GD. Brain metastases in patients with renal cell carcinoma: prognostic and treatment. J Clin Oncol 1984; 2:169.

36. Swanson DA, Orovan WL, Johnson DE, Giacco G. Osseous metastases secondary to renal cell carcinoma. Urology 1981; 18:556.

37. Orr S, Aisner J. Performance status assessment among oncology patients: a review. Cancer Treat Rep 1986; 70:1423.

38. Henry-Amar M, Friedman S, Hayat M, et al. Erythrocyte sedimentation rate predicts early relapse and survival in early-stage Hodgkin disease. Ann Intern Med 1991; 114:361.

39. Ljungber B, Stenling R, Roos G. Prognostic value of deoxyribonucleic acid content in metastatic renal cell carcinoma. J Urol 1986; 136:801.

3

von Hippel-Lindau Disease

Clinical and Biologic Features

Andrew C. Novick

The Cleveland Clinic Foundation, Cleveland, Ohio

I. INTRODUCTION

In 1885, Pye-Smith described a patient with a cerebellar cyst, pancreatic cyst, and multiple renal cysts (1). In 1894, Collins reported on a similar patient with retinal angiomas (2). In 1904, von Hippel, a German ophthalmologist, described a group of patients with retinal hemangioblastomas and noted that some also had central nervous system and visceral lesions (3). In 1921, Brandt reported necropsy findings in one of von Hippel's patients that indicated the presence of cysts and hypernephromas (4). In 1926, Lindau, a Swedish pathologist, studied 40 patients with similar findings and formally associated this constellation of lesions into a single disease entity that currently bears his name (5).

von Hippel-Lindau disease (VHLD) is one of the phakomatoses, a term derived from the Greek word *phakos*, meaning birthmark or spot. It has now been redefined to include diseases with multiple lesions arising predominantly from one germ layer. Examples include the lesions of tuberous sclerosis and von Ricklinghausen's disease, which are primarily ectodermal in origin, in contrast to the lesions of VHLD, which are primarily mesodermal in origin (6). More than 30 manifestations of VHLD have been described, although only some of these produce clinically significant disease.

II. DIAGNOSIS AND SCREENING

The most common lesions in VHLD are retinal angiomas, hemangioblastomas of the cerebellum and spinal cord, cysts and angiomas of
visceral organs (liver, pancreas, and lung), renal cell carcinoma, and pheochromocytoma. Less frequently encountered lesions include epididymal cyst,
epididymal adenoma, and adrenocortical adenoma or hyperplasia (7).

The diagnosis of VHLD is established by the demonstration of two or more
major manifestations or one major manifestation in a patient with a positive
family history. Although spontaneous cases can arise, VHLD is considered to
be transmitted in an autosomal dominant pattern with almost complete penetrance by the age of 60 years (6).

Since the number and location of lesions in VHLD are variable, all
potentially affected organ systems should be screened for involvement by
appropriate physical or radiographic examination upon suspicion of the diagnosis (8,9). It is important to screen the central nervous system since cerebellar tumors represent a major cause of death. It is also important to screen the
kidneys because of the high incidence of renal cell carcinoma, which is
usually asymptomatic. Complete screening for VHLD should include a physical, neurologic, and ophthalmologic examination, computed tomography or
magnetic resonance imaging of the skull, computed tomography or ultra-
sonography of the abdomen, and a plasma catecholamine assay. Siblings and
first-degree relatives of affected patients should be screened in this manner.
Considering the autosomal dominant nature of hereditary transmission, 50%
of siblings, 50% of offspring, and one parent is expected to have VHLD (7).
Affected individuals who have yet to bear children should be advised of the
risk of transmission to offspring.

III. CLINICAL FEATURES

Patients with VHLD typically present as young adults with dizziness, ataxia,
signs of increased intracranial pressure, or visual disturbances owing to
tumors of the cerebellum and retina. Often, no clinical symptoms are associated with the other manifestations of VHLD. The diagnosis of VHLD should
always be considered if a retinal angioma, central nervous system hemangioblastoma, or pheochromocytoma is newly diagnosed. In a recent study,
50% of affected individuals had involvement of only one organ at the time of
diagnosis (9).

The most comprehensive clinical study thus far was reported by Maher and
associates from Cambridge University (10). These investigators studied the
clinical features and survival of 152 patients with VHLD. The age at onset

varied from 4 to 68 years, with a mean of 26.3 years. Retinal angioma was the most frequent presenting manifestation. In the overall series, the most common manifestations were retinal angioma (59%), cerebellar hemangioblastoma (59%), renal cell carcinoma (28%), spinal cord hemangioblastoma (13%), and pheochromocytoma (7%). Renal, pancreatic, and epididymal cysts were frequent findings, but their exact incidence was not accurately assessed. Life table analysis indicated that renal cell carcinoma would develop eventually in most long-term survivors. The median actuarial survival was 49 years, with renal cell carcinoma the leading cause of death, followed by cerebellar hemangioblastoma.

In a recent study by Neumann and Wiestler (9), a clustering of VHLD-associated lesions was observed in members of affected families. VHLD families with a high incidence of pheochromocytoma were at high risk for developing retinal and central nervous system lesions but only rarely developed renal lesions. By comparison, there was a high association between renal cell carcinoma and central nervous system hemangioblastomas among affected family members. These data suggest that the vascular lesions of VHLD (retinal angioma and central nervous system hemangioblastoma) are core features and pheochromocytoma at one end of the spectrum and renal or pancreatic lesions at the other end are unlikely to develop in the same family. Newmann and Weistler suggested that a complex genetic locus with a linear arrangement of different adjacent transcription units may be responsible for these patterns of family expression.

IV. RENAL CELL CARCINOMA IN VHLD

Renal cell carcinoma (RCC) has been reported in up to 45% of patients with VHLD (7,11,12). Recent cytogenetic and molecular studies have demonstrated loss of genetic material from chromosome 3 in most cases of sporadic RCC, and it has been hypothesized that the lost material may contain a gene that when present is capable of preventing tumor formation (13). Studies in patients with RCC and VHLD have demonstrated deletions from the same area of chromosome 3 as in sporadic RCC (14,15).

RCC in VHLD differs from its sporadic counterpart in that the diagnosis is made at a younger age and there are usually multiple bilateral renal tumors. Although these are generally low-stage tumors, they are capable of progression with metastasis and represent a major cause of death in patients with VHLD (7). Histopathologically, RCC in VHLD is characterized by both solid tumors and renal cysts that contain either frank RCC or a lining of hyperplastic clear cells representing incipient RCC (16–18). Therefore, adequate surgical treatment of localized RCC in VHLD requires excision of all solid and cystic renal lesions.

Surgical treatment is indicated for patients with VHLD and localized bilateral RCC to prevent tumor progression and metastasis. The early results of nephron-sparing surgery in this setting have been promising (17,19–21). However, we recently reviewed the long-term outcome of nephron-sparing surgery in nine patients with localized bilateral RCC and VHLD (22). Only one of these patients has remained free of malignancy postoperatively. One patient died of metastatic RCC, and the remaining seven patients developed local recurrence of malignancy in the operated kidney; a second renal operation was done in six of these patients. The postoperative time to detection of local tumor recurrence ranged from 24 to 92 months, with a mean of 61 months. In view of the multicentric nature of RCC in VHLD, some of these local recurrences may alternatively be a manifestation of residual microscopic renal malignancy that was not removed at the time of surgery.

These data indicate that the results of nephron-sparing surgery in patients with RCC and VHLD are less satisfactory than in patients with sporadic RCC (23). If nephron-sparing surgery is done for localized RCC in VHLD, patients should be advised of the importance of close postoperative surveillance and the likely need for repeat renal surgery. Bilateral nephrectomy with subsequent chronic dialysis and renal transplantation is an alternative approach that is more likely to be curative of localized RCC in this setting (24,25). The long-term outcome with this approach is not known, since few patients with VHLD have undergone renal transplantation. When considering treatment options for RCC in VHLD, it is also appropriate to consider that, in some patients, extensive central nervous system involvement may render the renal malignancy of secondary importance as a determinant of longevity.

REFERENCES

1. Pye-Smith PH. Cysts of the cerebellum with numerous small cysts in the pancreas and kidneys. Trans Pathol Soc Lond 1985; 36:17.
2. Collins ET. Some unusual forms of intraocular neoplasms. Trans Ophthalmol Soc UK 1894; 14:141.
3. von Hippel E. Ueber eine sehr seltene Erkrankung de Netzhaut: klinische Beobachtungen. Arch Ophthalmol 1904; 59:83.
4. Brandt R. Zur Frage der Angiomatosis retinae. Arch Ophthalmol 1921; 106:127.
5. Lindau A. Studien uber Kleinhirncysten: Bau, Patholgenese and Beziehungen zur Angiomatosis Retinae. Acta Pathol Microbiol Scand Suppl 1926; 1:1.
6. Melmon KL, Rosen SW. Lindau's disease. Review of the literature and study of a large kindred. Am J Med 1964; 36:595.

7. Horton WA, Wong V, Eldrich R. von Hippel-Lindau disease: clinical and pathological manifestations in nine families with 50 affected members. Arch Intern Med 1976; 136:769.

8. Choyke PL, Filling-Katz MR, Shawker TH, et al. von Hippel-Lindau disease: radiologic screening for visceral manifestations. Radiology 1990: 174:815.

9. Newmann HPH, Wiestler OD. Clustering of features of von Hippel-Lindau syndrome: evidence for a complex genetic locus. Lancet 1991; 337:1052.

10. Maher ER, Yates JRW, Harries R, et al. Clinical features and natural history of von Hippel-Lindau's disease. Q J Med 1991; 283:1151.

11. Richards RD, Mebust WK, Schimke RN. A prospective study of von Hippel-Lindau's disease. JAMA 1961; 178:280.

12. Christoferson LA, Gustafson MB, Petersen AG. von Hippel-Lindau's disease. JAMA 1961; 178:280.

13. Yoshida MA, Ohyashiki K, Ochi H, et al. Rearrangement of chromosome 3 in renal cell carcinoma. Cancer Genet Cytogenet 1986; 19:351.

14. King CR, Schimke RN, Arthur T, et al. Proximal 3p deletion in renal cell carcinoma cells from a patient with von Hippel-Lindau disease. Cancer Genet Cytogenet 1987; 27:345.

15. Seizinger BR, Rouleau GA, Ozelius LJ, et al. von Hippel-Lindau disease maps to the region of chromosome 3 associated with renal cell carcinoma. Nature 1988; 332:268.

16. Loughlin KR, Gittes RF. Urological management of patients with von Hippel-Lindau disease. J Urol 1986; 136:789.

17. Spencer WF, Novick AC, Montie JE, Streem SB, Levin HS. Surgical treatment of localized renal cell carcinoma in von Hippel-Lindau's disease. J Urol 1988; 139:507.

18. Christenson PJ, Craig JP, Bibbo MC, O'Connell KJ. Cysts containing renal cell carcinoma in von Hippel-Lindau's disease. J Urol 1982; 128:798.

19. Pearson JC, Weiss J, Tanagho EA. A plea for conservation of kidneys in renal adenocarcinoma associated with von Hippel-Lindau disease. J Urol 1980; 124:910.

20. Malek RS, Omess PJ, Benson RC, Zincke H. Renal cell carcinoma in von Hippel-Lindau syndrome. Am J Med 1987; 82:236.

21. Das S, Egan RM, Awar AD. von Hippel-Lindau syndrome with bilateral synchronous renal cell carcinoma. Urology 1981; 18:599.

22. Novick Streem SB. Long-term follow-up after nephron-sparing surgery for renal cell carcinoma in von Hippel-Lindau's disease. In Press.

23. Novick AC, Streem SB, Montie JE, et al. Conservative surgery for renal cell carcinoma: a single-center experience with 100 patients. J Urol 1989; 141:835.

24. Fetner CD, Barilla DE, Scott T, Ballard J, Peters P. Bilateral renal cell carcinoma in von Hippel-Lindau syndrome: treatment and staged bilateral nephrectomy and hemodialysis. J Urol 1977; 117:534.

25. Peterson GJ, Codd JE, Cuddihee RE, Newton WT. Renal transplantation in von Hippel-Lindau disease. Arch Surg 1977; 112:841.

III

The Molecular Biology of Renal Cell Carcinoma

4

Molecular Studies of Sporadic and Familial Renal Cell Carcinoma

James R. Gnarra, Patrick Anglard*, Gladys M. Glenn, and W. Marston Linehan

National Cancer Institute, National Institutes of Health, Bethesda, Maryland

Kalmon Tory, Farida Latif, Michael I. Lerman, and Berton Zbar

National Cancer Institute–Frederick Cancer Research and Development Center, National Institutes of Health, Frederick, Maryland

I. INTRODUCTION

Specific chromosomal abnormalities have been associated with several cancer types. The association of numerous specific chromosomal translocations with certain neoplasias and subsequent protooncogene activation is well documented (1). It has recently become appreciated that deletions on specific chromosomes are consistently associated with certain cancers and are likely to result in inactivation of a class of genes known as tumor suppressor genes (2). The normal role of cellular protooncogenes is to positively regulate cell growth, but the normal role of tumor suppressor genes is thought to negatively regulate cell growth. Thus, mutations that activate cellular protooncogenes or inactivate tumor suppressor genes, either individually or together, can lead to a transformed phenotype.

---

* Current affiliation: Institut de Chimie Biologique, Strasbourg, France

Evidence indicating the existence of tumor suppressor genes is actually quite old. Malignant cells can be converted from a tumorigenic phenotype to a nontumorigenic phenotype through somatic cell fusion with normal cells, through fusion of two tumor cells of different origin, or through the introduction of specific chromosomes by microcell fusion. Such results indicate that the tumor cell lost a specific genetic function that could be complemented and are in support of tumorigenesis being linked to a recessive mechanism.

In the tumor suppressor gene model for sporadic and familial cancers, as few as two mutations can lead to cellular transformation. In familial cancer, a germ line mutation is inherited, and although this mutation does not itself induce transformation, it appears to predispose each cell to a second, transforming mutation. Also, although inheritance appears as an autosomal dominant mutation, the heterozygous state does not appear to have an altered phenotype. Sporadic cancers are thought to arise from two mutations in the same gene, except that these events occur in the same somatic cell. In either familial or sporadic cancer, the second mutation involves the normal allele in a manner that unmasks the mutant allele.

Several candidate tumor suppressor genes have been recently identified: RB1, the retinoblastoma gene, on chromosome 13q; WT1, associated with Wilms' tumor and the Beckwith-Wiedemann syndrome, on 11p; the MCC and FAP genes on 5q, as well as the DCC gene on 18q, associated with colorectal carcinoma; and the neurofibromatosis gene on 17q; and the p53 gene on 17p, involved in the Li-Fraumeni syndrome as well as many other cancer types. In each case, mutation of a specific gene appears associated with initiation of malignancy.

Renal cell carcinoma (RCC) comprises 2% of all human malignancies and is the most common malignancy in the adult kidney. Nearly twice as many men as women are affected, and a relationship exists with cigarette smoking (3,4). Renal cell carcinoma occurs in both sporadic and hereditary forms, with the sporadic form usually manifesting during the sixth or seventh decade in life; the familial form is often seen much earlier (5). It is commonly believed that these tumors arise from epithelial cells of the proximal convoluted tubule of the kidney.

II. ROLE OF CHROMOSOME 3 IN KIDNEY CANCER

Cytogenetic studies of kidney tumors indicate the short arm of chromosome 3 as the most frequent site of nonrandom aberrations in sporadic RCC (6–8). In addition, a large kindred with a constitutional 3:8 chromosomal translocation

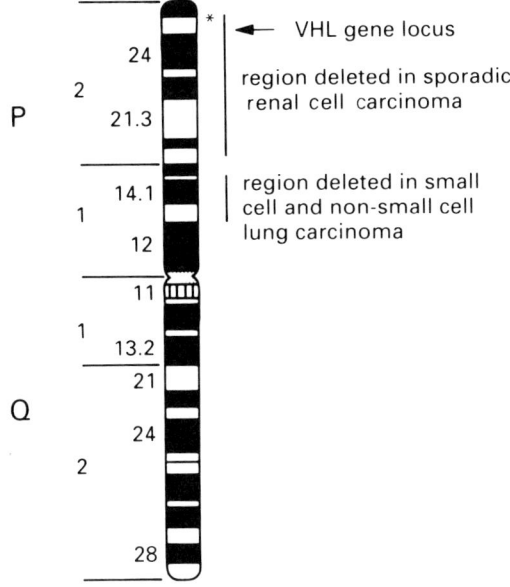

region deleted in sporadic renal cell carcinoma

region deleted in small cell and non-small cell lung carcinoma

Chromosome 3

Figure 1 Representation of human chromosome 3 showing common sites of genetic deletions in RCC and lung cancer.

has been extensively studied (9). Members of the kindred carrying t(3:8) developed RCC by 37 years of age, but members of a corresponding age not carrying the translocation did not develop RCC. The translocation breakpoint in these individuals was localized to 3p14.2. Subsequent karyotypic analysis of these renal tumors demonstrated that in the tumor derivative chromosome 8 was lost (10). A second family affected by RCC was also described. When tumor cells from affected by RCC was also described. When tumor cells from affected family members were examined cytogenetically, chromosome 3:11 translocations were noted with a breakpoint similarly localized to the 3p13–14 region (11). However, these individuals did not carry constitutional translocations; t(3:11) was consistently seen only in their tumors. Therefore, it appears that these individuals had a genetic predisposition to such a translocation.

Chromosome 3p deletions have been identified in several human cancers in addition to sporadic and hereditary RCC (see Figure 1). These include small cell lung carcinoma, non–small cell lung carcinoma, and carcinomas of the head and neck, breast, ovary, and cervix (1,12,13).

Table 1 Polymorphic Loci on Chromosome 3p

Location	Symbol	Probe	Enzyme	Allele size (kb)
3p26.1	D3S18	c162-1	BamHI	8.7;4.7
3p25	RAF1	p627	BglI	3.5;3.3
				4.0;3.3
			TaqI	6.3;6.8
3p24–25	D3S588	LIB 12–69	HindIII	7.2;6.5
				5.9;5.0
3p24	THJRB	pH302B	HindIII	7.0;5.5
3p21	DNF15S2	pH3H2	HindIII	2.0;2.3
3p21	D3S32	pEFD145.1	TaqI	9.0;4.0
3p14.2–21	D3S2	p12.32	MspI	2.9;1.6 + 1.3
3p	D3S607	LIB 31–39	HinfI	Variable

Source: Modified from Anglard et al., Cancer Res 1992; 16.

III. SPORADIC RENAL CELL CARCINOMA

Based on cytogenetic studies like those just described, chromosome 3p has been extensively analyzed in RCC. Restriction fragment length polymorphism (RFLP) studies using tumor tissue from patients with renal cell carcinoma were performed with ordered, polymorphic 3p probes (Table 1) (14). High-molecular-weight DNA was isolated from primary RCC tumors and adjacent normal kidney tissue from patients operated on in the National Cancer Institute (NCI) Surgery Branch. The DNA was digested with appropriate restriction enzymes, the fragments were separated by agarose gel electrophoresis, and the DNA fragments transferred to nylon membranes. Hybridization of paired normal tissue- and tumor-derived DNA samples was performed using chromosome 3p DNA probes. The basis for such DNA analysis is that many genomic alleles differ in sequence such that a particular restriction endonuclease recognition site or the spacing between two adjacent sites is altered. Therefore, when DNA from different individuals is Southern hybridized with a given probe, polymorphisms in restriction fragment patterns may be noted. Such restriction fragment length polymorphisms serve as markers for that allele. An example of RFLP analysis is shown in Figure 2.

Loss of heterozygosity (LOH) was noted in the 3p21–26 region in tumors from 51 of 58 (88%) evaluable patients (15). The frequency of loss of 3p

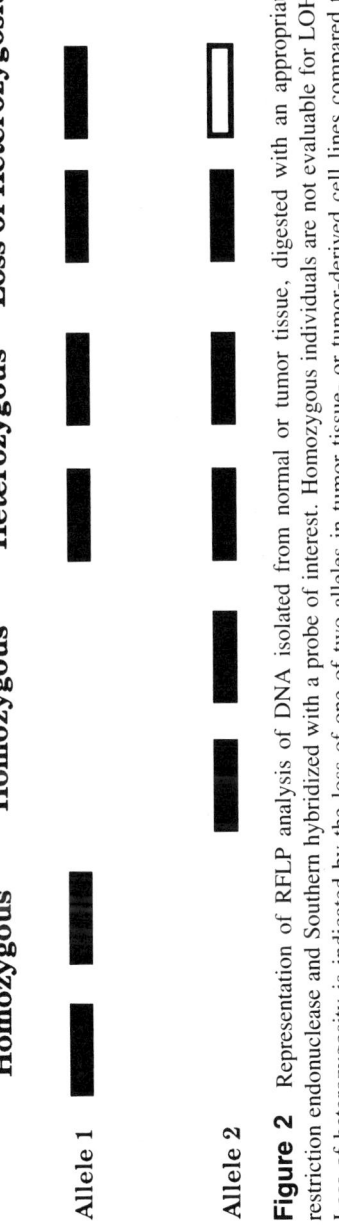

Figure 2 Representation of RFLP analysis of DNA isolated from normal or tumor tissue, digested with an appropriate restriction endonuclease and Southern hybridized with a probe of interest. Homozygous individuals are not evaluable for LOH. Loss of heterozygosity is indicated by the loss of one of two alleles in tumor tissue- or tumor-derived cell lines compared to matched normal tissue. LOH occurs in 88% of individuals with RCC.

sequences in RCC was greater than the reported frequency of loss of sequences on 11p in bladder carcinoma (42% LOH) or Wilms' tumor (55% LOH). These results showing an extremely high frequency of LOH in RCC suggest the presence of a tumor suppressor gene in the 3p21–26 region that may be responsible for initiation of this malignancy.

IV. ESTABLISHMENT OF RCC CELL LINES

To better understand the process of RCC disease initiation, RCC cell lines were established (16). Such cell lines, free of contaminating normal kidney cells or infiltrating lymphocytes, which complicate RFLP analyses of solid tumors, would provide a resource to more precisely localize, identify, and clone the RCC disease gene. Thus far, 42 renal cell carcinoma cell lines have been generated from patients with advanced disease (16). Most of these patients underwent nephrectomy in the NCI Surgery Branch. That tumor specimens in culture were fresh specimens from patients with advanced disease probably accounted for a relatively high success rate (18 of 24; 75%) of cell line establishment. In contrast, the success rate for cryopreserved tumors was 35% (17 of 48 attempts). These cell lines are very useful for gene localization studies, since in most cases normal, matched tissue is also available for analysis.

Molecular and cellular analyses of 35 of the 42 cell lines have been performed (16). In 25 of 30 evaluable cell lines there was LOH at one or more of the polymorphic loci tested (Table 1) (16). Of the 30 cell lines 2 were derived from tumors with papillary histology, and neither of these lines demonstrated 3p LOH. These results are in accord with earlier studies demonstrating no 3p LOH in papillary kidney tumors (17). Loss of heterozygosity was demonstrated in 25 of 28 (89%) RCC cell lines derived from nonpapillary tumors. No deletions were detected in the remaining 5 evaluable cell lines. Analysis of the genotype of one particular cell line, UOK 114, provided further information concerning the location of the tumor suppressor gene on chromosome 3p. In this line LOH was determined at the proximal loci, DNF15S2 and THRB. However, both sets of alleles at the D3S18 locus were retained, implying that the location of a gene important in RCC is proximal to D3S18.

Of the RCC cell lines tested 14 were derived from solid renal tumors that were previously analyzed on the short arm of chromosome 3 (see earlier). In each instance, the same 3p genotype was found in both the solid tumor and the corresponding RCC cell lines.

V. TUMOR HISTOLOGY AND CHROMOSOME 3p ANALYSIS

Previous reports demonstrated a lower incidence of chromosome 3p allelic deletion in granular cell variants of RCC (18). It was therefore suggested that LOH on chromosome 3p may be specific to the clear cell phenotype. However, most of the RCC tumors examined in these studies were composed of mixed cell populations, containing both clear and granular cells. If only clear cells showed 3p deletions, this would imply the coexistence of cells with two different genotypes in the same tumor, one population carrying 3p LOH and one with an intact chromosome 3. To better understand the relationship between cellular phenotype and genotype, cell lines were examined that were derived from nine mixed types of RCC (containing both clear and granular cells), including four with 3p deletions, four without 3p deletions, and one line that was not evaluable because no normal DNA was available. Each line was injected subcutaneously in nude mice: each had a characteristic morphology in culture, but in each instance the histopathology of the tumor that formed in nude mice was similar to that of the patient's original tumor. In addition, of five cell lines derived from tumors with granular features, three (UOK 105, 117, and 127) had deletions on chromosome 3p and two (UOK 120 and 124) did not. Like the parental tumor, all the nude mouse tumors formed from these cell lines contained granular cells. Therefore, deletions on chromosome 3p did not correlate with either the granular or the clear cell phenotype. The similar histopathology of the original human and nude mice tumors suggests that the different phenotypic variants of RCC—clear, granular, and sacromatoid—may have a common cellular origin.

VI. FAMILIAL RENAL CELL CARCINOMA

As discussed, familial forms of RCC exist. Family members having constitutional translocations involving 3p develop RCC relatively early in life. Another type of familial RCC is seen in individuals with von Hippel-Lindau disease (VHLD). VHLD is an autosomal dominant disorder with varying penetrance that features renal cancers and multiple benign cysts of the kidneys, pancreas, and testes, as well as pheochromocytoma and central nervous system hemangioblastomas (19–21).

Renal cell carcinoma tissue from VHLD patients was analyzed by RFLP analysis to determine if these tumors carried a genetic lesion in the same location as identified in sporadic RCC. Loss of heterozygosity on chromosome 3p was noted in 15 of 15 tumors tested (22). Multiple RCC tumors taken from the same individual showed loss of the same chromosome 3p alleles, demonstrating that the same chromosome was deleted in each tumor. Haplotypic analyses demonstrated that in each instance, the wild-type allele, inherited from the nonaffected parent, was deleted. These results led to the initiation of a clinical trial in which 500 members in 42 kindreds of patients affected with VHLD were evaluated by RFLP linkage analysis. Linkage of the VHLD gene to RAF1 (23), a protooncogene at 3p25, was confirmed, and linkage to D3S18, an anonymous marker at 3p26, was demonstrated (Figure 1) (24). Two-point linkage analysis determined a recombination frequency between VHLD and RAF1 as 0.06 and between VHLD and D3S18 as 0.04. In addition, a prospective trial was initiated to evaluate whether presymptomatic detection of VHLD by RFLP analysis could be performed. In asymptomatic, at-risk family members there was significant concordance between DNA polymorphism analysis and clinical evaluation (25).

Like most cases of sporadic RCC, kidney specimens obtained from patients carrying t(3:8) do not show the histopathologic evidence of benign renal cysts seen in VHLD. In addition, members of these kindreds show none of the clinical features of VHLD other than RCC. Last, although patients carrying t(3:8) lose the derivative chromosome 8 in their tumors, renal cancers seen as part of VHLD show LOH involving the chromosome 3 that was inherited from the unaffected parent. Therefore, there appear to be two types of hereditary kidney cancer: one is identified by balanced, reciprocal chromosomal translocations involving chromosome 3p; the other, VHLD, is identified by chromosome 3p deletions. Both involve the same region of chromosome 3p, however, implying that similar genes may be responsible for the resultant tumors.

VII. FUTURE PLANS: IDENTIFICATION OF THE RCC DISEASE GENE

Molecular analysis of individuals with VHLD allowed localization of the VHLD gene locus to a 6–8 cm region at 3p25–26. Using markers closest to the VHLD gene as starting points, chromsomal walking utilizing yeast artificial chromosomes and cosmid libraries will allow analysis of genes contained within this region.

REFERENCES

1. Solomon E, Borrow J, Goddard AD. Chromosome aberrations and cancer. Science 1991; 254:1153–60.

2. Weinberg RA. Tumor suppressor genes. Science 1991; 254:1138–46.
3. La Vecchia C, Negri E, D'Avanzo B, Franceschi S. Smoking and renal cell carcinoma. Cancer Res 1990; 50:5231–3.
4. Yu MC, Mack TM, Hanisch R, Cicioni C, Henderson BE. Cigarette smoking, obesity, diuretic use, and coffee consumption as risk factors for renal cell carcinoma. J Natl Cancer Inst 1986; 77:351–6.
5. Linehan WM, Shipley W, Longo D. Cancer of the kidney and ureter. In: De Vita VT, Hellman S, Rosenberg SA, eds. *Cancer principles and practice of oncology*, Philadelphia: J.B. Lippincott, 1989; 979–1007.
6. Nordenson I, Ljungberg B, Roos G. Chromosomes in renal carcinoma with reference to intratumor heterogeneity. Cancer Genet Cytogenet 1988; 32:35–41.
7. Yoshida MA, Ohyashiki K, Ochi H, et al. Rearrangement of chromosome 3 in renal cell carcinoma. Cancer Genet Cytogenet 1986; 19:351–4.
8. Weaver DJ, Michalski K, Miles J. Cytogenetic analysis in renal cell carcinoma: correlation with tumor aggressiveness. Cancer Res 1988; 48:2887–9.
9. Cohen AJ, Li FP, Berg S, et al. Hereditary renal-cell carcinoma associated with a chromosomal translocation. N Engl J Med 1979; 301:592–5.
10. Li FP, Decker JH, Zbar B, et al. Renal cell carcinomas in a family with a constitutional 3:8 translocation: clinical follow-up and genetic analyses of tumors. Genomics (In Press).
11. Pathak S, Strong LC, Ferrell RE, Trindade A. Familial renal cell carcinoma with a 3:11 chromosome translocation limited to tumor cells. Science 1982; 217: 939–41.
12. Brauch H, Johnson B, Hovis J, et al. Molecular analysis of the short arm of chromosome 3 in small-cell and non–small-cell carcinoma of the lung. N Engl J Med 1987; 317:1109–13.
13. Ali IU, Lidereau R, Callahan R. Presence of two members of c-cebA receptor gene family (c-erbAB and c-erbA2) in smallest region of somatic homozygosity on chromosome 3p21-p25 in human breast carcinoma. J Natl Cancer Inst 1989; 81:1815–20.
14. Lerman MI, Latif F, Glenn GM, et al. Isolation and regional localization of a large collection (2,000) of single copy DNA fragments on human chromosome 3 for mapping and cloning tumor suppressor genes. Hum Genet 1991; 86:567–77.
15. Anglard P, Brauch TH, Weiss GH, et al. Molecular analysis of genetic changes in the origin and development of renal cell carcinoma. Cancer Res 1991; 51:1071–7.
16. Anglard P, Trahan E, Liu S, et al. Molecular and cellular characterization of human renal cell carcinoma cell lines. Cancer Res 1992; 52:348–56.
17. Kovacs G, Wilkens L, Papp T, de Riese W. Differentiation between papillary and nonpapillary renal cell carcinomas by DNA analysis. J Natl Cancer Inst 1989; 81:527–30.
18. Ogawa O, Kakehi Y, Ogawa K, Koshiba M, Sugiyama T, Yoshida O. Allelic loss at chromosome 3p characterizes clear cell phenotype of renal cell carcinoma. Cancer Res 1991; 51:949–53.

19. Malek RS, Omess PJ, Benson RC. Renal cell carcinoma in von Hippel-Lindau syndrome. Am J Med 1987; 82:236–8.

20. Daniel LN, Linehan WM. Genetics of renal cell carcinoma. Semin Urol 1989; 7:258–63.

21. Glenn GM, Choyke PL, Zbar B, Linehan WM. von Hippel-Lindau disease: clinical aspects and molecular genetics. In: EE Anderson, (ed.) *Problems in urologic surgery: benign and malignant tumors of the kidney*, Philadelphia: J.B. Lippincott, 1990; 312–30.

22. Zbar B, Brauch H, Talmadge C, Linehan M. Loss of alleles of loci on the short arm of chromosome 3 in renal cell carcinoma. Nature 1987; 327:721–4.

23. Seizinger BR, Rouleau GA, Ozelius LJ, Lane et al. von Hippel-Lindau disease maps to the region of chromosome 3 associated with renal cell carcinoma. Nature 1988; 332: 268–9.

24. Hosoe S, Brauch H, Latif F, et al. Localization of the von Hippel-Lindau disease gene to a small region of chromosome 3. Genomics 1990; 8:634–40.

25. Glenn GM, Linehan WM, Hosoe S, et al. Screening for von Hippel-Lindau disease by DNA-polymorphism analysis. JAMA; in press.

5

Oncogenes in Renal Cell Carcinoma

Osamu Yoshida, Osamu Ogawa, Jun Takenawa, and Jun Fujita

Kyoto University, Kyoto, Japan

I. INTRODUCTION

It is currently accepted that a variety of genetic aberrations is responsible for the genesis and progression of human cancers. Since 1979, when it was demonstrated that DNA derived from cancer cells can transform recipient normal cells by DNA transfection (1), dominant oncogenes have been a central theme of the molecular biology of human carcinogenesis. Of the many important investigations into these oncogenes, the most significant breakthrough was the realization that viral oncogenes have homology to normal cellular genes (protooncogenes). These protooncogenes apparently code for essential proteins involved in the signal transduction network from cell membrane to nucleus; including growth factors, growth factor receptors, protein kinases, and so forth (2). The cell cycle is under finely tuned control, modulated by extracellular stimuli. To maintain normal cell growth and development, it is necessary that the signal transduction network function appropriately. Although the biochemical mechanisms underlying cell proliferation and differentiation remain unclear, it seems possible that certain perturbations of the transduction network result in the activation of the protooncogenes and convert susceptible normal cells to malignant cells.

In this chapter, the possible roles of the oncogenes in the development of renal cell carcinomas (RCC) are discussed with reference to previous reports.

II. GROWTH FACTORS AND GROWTH FACTOR RECEPTORS

The interaction between the internal milieu of the cell and the growth factor receptors has been regarded as one of the most important mechanisms governing the development and differentiation of normal organs and regeneration. That some viral oncogenes encode for proteins homologous to known growth factors and their receptors suggests that abnormalities in the structure or expression of these genes may be responsible for human carcinogenesis (3). In addition, that media from cultured tumor cells contain polypeptide growth factors, and furthermore that the tumor cells often possess functional receptors, indicates the possibility that these growth factor–receptor interactions and autocrine mechanisms may participate in the progression of a variety of human tumors (4).

A. Epidermal Growth Factor Receptor

The v-*erb*B oncogene is a truncated version of the epidermal growth factor (EGF) receptor (EGFR) gene. Previous cytogenetic studies reported that the trisomy of chromosome 7, on which the EGFR gene is mapped, is one of the most frequent chromosomal changes in RCC (5). This may correlate with the malignant potential of RCC. To determine if there is an amplification or rearrangement of the EGFR gene, we performed Southern blot analyses of this gene in 45 normal kidney-RCC pairs, including four specimens from metastatic lesions. We did not detect any rearrangement or amplification of the EGFR gene in primary tumors or in metastatic tumors, as shown in Figure 1. However, several investigators have demonstrated the enhanced expression of EGFR mRNA and suggested a correlation between tumor stage and the increased level of EGFR mRNA (6,7). Although our observations as well as those of other previous studies (8,9) suggest that amplification and rearrangement of the EGFR gene are infrequent genetic events in the genesis of RCC, other molecular mechanisms may be implicated in the enhanced expression of the EGFR gene.

B. Transforming Growth Factor α

Several growth factors have been identified not as classic oncogene products, but as important molecules that enhance the proliferation of cancer cells. Transforming growth factor α (TGF-α) is a secreted polypeptide that was discovered in the medium of certain retrovirus-transformed fibroblasts (10). TGF-α shares about 30% structural similarity to EGF, being a potent ligand of the EGF receptor. In addition, TGF-α is reported to be capable of inducing

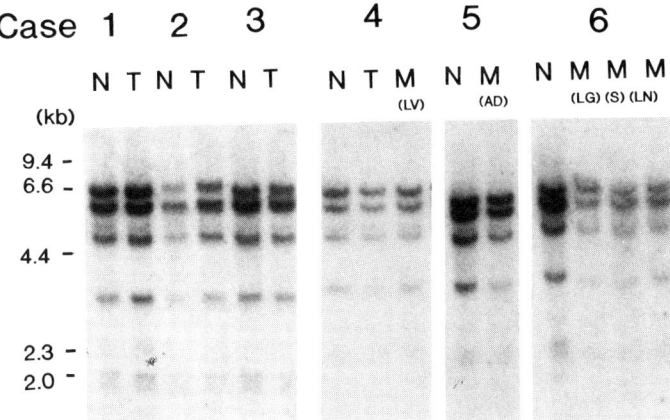

Figure 1 Southern blot analysis of the EGFR gene in six representative cases of renal cell carcinoma. DNA from each tumor specimen and each normal kidney specimen (10 μg) was digested with EcoR1, and the resulting fragments were electrophoresed through agarose gels. After membrane transfer, the membrane was hybridized with an EGFR(pE7) probe. Lane N, normal kidney; lane T, primary tumor; lane M, metastatic tumor (the letters in parentheses indicate the site of metastasis: AD, adrenal gland; LV, liver; LG, lung; S, spleen; LN, lymph node). Neither amplification nor rearrangement could be detected in either the primary or the metastatic tumors.

neovascularization (11). Derynck et al. (12) demonstrated that TGF-α mRNA was transcribed in a variety of solid human tumors, especially in squamous carcinomas and RCC. Recently, northern hybridization studies demonstrated an enhanced expression of TGF-α in all RCC examined (13,14). These findings, together with the enhanced expression of EGFR mRNA in RCC, suggest that a TGF-α–EGFR interaction may play an important role in the progression of RCC.

C. Interleukin-6

Interleukin-6 (IL-6), originally identified as a T cell-derived lymphokine, is now considered an autocrine growth factor derived from RCC in vitro (15).

To demonstrate the role of IL-6 in RCC in vivo, we preformed northern hybridization studies of IL-6 and the IL-6 receptor in 43 primary RCC (16). IL-6 expression could be detected in 22 of the 43 cases (51%), and the enhanced expression of IL-6 (compared to the normal kidney) was demon-

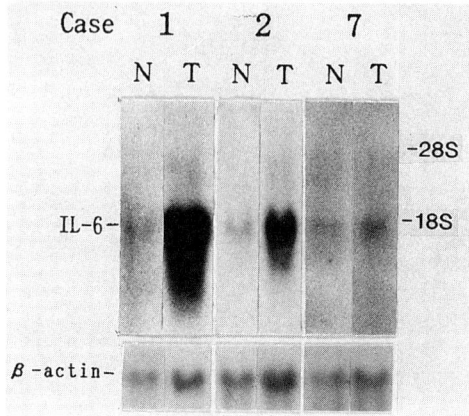

Figure 2   Northern blot analysis of IL-6 gene expression in renal cell carcinomas: T, primary tumor; N, normal kidney. The enhanced expression of IL-6 was demonstrated in cases 1 and 2.

strated in 10 cases (23%; Fig. 2). To study the relationship between IL-6 expression and the histopathologic and clinical findings, we performed statistical analyses on 28 RCC patients for whom clinical data was available. These patients were grouped on the basis of the tumor-normal ratio of IL-6 expression (≤ 1.0 or >1.0). Analyses of the clinical data between the two groups showed that the enhanced IL-6 expression correlated with the clinical stage, with the level of serum C-reactive protein, and especially with the degree of lymph node metastasis (Tables 1 and 2). Immunohistochemical study using an anti-IL-6 antibody indicated that RCC cells, rather than other nonneoplastic

Table 1   Correlation of Tumor-Normal Ratio of IL-6 Gene Expression and Pathologic Stage

Tumor-normal ratio (no. cases)	Pathologic stage								
	Tumor			Node[a]			Metastasis		
	T1+T2	T3+T4	TX	N^-	N^+	NX	M^-	M^+	MX
>1 (7)	5	2	0	2	5	0	3	4	0
≤ 1 (21)	11	6	4	14	3	4	14	3	4

[a]Statistically significant ($P < 0.05$).

Table 2 Correlation of Tumor-Normal Ratio of IL-6 Gene Expression
and Clinical Findings

Tumor-normal ratio (no. cases)	Clinical findings[a]	
	CRP[b] (mg/ml)	ESR (1 h) (mm)
>1 (7)	2.91 ± 3.27[c]	60.2 ± 49.4
≤1 (21)	0.57 ± 1.19	30.5 ± 32.8

[a] CRP, serum C-reactive protein; ESR (1 h), erythrocyte sedimentation rate at 1 h.
[b] Statistically significant ($P < 0.05$).
[c] Data represent mean ± standard deviation.

cells, were responsible for the expression of IL-6 (data not shown). In
addition, northern blot analysis of the IL-6 receptor showed that the expression of the IL-6 receptor was detectable in 11 of the 43 patients (26%; data not
shown). However, coexpression of both IL-6 and its receptor was detected in
only 1 patient. Although additional studies are necessary to define the role of
IL-6 in the tumorigenesis of RCC in vivo, our study suggests the possibility
that the level of IL-6 expression may be a predictor of the malignant potential
of the RCC.

III. THE PROTEIN KINASES

Many oncogenes belong to a characteristic gene family that encodes the
protein kinases. It is widely accepted that protein phosphorylation can regulate enzyme function, and therefore the products of this gene family are
considered involved in the signal transduction network.

In human malignancy, this type of oncogene is presumably implicated in
the genesis of chronic myelogeneous leukemia (CML). The Philadelphia
chromosome (Ph1) can be detected in more than 95% of CML cases. This is
an abnormal chromosome made by the reciprocal exchange or translocation of
genetic material between chromosome 9 and chromosome 22, on which the
c-*abl* and the *bcr* genes, respectively, are located. As a consequence of this
recombination, the *bcr/abl* fusion mRNA translates into a fusion protein with
increased autophosphorylation activity compared to the normal *abl* protein
(17).

Although a few studies have been reported so far, the specific, abnormal
expression of this type of oncogene in RCC has not been identified yet (6,18).

IV. *myc* AND OTHER NUCLEAR ONCOGENES

The products of some protooncogenes, including those in the *myc* family, are located in the nucleus and are believed to have important roles in the regulation of transcription or the processing of RNA. In the case of Burkitt's lymphoma, the level of *myc* gene expression is enhanced by translocated immunoglobulin enhancer sequences (19). Furthermore, the gene amplification of N-*myc* is demonstrated in high-stage neuroblastomas (20), indicating that the overexpression of *myc* gene products is related to the progression of neuroblastomas.

In an early cytogenetic study, a translocation of c-*myc* was reported in hereditary RCC (21). In addition, Yao et al. (6) demonstrated enhanced expression of the c-*myc* genes in 11 of 15 RCC (73%). However, further studies are necessary to determine whether the differences in the expression of c-*myc* are the consequence or cause of the malignant state, because c-*myc* genes are expressed at high levels in a variety of human cancers (22).

V. THE *ras* FAMILY

The *ras* genes encode for proteins that possess GTPase activity, with a molecular weight of about 21,000 (p21). It has been suggested that this protein is actively a G protein and has important functions in transmembranous signal transduction. These genes can become activated by mutations in the codons for amino acids 12, 13, or 61 and/or by overexpression (23). Point mutational activation of the *ras* genes has been detected in pancreatic and colon cancers with high frequency (24,25), and these findings suggest that this type of activation may play an important role in the initiation and/or progression of some human cancers. Fujita et al. (18) reported a point mutation of the Ha-*ras* gene in 1 of 15 RCC cases by using the NIH/3T3 transfection assay. Recently, Nanus et al. (26) detected the Ha-*ras* mutation in only one metastatic RCC in 51 primary and metastatic RCC (including three oncocytomas) using the polymerase chain reaction. These observations suggest that the point mutational activation of the *ras* genes may not play a significant role in the genesis of RCC.

VI. TUMOR SUPPRESSOR GENES

In a variety of human tumors, several specific chromosomal losses have been reported (27). It is now becoming clear that an accumulation of these losses at specific chromosomal loci, for which inactivating mutations elicit tumorigenesis, is also necessary for neoplastic conversion. At present, several

Table 3 Tumor Suppressor Genes Associated with Human Cancers

Gene	Map location	Type of cancer
MCC	5q21	Colorectal carcinoma (FAP[a])
WT1	11p13	Wilms' tumor (WAGR[b] complex), rhabdomyosarcoma, bladder carcinoma
RB1	13q14	Retinoblastoma, osteosarcoma, breast carcinoma, small cell lung carcinoma
p53	17p13	Colorectal carcinoma, small cell lung carcinoma, bladder carcinoma
NF1	17q	Neurofibroma
DCC	18q21	Colorectal carcinoma

[a] Familial adenomatous polyposis.
[b] Wilms' tumor, aniridia, genitourinary abnormality, and mental retardation.

genes have been identified as candidates for this additional major class of tumorigenic suppressor gene (Table 3).

In human RCC, recent restriction fragment length polymorphism (RFLP) analyses have demonstrated frequent losses at the chromosome 3p loci (28), suggesting that these putative tumor suppressor gene(s) locate on the chromosome 3p. Furthermore, additional high and frequent losses at other chromosomal loci suggest that several chromosomal loci are responsible for the tumorigenesis of RCC (29). We examined 35 Japanese patients with sporadic RCC by RFLP study to assess the incidence of the chromosome 3p rearrangement. In agreement with other studies, the allelic loss at 3p was demonstrated with high frequency in our study (Table 4). In addition, we demonstrated that this type of chromosomal rearrangement is specific to the clear cell type of RCC, suggesting that the type of 3p rearrangement can differentiate the histopathologic subtypes of RCC (30).

VII. CONCLUSION

Despite the intense investigation into the oncogenes and their products, surprisingly little is known about the precise mechanism of neoplastic conversion, in which some oncogenes undoubtedly play important roles. There is no definitive evidence that the activation of these protooncogenes is responsible for the genesis or progression of the tumors. RCC is an interesting tumor in both genetic and clinical aspects, because RCC has strange biologic properties. For example, RCC shows spontaneous regression of its distant metastatic sites after the removal of the original tumor in rare instances and often shows

Table 4 Histopathologic Features and Loss
of Heterozygosity on Chromosome 3p

	No. cases with LOH/ no. informative cases[a]	%
All cases	16/30	53
Cell type[b]		
Clear cell	12/16	75
Granular cell	1/7	14
Mixed cell	2/5	40
Other	1/2	50
Configuration		
Papillary	0/3	0
Nonpapillary	16/27	60

[a] Allelic loss was tested using the following seven polymorphic probes: p627, pBH302, pH3H2, pHF-12-32, B67, pMS1-37, and pEFD145.1.
[b] Clear versus granular ($P < 0.01$).

late recurrence many years after the curative operation. Besides the immunologic mechanisms, genetic mechanisms that involves another oncogene, for example an autocrine mechanism, may be implicated in the strange characteristics of RCC.

In the near future, a putative suppressor gene located on chromosome 3p will be isolated and characterized. Through close investigation of this gene, new insights may occur into the role of oncogenes in the genesis or progression of RCC. This may provide new clinical applications of molecular analysis for the diagnosis and prognosis of RCC.

REFERENCES

1. Shih C, Shilo B-Z, Goldfarb MO, Dannenberg A, Weinberg RA. Passage of phenotypes of chemically transformed cells via transfection of DNA and chromatin. Proc Natl Acad Sci USA 1979; 76:5714–8.
2. Bishop JM. The molecular genetics of cancer. Science (Wash 1987); 235: 305–11.
3. Heldin C-H, Westermark B. Growth factors: mechanism of action and relation to oncogenes. Cell 1984; 37:9–20.
4. Sporn MB, Roberts AB. Autocrine growth factors and cancer. Nature (Lo 1985); 313:745–7.

5. Weaver DJ, Michalski K, Miles J. Cytogenetic analysis in renal cell carcinoma: correlation with tumor aggressiveness. Cancer Res 1988; 48:2887–9.

6. Yao M, Shuin T, Misaki H, Kubota Y. Enhanced expression of c-*myc* and epidermal growth factor receptor (C-*erb*B-1) genes in primary renal cancer. Cancer Res 1988; 48:6753–7.

7. Weidner U, Peter S, Strohmeyer T, Hussnätter R, Ackermann R, Sies H. Inverse relationship of epidermal growth factor receptor and HER2/*neu* gene expression in human renal cell carcinoma. Cancer Res 1990; 50:4504–9.

8. Gomella LG, Anglard P, Sargent ER, Robertson CN, Kasid A, Linehan WM. Epidermal growth factor gene analysis in renal cell carcinoma. J Urol 1989; 143:191–3.

9. Ishikawa J, Maeda S, Umezu K, Sugiyama T, Kamidono S. Amplification and overexpression of the epidermal growth factor receptor gene in human renal-cell carcinoma. Int J Cancer 1990; 45:1018–21.

10. De Larco JE, Todaro GJ. Growth factors from urine sarcoma virus-transformed cells. Proc Natl Acad Sci USA 1978; 75:4001–5.

11. Derynck R. Transforming growth factor α. Cell 1988; 54:593–5.

12. Derynck R, Goeddel DV, Ullrich A, et al. Synthesis of messenger RNAs for transforming growth factors α and β and the epidermal growth factor receptor by human tumors. Cancer Res 1987; 47:707–12.

13. Mydlo JH, Michaeli J, Cordon-Cardo C, Goldenberg AS, Heston WDW, Fair WR. Expression of transforming growth factor α and epidermal growth factor receptor messenger RNA in neoplastic and nonneoplastic human kidney tissue. Cancer Res 1989; 49:3407–11.

14. Petrides PE, Bock S, Bovens J, Hofmann R, Jakse G. Modulation of pro-epidermal growth factor, protransforming growth factor α an epidermal growth factor receptor gene expression in human renal carcinomas. Cancer Res 1990; 50:3934–9.

15. Miki S, Iwano M, Miki Y, et al. Interleukin-6 (IL-6) functions as an in vitro autocrine growth factor in renal cell carcinoma. FEBS Lett 1989; 250:607–10.

16. Takenawa J, Kaneko Y, Fukumoto M, et al. Enhanced expression of inter-leukin-6 in primary human renal cell carcinomas. J Natl Cancer Inst 1991; 83:1668–1672.

17. Shtivelman E, Lifshitz B, Gale RP, Canaani E. Fused transcript of *abl* and *bcr* genes in chronic myelogenous leukaemia. Nature 1985; 315:550–4.

18. Fujita J, Kraus MH, Onoue H, et al. Activated H-*ras* oncogenes in human kidney tumors. Cancer Res 1988; 48:5251–5.

19. Croce CM, Nowell PC. Molecular basis of human B cell neoplasia. Blood 1985; 65:1–7.

20. Seeger RC, Brodeur GM, Sather H, et al. Association of multiple copies of the N-*myc* oncogene with rapid progression of neuroblastomas. N Engl J Med 1985; 313:1111–6.

21. Drabkin HA, Bradley C, Hart I, Bleskan J, Li FP, Patterson D. Translocation of

c-*myc* in the hereditary renal cell carcinoma associated with a t(3;8) (p14.2;q24.13) chromosomal translocation. Proc Natl Acad Sci USA 1985; 82:6980–4.

22. Slamon DJ, deKernion JB, Verma IM, Cline MJ. Expression of cellular oncogenes in human malignancies. Science 1984; 224:256–62.

23. Bos JL. The *ras* gene family and human carcinogenesis. Mutat Res 1988; 195:255–71.

24. Almoguera C, Shibata D, Forrester K, Martin J, Arnheim N, Perucho M. Most human carcinomas of the exocrine pancreas contain mutant c-K-*ras* genes. Cell 1988; 53:549–54.

25. Bos JL, Fearon ER, Hamilton SR, et al. Prevalence of *ras* gene mutations in human colorectal cancers. Nature 1987; 327:293–7.

26. Nanus DM, Mentle IR, Motzer RJ, Bander NH, Albino AP. Infrequent *ras* oncogene point mutations in renal cell carcinoma. J Urol 1990; 143:175–8.

27. Sager R. Tumor suppressor genes: the puzzle and the promise. Science 1989; 246:1406–12.

28. Zbar B, Brauch H, Talmadge C, Linehan M. Loss of alleles of loci on the short arm of chromosome 3 in renal cell carcinoma. Nature 1987; 327:721–4.

29. Morita R, Ishikawa J, Tsutsumi M, et al. Allelotype of renal cell carcinoma. Cancer Res 1991; 51:820–3.

30. Ogawa O, Kakehi Y, Ogawa K, Koshiba M, Sugiyama T, Yoshida O. Allelic loss at chromosome 3p characterizes clear cell phenotype of renal cell carcinoma. Cancer Res 1991; 51:949–53.

6

Oncogene-Induced Transformation of Human Kidney Proximal Tubule Cells

David M. Nanus and Anthony P. Albino

Memorial Sloan-Kettering Cancer Center, New York, New York

I. INTRODUCTION TO THE HUMAN RENAL CELL SYSTEM

Numerous studies have implicated a role in carcinogenesis for dominant-acting oncogenes, activated by mutation, chromosomal rearrangements, insertion of a nearby promoter element, gene amplification, and enhanced transcription (1). Other studies indicate that tumorigenicity also behaves as a recessive trait, in that dominant genetic elements (tumor suppressor genes) must first be inactivated in various ways, such as gene or chromosomal deletion, rearrangement, or mutation, for the cell to become neoplastic (2). The supposition that normal progenitor cells require a specific series of gene activations and inactivations to complete the transformation process is being confirmed at the molecular level (3,4). Moreover, since it is likely that the series of genetic defects required for neoplastic transformation would differ depending upon the tumor type and the differentiation program of the corresponding normal progenitor cell, present research is focusing on (1) genetic changes common to all members of a specific neoplasm; (2) genetic alterations that correlate with other biologic characteristics, such as tumor stage, differentiation status, and clinical responsiveness; (3) the temporal sequence of alterations; and (4) the biologic and biochemical functions of the permuted genes. These types of studies require a source of well-defined normal and malignant tissues in which to assess the status of specific genes, as well as an in vitro cell culture system in which genetic elements can be introduced and tested for effects on both the normal and abnormal cell. The human renal cell system provides a prototypical experimental system for analyzing the impact of oncogenes in renal carcinogenesis.

The ability to culture cells from both renal cell carcinomas (RCC) and human kidney allows a direct comparison of the normal and malignant phenotypes (5). At the Memorial Sloan-Kettering Cancer Center (MSKCC) we have to date established over 50 RCC cell lines (SK-RC) and derived numerous short-term cultures of human kidney cells from fresh nephrectomy specimens (5). The biologic characteristics of these cultured normal and malignant kidney cell have been well defined (see Table 1) (5–7). These studies have clarified two important points.

First, normal kidney cells exhibit a biologic phenotype characteristic of other short-term cultures of nonmalignant human epithelial cells. In culture, the normal kidney cell shows: (1) a limited proliferative capacity, which is marked by rapid growth up to passage 2, followed by a sharp decline in growth capacity and eventual senescence by passage 4 or 5 (i.e., by 8–10 generations); (2) contact inhibition upon confluence; (3) anchorage-dependent growth; (4) an inability to form tumors upon injection into athymic mice; (5) a diploid karyotype; and (6) the absence of nonrandom chromosomal abnormalities. In contrast, the characteristic phenotype of cultured RCC cells includes a sustained and essentially unlimited growth capacity, a lack of contact inhibition and anchorage dependence, a capacity to form tumors in athymic mice, an aneuploid karyotype, and nonrandom chromosomal abnormalities (8).

Second, cultured normal kidney cells represent the true progenitor cell of RCC. The confirmation of this involved numerous studies with monoclonal antibodies generated against cell glycoproteins, glycolipids, and blood group antigens of normal and malignant renal cells (see Reference 9 for review), which indicated that over 90% of cultured normal human kidney cells and over 90% of RCC are of proximal tubule derivation.

These two key elements of the in vitro renal cell system provide a testable hypothesis, namely that transformation experiments with normal proximal tubule (PT) cells would have a direct relationship to events occurring in vivo. Here, we briefly review some of the studies that have attempted to define the role of specific oncogenes in the transformation of the human PT cell.

Table 1 Comparison of Characteristics of Kidney Cells[a]

Phenotypic trait	Normal kidney	PT-SV cells	PT-Ha cells	PT-Ki cells	PT-src cells	RCC cells
Proximal tubule phenotype[b]	+	+	+	+	+	+
Ganglioside expression[c]	−	+	+	+	−	10%
Proliferative capacity[d]	Low	High	High	High	High	High
Contact inhibition	+	−	−	−	−	−
Immortality[e]	−	−	+	+	+	+
Anchorage dependence[f]	+	+	+	+/−	−	−
Tumorigenicity[g]	−	−	+	+	+	+
Karyotype	Diploid	Hyperdiploid	Aneuploid	Aneuploid	Aneuploid	Aneuploid
Nonrandom chromosomal abnormalities	No	No	Yes	Yes	Yes	Yes

[a] Presence (+) or absense (−) of phenotype trait.

[b] Exhibiting expression of cell surface antigens characteristic of the proximal tubule portion of the nephron, specifically, adenosine deaminase binding protein and antigens defined by MAb S4/URO-2, F23/URO-3, T43/URO-10, and AJ8 (which detects the CALLA antigen), and lack of expression of distal tubule marker Tamm-Horsfall protein.

[c] Expression of GD3 ganglioside, which is present in 10% of renal cancers.

[d] Ability to proliferate beyond passage 5 and to be subcultured at a low-seeding density (i.e., <100 cells per cm²).

[e] Having an immortalized phenotype.

[f] Ability to form colonies in semisolid media.

[g] Ability to form tumors in athymic mice.

II. TRANSFORMATION OF PROXIMAL TUBULE CELLS BY SIMIAN VIRUS 40

The effects of simian virus 40 (SV40) on primary cultures of human epithelial cells has been frequently studied (10–12). SV40 is a potent DNA tumor virus that encodes several genes, including the large (T) antigen, a nuclear phosphoprotein (13). Large T antigen is responsible for SV40-induced transformation, in part as a result of its ability to form complexes with host-encoded polypeptides that regulate cell division (e.g., p53 and retinoblastoma genes) (14,15). SV40 can induce the single-step malignant transformation of cultured rodent cells, but the typical effect on human cells is to induce morphologic alterations and a prolonged life span, but not neoplastic transformation (10). Continued culture of these partially transformed, nonneoplastic human cells results in a phenomenon in which the cells enter a crisis phase, which is usually followed by senescence and cell death. Infrequently, however, some cells survive this phase to yield an immortal but still nontumorigenic cell line (16,17). The complete neoplastic transformation of SV40-immortalized, nontumorigenic human cells can often be achieved by the addition of complementing oncogenes (e.g., members of the *ras* gene family or tyrosine kinases) (16,18–20). These results indicate the requirement for multiple independent events in the transformation of human epithelial cells.

We observed a similar series of events upon introducing SV40 into normal PT cells via a retroviral vector. Initially, PT cells expressing SV40 large T antigen (termed PT-SV) exhibited an altered morphology compared to uninfected PT cells and PT cells infected with a retrovirus that contained no oncogene. PT-SV cells were slightly smaller than control cells and grew to a higher density, eventually forming densely packed colonies of cells. Immunoprecipitation studies with monoclonal antibody (MAb) specific for large T antigen (Ag) confirmed the presence of this antigen in PT-SV cells (Figure 1). Cell surface antigenic analysis showed that PT-SV cells continued to express the entire complement of PT surface antigens displayed on control cultures of PT cells. However, a possibly critical alteration in PT-SV cells involved the novel cell surface expression of the disialoganglioside GD3. GD3 is normally not expressed by PT cells but is expressed on a subset ($\sim$ 10%) of cultured and noncultured RCC (7,21). Expression of GD3 is associated with malignant transformation in other tumor types, most notably malignant melanomas and gliomas (21,22). The precise impact of GD3 in the transformation process is obscure, but it has been shown to have a wide range of biologic roles, including involvement in cellular adherence and membrane permeability (23).

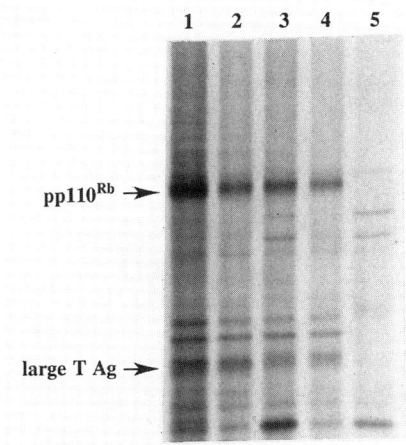

Figure 1 Immunoprecipitation of SV40-infected PT cells. Short-term cultures of PT cells were infected with SV40-containing retrovirus, labeled with [^{35}S]-methionine, and immunoprecipitated with MAb PAb419 (Oncogene Science, New York), as described (14). Note the precipitation of SV40 large T Ag and coprecipitation of the Rb gene product (arrows). Lanes 1–4, four individual SV40-infected PT cells lines; lane 5, SK-RC-44 (negative control).

PT-SV cells were also examined for a range of biologic traits characteristic of normal PT cells and RCC (Table 1). PT-SV cells exhibited a marked increase in proliferative capacity and a loss of contact inhibition, two phenotypic characteristics of cultured RCC cells. Cytogenetic analyses of two independent SV-40-infected PT cultures revealed a hyperdiploid karyotype, but in contrast to RCC, nonrandom chromosomal abnormalities were not present. Moreover, analogously to normal PT cells, PT-SV cells were both anchorage dependent, being unable to grow in soft agar assays, and nontumorigenic in athymic mice. After approximately 20 passages in culture (i.e., 3 months), PT-SV cells underwent a distinct change in morphology and entered a crisis stage, after which the cells became senescent. Identical experiments with six independent normal human PT cultures resulted in similar results. Thus, reminiscent of other human epithelial cell cultures, introduction of SV40 into PT cells results in a deregulation of growth control characterized by a marked increase in proliferation but not succeeded by cellular immortalization or neoplastic transformation.

It is clear that the introduction of SV40 into normal human cells usually results in the partial transformation of human cells and only rarely in the development of a fully transformed neoplastic cell. A putative mechanism for SV40-induced growth stimulation may be the association of the large T Ag with the Rb gene product (15). In immunoprecipitation studies of PT-SV cells, we determined that large T Ag coprecipitated with the Rb gene product (Figure 1), indicating that this mechanism may be active in SV40-transformed PT cells. It is likely that the completion of the transformation process in PT cells involves the occurrence of an unknown number of specific chromosomal and genetic abnormalities. A hallmark of SV40 infection is the induction of a range of karyotypic abnormalities, including aneuploidy and chromosomal rearrangement, the effects of which are unknown, but presumably, in our experiments with PT cells the critical defects were not generated. It is the rare SV40-transformed cell that completes the neoplastic conversion process in which this presumptive critical genetic defect has occurred. One interpretation of these data is that there is synergism between the introduced SV40 oncogene and undefined oncogenes activated spontaneously in the cell by acquired genetic defects. Deciphering any nonrandom chromosomal defects and the genes involved that lead to the neoplastic transformation of SV40-infected cells would provide insight into the transformation process of that particular cell type.

III. TRANSFORMATION OF PROXIMAL TUBULE CELLS BY THE *ras* ONCOGENE

Derangement of *ras* oncogenes has been implicated in the pathogenesis of a wide range of human malignancies, including cancers of the genitourinary tract (24). Members of the *ras* gene family, that is, c-Ha-*ras* (Harvey), c-Ki-*ras* (Kirsten), and N-*ras*, encode a homologous guanosine triphosphate-diphosphate (GTP/GDP) binding protein with a molecular weight of 21,000 (p21) (25). Although the precise function of p21 protein is unknown, evidence suggests that it is involved in the process of signal transduction across cellular membranes (26). Spontaneous mutation of the *ras* genes by a single nucleotide substitution in codons 12, 13, or 61 alters the *ras* p21 protein, converting it to one with transforming potential (24,25). The prevalence of transforming *ras* genes activated by somatic mutation in human tumors has ranged from essentially 0 [e.g., in esophageal tumors (27)] to 95% [e.g., in pancreatic carcinomas (28)]. Consequently, the involvement of *ras* genes in the initiation, maintenance, and metastasis of individual tumor types may be fundamentally different. To investigate the relationship of *ras* oncogenes and renal cell carcinogenesis we performed two studies. First, we introduced the viral Ki-*ras* and Ha-*ras* oncogenes into normal human renal PT cells via an amphotropic retroviral vector and determined the biologic, antigenic, and genetic effects on these cells (7). Second, we analyzed the frequency of *ras* point mutations in cultured and noncultured RCC (29).

Infection of PT cells with either the viral Ha-*ras* or Ki-*ras* oncogene consistently resulted in a transient increase in the growth rate. The *ras*-infected PT cells survive at least two to four more generations longer than uninfected cells or cells infected with a control virus that does not contain an oncogene. Like control cells, however, *ras*-containing PT cells eventually become senescent. In two separate experiments, Ha-*ras*- and Ki-*ras*-infected PT cells (PT-Ha and PT-Ki) continued to replicate well beyond passage 5. Long-term growth studies of these cell cultures indicate that they are immortal. Analysis of the surface antigenic phenotype of these cells confirmed the expression of normal PT surface antigens, as well expression of a RCC marker, GD3. Biologic analysis indicated that PT-Ki and PT-Ha cells possessed a characteristic RCC phenotype (Table 1), which included an altered morphology, increased growth capacity, loss of contact inhibition, tumorigenicity in athymic mice, and an aneuploid karyotype. Interestingly, however, although PT-Ha or PT-Ki cells were neoplastic, they also maintained an anchorage-dependent requirement for growth, being unable to form colonies in soft agar. Cytogenetic analysis of PT-Ki cells karyotyped at passage 3 showed that 92% of the cells were 46XY,-21, + der(21)t(1;21)(q21;q22), and PT-Ha cells karyotyped at passage 4 showed that 50% were 45XY,-21. At passage 23 (approximately 8 months in culture), PT-Ki cells acquired the capacity for anchorage-independent growth and could then form colonies in soft agar with an efficiency of approximately 10%. Karyotypic analysis of these cells and five soft agar clones revealed that 100% of the cells still possessed the marker chromosome + der(21)t(1;21)(q21;q22). In addition, several other nonrandom karyotypic abnormalities were present in the soft agar clones that are commonly observed in noncultured RCC (30,31). These included − 5, 5q+ , + 7, − 18, and − Y (7). Chromosomal analysis of the PT-Ki cells at passage 57 revealed the persistence of the marker chromosome and abnormalities involving chromosome 3q [47,XY,-3,-21, + der(3)t(3;?)(q27;?), + der(21)t(1:21)(q21:q22), + 20].

Several conclusions can be drawn from these experiments. First, that alterations of chromosome 21 were among the earliest nonrandom chromosomal defects observed in two individual cell lines transformed by *ras* oncogenes suggests that disruption of a specific gene(s) on chromosome 21 (possibly in the region of the 1:21 translocation observed in PT-Ki cells) may play an early and pivotal role in the transformation of the PT cell. To test this possibility, we analyzed PT-Ha cells, PT-Ki cells, and cultured and noncultured RCC for abnormalities on chromosome 21 by Southern blotting. However, to date we have been unable to detect any deletions, rearrangements, or reduction to hemi- or homozygosity in these DNAs using 10 chromosome 21-specific probes. Second, in our experimental model, sequential karyotyping revealed the generation of specific chromosomal abnormalities, most of which have been reported to occur spontaneously in RCC in vivo. These included abnormalities of chromosomes 3q, 5, 7, 18, and Y. Since these *ras*-transformed PT cells were already malignant, this set of chromosomal abnormalities must be secondary events in renal cell transformation. Finally, the combination of an activated *ras* gene and specific chromosomal alterations can induce in normal human PT cells the fully transformed phenotype characteristic of RCC. This conclusion led us to ask about the role of the *ras* oncogene in RCC in vivo.

We assessed the incidence of naturally occurring activating mutations in the three functional *ras* genes (N-, Ki-, and Ha-*ras*) at codons 12, 13, and 61 in both cultured and noncultured primary and metastatic RCC using polymerase chain reaction (PCR) and oligonucleotide hybridization. This study detected a frequency rate for *ras* mutations of 2% in RCC (29). Thus, this low frequency of *ras* gene mutations suggests that *ras* oncogenes play a minor role in the pathogenesis of RCC, although it is possible that other undetected perturbations in these genes may contribute to RCC oncogenesis. At present, we presume that there are multiple pathways by which the PT cell can progress toward transformation, and *ras* may interdict one of the pathways that are actually disturbed in RCC.

IV. TRANSFORMATION OF PROXIMAL TUBULE CELLS BY THE *src* ONCOGENE

The *ras* oncogene is a p21 GTP binding protein capable of transforming human and animal cells. It is normally located on the inner cytoplasmic membrane and is involved in signal transduction (25,26). Another class of potent transforming genes are the *src* family of protein tyrosine kinases (3). The v-*src*-encoded protein (pp60^{v-src}) has transforming potential that correlates closely with v-*src*-specific tyrosine protein kinase activity (32,33). Like *ras*, *src* is normally located on the inner cytoplasmic membrane and is believed to be involved in signal transduction (26). Furthermore, recent studies suggest that *ras* and *src* may normally cooperate in signal transduction through p21^{ras} GTPase-activating proteins (GAP) (26,34,35). Consequently, to determine the specific effects of an activated tyrosine kinase on the biologic and genetic phenotype of cultured normal human PT cells, we introduced the v-*src* oncogene. Small colonies of rapidly proliferating cells appeared in the culture 8 weeks following infection with v-*src*, which possessed a well-defined epithelial morphology, similar to that seen in cultured renal cancers (5). These morphologically distinct cells, PT-*src*, displayed an increased growth capacity with a doubling time of 58 h, which has been maintained for >50 passages (30 months). PT-*src* cells possessed high levels of pp60^{v-src} kinase activity as determined by an in vitro kinase assay and expressed surface antigens characteristic of the PT portion of the human nephron (36). The biologic phenotype of PT-*src* cells was very similar to that of PT-*ras* cells. PT-*src* cells were immortal, were not contact inhibited, and were anchorage independent, tumorigenic, and aneuploid (Table 1). Karyotypic analysis of PT-*src* cells immediately following the outgrowth of proliferating cells at passage 6 revealed a highly abnormal karyotype containing a deletion of chromosome 3p involving bands 3p14–23. Southern blotting analysis confirmed deletion of this region (36). Loss of genetic material at this location is the most common nonrandom chromosomal abnormality reported in RCC (30,31). In addition to the deletions at chromosome 3p, PT-*src* cells showed abnormalities involving chromosomes 5, 7, 17, 18, and Y, defects are also observed in noncultured RCC.

These experiments indicate that introduction of an activated v-*src* gene into normal PT cells can induce a transformed cell with many of the features prominent in cultured and noncultured RCC. An obvious question in light of these results is to what extent c-*src* is involved in the pathogenesis of human renal cancers. One study, designed to detect an increase in *src*-specific tyrosine kinase activity, failed to find any in two noncultured RCC (37). In a similar study we were also unable to detect increased *src*-related tyrosine kinase activity in four cultured RCC (36). Although v-*src* tyrosine kinase activity is believed to be necessary for transformation, the mechanism by which tyrosine phosphorylation mediates the events leading to cellular transformation remains uncertain (32,33,38). Thus, it remains to be determined precisely how v-*src* mediates cellular transformation in cultured PT cells and whether human c-*src* actually plays a fundamental role in renal carcinogenesis in vivo. What is clear is that pp60^{v-src} triggers a cascade of events that affect a wide range of normal cellular characteristics in the human PT cell. A simplistic model could argue that v-*src* not only stimulates and sustains the deregulated growth of PT cells but also sets in motion structural or biochemical alterations that result in aberrant control of the cell's genetic machinery, one outcome being the acquisition of secondary genetic changes that play some critical role in the induction of a transformed phenotype. A potential candidate is the induction of defects of chromosome 3p both in vivo and in vitro in *src*-transformed PT cells. If the deletion of genes on 3p is primarily responsible for kidney cell transformation, then the occurrence of earlier abnormalities in other genes may be dispensable. A second possibility is that, although c-*src* may not be involved in RCC, other *src*-related tyrosine kinases, such as c-*yes*, c-*fgr*, *lck*, *fyn*, and *hck*, may be. Ongoing studies re examining the status of these genes in RCC. It may well be that, despite that increased phosphorylation of tyrosine by protein kinases can lead to oncogenic transformation, the cause of this deregulation in phosphorylation may not be defective protein tyrosine kinases, such as c-*src*. An alternative pathway for the regulation of protein phosphorylation involves enzymes that normally inactivate proteins by removing the phosphate moieties. This group of enzymes, the protein tyrosine phosphatases (PTP) (39), can cause transformation by being underexpressed (39). The loss of PTP activity could result in a substrate being permanently phosphorylated and thus in an active, stimulatory mode, leading to, among other abnormalities, cell transformation. It is intriguing to note that the receptor protein tyrosine phosphatase γ is located at 3p21 (40), a chromosomal region frequently deleted in RCC (31,41).

V. SUMMARY

In summary, it is clear that viral *ras* and *src* oncogenes have a pronounced effect on PT cells, affecting cellular processes that appear to be necessary for progression to a full malignant phenotype (e.g., cell proliferation, chromosomal instability, and gene deletions). More important, these alterations observed in vitro reflect events associated with the tumor progression of RCC in vivo. There is as yet no convincing evidence implicating either activated *ras* or *src* genes in the development of RCC, however. If either oncogene is directly involved in RCC, it appears not to be by mechanisms described in other tumors, such as mutations in *ras* and increased tyrosine kinase activity in *src*. One possibility is that v-*ras* and v-*src* oncogenes mimic or intersect other overlapping pathways, those that are actually perturbed during the transformation of the human PT cell. Moreover, based on our in vitro experiments, these as yet undefined pathways are likely to involve defects in the processes that are crucial to signal transduction (3,26). In conclusion, the in vitro PT cell model described here provides a valuable experimental system with which to analyze the effects of oncogenes on the normal functioning of the PT cell, as well as determining the role of these genes in the pathogenesis of RCC.

ACKNOWLEDGMENTS

This work was supported in part by the National Kidney Foundation Young Investigator Award (Nanus) and American Cancer Society Clinical Oncology Career Development Award No. 91-260 (Nanus).

REFERENCES

1. Bishop JM. Molecular themes in oncogenesis. Cell 1991; 64:235–48.
2. Marshall CJ. Tumor suppressor genes. Cell 1991; 64:313–26.
3. Hunter T. Cooperation between oncogenes. Cell 1991; 64:249–70.
4. Liotta LA, Steeg PS, Stetler-Stevenson WG. Cancer metastasis and angiogenesis: an imbalance of positive and negative regulation. Cell 1991; 64:327–36.
5. Ebert T, Bander NH, Finstad CL, Ramsawak RD, Old LJ. Establishment and characterization of human renal cancer and normal kidney cell lines. Cancer Res 1990; 50:5531–6.
6. Bander NH. Study of the normal human kidney and kidney cancer with monoclonal antibodies. Uremia Invest 1985; 8:263–73.
7. Nanus DM, Ebrahim SA, Bander NH, et al. Transformation of human kidney proximal tubule cells by *ras*-containing retroviruses. Implications for tumor progression. J Exp Med 1989; 169:953–72.
8. Ebert T, Bander NH. Kidney-derived cell lines. Semin Urol 1989; 7:247–51.
9. Bander NH. Monoclonal antibodies in urologic oncology. Cancer 1987; 60:658–67.
10. Chang SE. In vitro transformation of human epithelial cells. Biochim Biophys Acta 1986; 823:161–94.
11. Harris CC. Human tissues and cells in carcinogenesis research. Cancer Res 1987; 47:1–10.
12. Rhim JS. Neoplastic transformation of human epithelial cells in vitro. Anticancer Res 1989; 9:1345–65.
13. Stahl H, Knippers R. The simian virus 40 large tumor antigen. Biochim Biophys Acta 1987; 910:1–10.
14. De Caprio JA, Ludlow JW, Figge J, et al. SV40 large tumor antigen forms a specific complex with the product of the retinoblastoma susceptibility gene. Cell 1988; 54:275–83.
15. Deppert W, Steinmayer T, Richter W. Cooperation of SV40 large T antigen and the cellular protein p53 in maintenance of cell transformation. Oncogene 1989; 4:1103–10.
16. Rhim JS, Yoo JH, Park JH, Thraves P, Salehi Z, Dritschilo A. Evidence for the multistep nature of in vitro human epithelial cell carcinogenesis. Cancer Res 1990; 50:5653S-7S.
17. Christian BJ, Loretz LJ, Oberley TD, Reznikoff CA. Characterization of human uroepithelial cells immortalized in vitro by simian virus 40. Cancer Res 1987; 47:6066–73.

18. Rhim JS, Jay G, Arnstein P, Price FM, Sanford KK, Aaronson SA. Neoplastic transformation of human epidermal keratinocytes by AD12-SV40 and Kirsten sarcoma viruses. Science 1985; 227:1250–2.

19. Rhim JS, Kawakami T, Pierce J, Sanford K, Arnstein P. Cooperation of V-oncogenes in human epithelial cell transformation. Leukemia 1988; 2: 151S–9S.

20. Christian BJ, Kao CH, Wu SQ, Meisner LF, Reznikoff CA. EJ/ras neoplastic transformation of simian virus 40-immortalized human uroepithelial cells: a rare event. Cancer Res 1990; 50:4779–86.

21. Thampoe IJ, Furukawa K, Vellve E, Lloyd KO. Sialyltransferase levels and ganglioside expression in melanoma and other cultured human cancer cells. Cancer Res 1989; 49:6258–64.

22. Traylor TD, Hogan EL. Gangliosides of human cerebral astrocytomas. J Neurochem 1980; 34:126–31.

23. Cheresh DA, Harper JR, Schulz G, Reisfeld RA. Localization of the gangliosides GD2 and GD3 in adhesion plaques and on the surface of human melanoma cells. Proc Natl Acad Sci U S A 1984; 81:5767–71.

24. Bos JL. *ras* Oncogenes in human cancer: a review. Cancer Res 1989; 49: 4682–9.

25. Barbacid M. *ras* Genes. Annu Rev Biochem 1987; 56:779–827.

26. Cantley LC, Auger KR, Carpenter C, et al. Oncogenes and signal transduction. Cell 1991; 64:281–302.

27. Hollstein MC, Smits AM, Galiana C, et al. Amplification of epidermal growth factor receptor gene but no evidence of *ras* mutations in primary human esophageal cancers. Cancer Res 1988; 48:5119–23.

28. Almoguera C, Shibata D, Forrester K, Martin J, Arnheim N, Perucho M. Most human carcinomas of the exocrine pancreas contain mutant c-K-*ras* genes. Cell 1988; 53:549–54.

29. Nanus DM, Mentle IR, Motzer RJ, Bander NH, Albino AP. Infrequent *ras* oncogene point mutations in renal cell carcinoma. J Urol 1990; 143:175–8.

30. Walter TA, Berger CS, Sandberg AA. The cytogenetics of renal tumors. Where do we stand, where do we go. Cancer Genet Cytogenet 1989; 43:15–34.

31. Anglard P, Tory K, Brauch H, et al. Molecular analysis of genetic changes in the origin and development of renal cell carcinoma. Cancer Res 1991; 51:1071–7.

32. Golden A, Brugge JS. The *src* oncogene. In Reddy EP, Skalka AM, Curran T, eds. The Oncogene Handbook. New York: Elsevier, 1988; 149–73.

33. Parsons JT, Weber MJ. Genetics of *src*: structure and functional organization of a protein tyrosine kinase. Curr Top Microbiol Immunol 1989; 147:79–127.

34. Anderson D, Koch CA, Grey L, Ellis C, Moran MF, Pawson T. Binding of SH2 domains of phospholipase C1, GAP, and *src* to activated growth factor receptors. Science 1990; 250:979–82.

35. Brott BK, Decker S, Shafer J, Gibbs JB, Jove R. GTPase-activating protein interactions with the viral and cellular *src* kinases. Proc Natl Acad Sci USA 1991; 88:755–9.

36. Nanus DM, Lynch SA, Rao PH, Anderson SM, Jhanwar SC, Albino AP. Transformation of human kidney proximal tubule cells by a *src*-containing retrovirus. Oncogene 1991; 6:2105–2111.

37. Rosen N, Bolen JB, Schwartz AM, Cohen P, DeSeau V, Israel MA. Analysis of pp60c-*src* protein kinase activity in human tumor cell lines and tissues. J Biol Chem 1986; 261:13754–9.

38. Hunter T. A tail of two *src*'s: mutatis mutandis. Cell 1987; 49:1–4.

39. Fischer EH, Charbonneau H, Tonks NK. Protein tyrosine phosphotases: a diverse family of intracellular and transmembrane enzymes. Science 1991; 253:401–6.

40. La Forgia S, Morse B, Levy J, et al. Receptor protein-tyrosine phosphatase gamma is a candidate tumor suppressor gene at human chromosome region 3p21. Proc Natl Acad Sci U S A 1991; 88:5036–40.

41. Presti JC Jr, Rao PH, Chen Q, et al. Histopathologic, cytogenetic, and molecular characterization of renal cortical tumors. Cancer Res 1991; 51:1544–52.

7

Targeted Bispecific Antibody-Dependent Cellular Cytotoxicity Against Renal Cancer

Reinder L. H. Bolhuis, Cor Lamers, E. Braakman, and Gerrit Stoter

Rotterdam Cancer Institute, Daniel den Hoed Cancer Center, Rotterdam, The Netherlands

G. J. Fleuren and J. van Dijk

University of Leiden, Leiden, The Netherlands

S. O. Warnaar

Academic Hospital Leiden, Rotterdam, The Netherlands

I. INTRODUCTION

Experimentally induced tumor cell in animals express "new antigens" on the surface of the membranes that are specific for the particular tumor and are immunogenic. Some investigators have also claimed the existence of human immunospecific cytotoxic T lymphocyte (CTL) reactivity against tumor cells, even in the absence of major histocompatibility complex (MHC) differences between tumor cells and effector lymphocytes, that is, no MHC restriction of immune recognition. With the possible exception of melanoma, thus far no tumor-specific cytotoxic T cells have been generated because of the lack of either immunogenic expression of tumor specific antigens or because of their absence.

Moreover, around 1970 it was found that lymphocytes derived from healthy individuals were also quite capable of directly killing cancer cells in vitro. After the initial applications of immunotherapy for the treatment of cancer at the end of the 19th century by Coley and others, who used anti-cancer vaccines consisting of bacteria, and again in the 1960s and early 1970s using such bacteria as bacillus Calmette-Guérin or *Corynebacterium parvum*, the call for highly purified biologic response modifiers (BRM) with better defined modes of action became stronger in the late 1980s with the advent of recombinant DNA technology, the production of monoclonal antibodies (MAb), and advancements in the field of cellular immunology.

Monoclonal antibodies selective for tumor cells have been produced and enabled immunologic diagnosis and, in some instances, immunotherapy. Because tumor-associated antigens (TAA) are selectively expressed by tumor cells and are absent or present in only low density on normal tissue, we produced bispecific MAb (bs-MAb) by somatic hybridization of two mouse hybridomas, one producing MAb against the T cell antigen CD3 and the other against the G250 renal cell carcinoma (RCC) TAA and the MOV-18 ovarian carcinoma TAA, respectively (1,2).

The CD3 antigen is physically associated with the T cell receptor (TCR) heterodimer. Binding of MAb to the TCR/CD3 complex in a cross-linked fashion results in delivery of a signal via CD3 that activates the T cell (for review, see Reference 3). This MAb-mediated activation of T lymphocytes mimics the activation that physiologically occurs upon recognition of antigen by TCR. Such anti-CD3 MAb can also induce cytolysis of target cells by CD3[+] T cells when IgG FcR[+] target cells are used (4–7). However, most tumor cells do not express IgG Fc receptors.

The bs-MAb mentioned earlier are able to bridge CTL to the tumor cells, thereby cross-linking the TCR, resulting in activation of the T lymphocytes, triggering of their lytic machinery, and lysis of the tumor cells. We tested the efficacy of cloned CTL for their ability to lyse RCC and ovarian carcinoma cell lines in vitro in the presence of relevant bs-MAb. We also studied the involvement of lymphocyte function antigen 1 (LFA-1) in the adhesion of CTL to target cells, to investigate their possible capacity to act as a costimulatory signal to the TCR (8). This question was addressed because of the heterogeneity of tumor cells with regard to their expression of cell surface molecules, that is, the intracellular adhesion molecule type 1 (ICAM-1), which serves as the counterstructure for LFA-1. Finally, we investigated whether bs-MAb-targeted CTL can recycle, that is, can enter into repeated lytic encounters with tumor cells.

II. RESULTS

A. bs-MAb-Induced Lysis of RCC

We tested four different preparations of bs-MAb that are selective for RCC cell lines and were produced by somatic hybridization of the anti-CD3 MAb (OKT3)-producing hybridoma (the IgG_{2a} isotype) with isotype switch variants of a hybridoma producing the G250 RCC TAA, that is, each clone producing a distinct isotype: IgG_1, IgG_{2a}, IgG_{2b}, or IgE, respectively. The resulting quadromas from the fusion were subcloned and tested by immunohisto-chemistry on frozen tissue sections for RCC-selective reactivity. On average, a minimum of three cloning steps was needed to stabilize production of the hybrid MAb. All stabilized quadromas, irrespective of the isotype combinations, were able to effectively lyse the RCC target cell line (A704) using the TCR $\alpha\beta^+CD3^+$ CTL clone D11 (Figure 1).

The bs-MAb CD3/G250 (IgG_{2a}/IgE) did not induce lysis of RCC. The control parental MAb did not induce lysis, as expected. That indeed the target cell lysis by CTL, which were targeted with the anti-RCC bs-MAb, is selective was demonstrated by including tumor cells of distinct histogenetic origins as target cells, that is, melanoma and T lymphoma (IgR39 and MOLT-4, respectively; Figure 2). Irrelevant bs-MAb not directed against

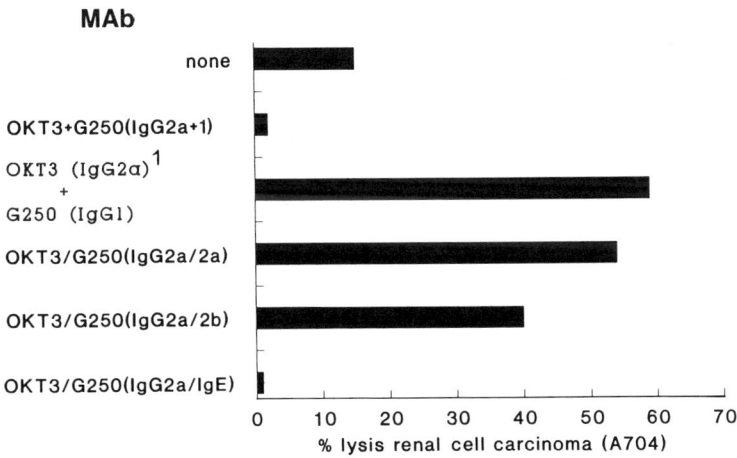

Figure 1 RCC cell lysis by a CTL clone in the presence of bispecific MAb.

target cells

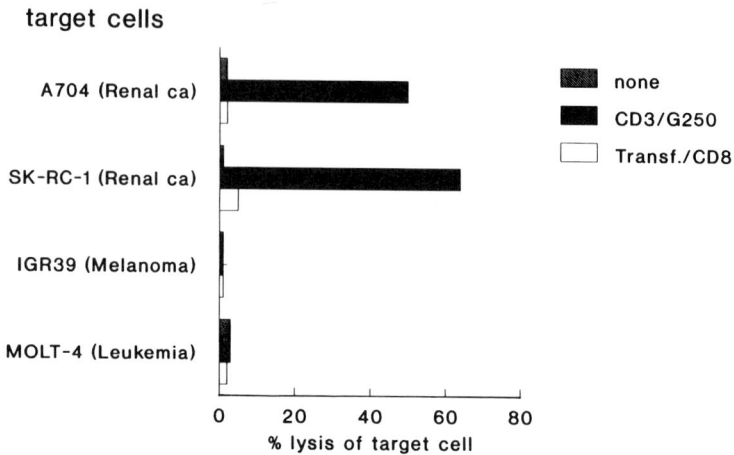

Figure 2 Tumor cell lysis by a CTL clone in the presence of bs-MAb CD3/G250 ($IgG_{2a}/1$).

CD3 and RCC TAA did not induce lysis of tumor cells (Figure 2). Only the relevant combination of RCC tumor cells, CTL, and the CD3/G250 bs-MAb resulted in RCC tumor cell death.

B. The LFA-1 Adhesion Molecule Costimulates the T Cell Receptor

LFA-1 is a transmembrane heterodimer and is expressed by most leukocytes (9). The function of LFA-1 in adhesion has been extensively studied. Recently, data have been published suggesting that LFA-1 is also involved in T cell activation. Its ligand is ICAM-1, a monomeric glycoprotein, which can be expressed by cells of many lineages, especially at specific differentiation stages or after exposure of cells to certain inflammatory mediators either in vitro or in vivo. Lysis-resistant Burkitt's lymphoma cells appear to express low levels of LFA-1, LFA-3, ICAM-1, and Epstein-Barr virus-positive B cells with a low resistance to lysis by specific CTL. These findings prompted us to study the role of LFA-1 in T lymphocyte activation and triggering of its lytic machinery via the TCR, making use of bs-MAb.

We tested a panel of histologically distinct tumor cell lines for their

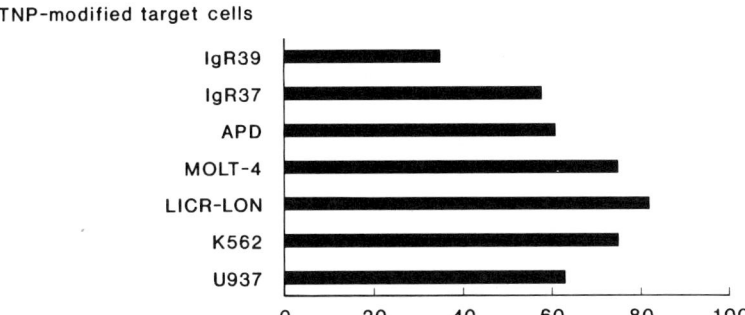

Figure 3 IgR39 melanoma cell line is relatively resistant to CD3-mediated lysis by a CTL clone.

susceptibility to lysis by TCR $\alpha\beta^+ CD3^+$ clones triggered via CD3, using bs-MAb produced by chemical cross-linking of the relevant MAb, that is, anti-CD3 MAb cross-linked to anti-DNP MAb. The different tumor cells were modified by trinitrophenol (TNP), a procedure that does not affect their susceptibility to lysis. This model system using TNP-modified tumor cells, in combination with a anti-CD3 × anti-DNP bs-MAb, circumvents the necessity to generate an array of distinct bs-MAb, each recognizing a particular TAA.

The melanoma-derived cell line IgR39 was known to have a relative resistance to CD3-mediated lysis by cloned TCR $\alpha\beta^+ CD3^+$ CTL (Figure 3) (8).

Increasing the concentration of the bs-MAb enhanced the level of lysis of the tumor cells. We tested many different cloned CTL, and the relative resistance of IgR39 melanoma cell to CD3-mediated CTL lysis remained unaffected. It was therefore concluded that the IgR39 melanoma cells could be either qualitatively or quantitatively distinct from melanoma or other types of tumor cells by a differential cell surface structure composition. Indeed, we found that these cells lacked the expression of ICAM-1, the ligand for LFA-1 on CTL (data not shown). In our screening procedure we have not yet found a particular melanoma tumor cell line to lack expression of LFA-1, but we have found histogenetically distinct tumor cell types also to lack LFA-1 and also to demonstrate relative resistance to lysis by CTL (data not shown).

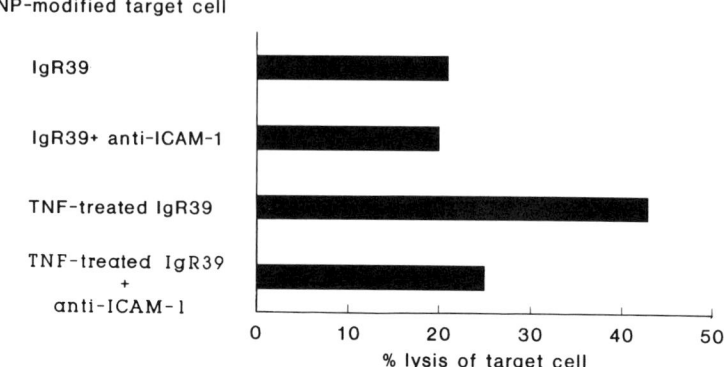

TNP-modified target cell

CTL: TCRab/CD3+8+ clone D11
heteroconjugate: 15 ng/mL

Figure 4   Anti-ICAM-1 MAb abolishes the increased susceptibility of TNF-treated IgR39 cell line to CD3-mediated lysis by CTL.

C. T Cell Necrosis Factor Induces ICAM-1 Expression on Tumor Cells, Rendering Them Susceptible to Lysis by CTL

T cell necrosis factor (tumor necrosis factor, TNF) has been known to induce ICAM-1 expression on many cell types, and indeed the IgR39 melanoma cells were induced to express ICAM-1 (data not shown). This ICAM-1 expression was accompanied by a simultaneous increase in susceptibility to CTL lysis triggered via CD3 by bs-MAb (Figure 4). That ICAM-1 indeed was the critical molecule determining the susceptibility to CD3 MAb-triggered CTL lysis, rather than modulation of the expression of an unknown cell surface molecule, was proven by the fact that the enhanced susceptibility to lysis of TNF-treated IgR39 cells was abrogated by the addition of anti-ICAM-1 MAb.

D. Anti-CD18 × anti-DNP Hetero–Cross-Linked Ab-Coactivated CD3-Mediated Lysis of ICAM-1⁻ Target Cells

When anti-CD18 × anti-DNP (dinitrophenol) bs-MAb was added to the ICAM-1⁻ melanoma tumor cells and anti-CD3 × anti-DNP–targeted CTL to

Table 1 Anti-CD18 × Anti-DNP Ab Coactivates Lysis of ICAM-1⁻ Target Cell by TCR αβ CTL[a]

Addition of Ab heteroconjugates	% Lysis of ICAM-1⁻ IgR39 by TCR αβ⁺ clones	
	Clone D11	Clone 75
—	1	0
aCD18 × aDNP	0	0
aCD3 × aDNP	37	37
aCD3 × aDNP + aCD18 × aDNP	70	68

[a] Effector-target (E/T) cell ratios of 7 (clone D11) and 14 (clone 75). Heteroconjugate concentration: aCD3 × aDNP, 25 μg/ml; aCD18 × aDNP, 25 μg/ml.

mimic the LFA-1/ICAM-1 interaction, indeed an increased susceptibility to lysis of the ICAM-1⁻ melanoma cells was observed (Table 1).

E. bs-Ab-Induced Anergy in CTL

For prolonged clinical efficacy of immunotherapy using bs-MAb, in combination with in vitro expanded CTL from cancer patients, it is important to establish whether bs-MAb-targeted CTL can enter multiple cycles of cytolysis. Bs-MAb-targeted CTL were incubated with the relevant tumor cells, in this case ovarian carcinoma cells, using bs-MAb that recognized both CD3 and the MOV-18 ovarian carcinoma TAA. As can be seen in Table 2, the ovarian carcinoma cells, as already illustrated for renal cell carcinoma and melanoma, are effectively lysed by a CD3/aMOV-18 bs-MAb-targeted CTL.

When the antiovarian carcinoma bs-MAb-targeted CTL were reisolated from ovarian cancer cells after varying time points and subsequently tested again in a 4 h cytotoxicity assay for their capacity to lyse ovarian carcinoma cells, *no* lysis of tumor cells was observed (Table 2). This could be due to the following: (1) the bs-MAb were modulated from the surface of the CTL; (2) the MOV-18 antigen was shed from the surface of the ovarian carcinoma cells, thereby abrogating the bridging capacity of the bs-MAb of CTL to the ovarian carcinoma cells; (3) the CTL became anergic after having been engaged in the lysis of a tumor cell; or (4) although there was still sufficient bs-MAb on the surface of the CTL, with a free binding site for MOV-18 antigen on the ovarian carcinoma cells, the TCR/CD3 structures that have been involved in signal transduction cannot thereafter transduce other signals. Therefore, newly synthesized TCR complexes at the CTL surface are required to transduce signals.

Table 2 Recycling Capacity of bs-MAb-Targeted CTL[a]

Preincubation		% Specific lysis of ovarian carcinoma cells	
bs-MAb[b]	Ovarian carcinoma cells	−	+[c]
None	−	0	68
None	+	0[d]	68
Anti-CD3 × anti-OVA-CA	−	55	67
Anti-CD3 × anti-OVA-CA	+	15	64

[a] CTL (TCR αβ/CD3[+] clone D11) were incubated with either medium or anti-CD3 × anti-OVA-CA bs-MAb (50 μg/ml) for 30 minutes. After washing, CTL were incubated with either medium or cocultured with an ovarian carcinoma cell line (IGROV). After 24 h CTL were harvested and tested for remaining cytotoxic activity on ^{51}CR-labeled OVA-CA cells in the absence or presence of soluble bs-MAb.
[b] Bs-MAb TR3 × MOV-18; F(ab')$_2$ fragments.
[c] Bs-MAb added in the CTX assay, final concentration 50 μg/ml.
[d] E/T ratio 27:1.

F. bs-MAb-Targeted CTL Can Recycle

We therefore added "fresh" soluble bs-MAb to the mixture of CTL and carcinoma cells. As can be seen from Table 1, such readdition of bs-MAb resulted in lysis of the carcinoma cell.

Because immunofluorescence analysis demonstrated that sufficient MAb remained on the surface of the CTL that was preincubated on the carcinoma cells (data not shown), together with the fact that CTL again lyse the tumor cells following addition of such bs-MAb, the MOV-18 binding site of the bs-MAb was occupied by shed MOV-18 antigen (data not shown), and we conclude that CTL can enter multiple cycles of lysis but that CD3/TCR complexes on the CTL, which have been formally engaged in signal transduction, cannot subsequently transduce signals and hence become anergic.

III. CONCLUDING REMARKS

Many preparations of bs-MAb have been produced against a wide variety of histogenetically distinct tumor cells. They have been shown to effectively induce lysis of the relevant tumor cells by targeted CTL, as shown here for RCC, melanoma, and ovarian cancer. Therefore, the use of bs-MAb in combination with highly cytolytic T lymphocytes endows originally MHC-restricted cytotoxic T lymphocytes with a MAb-dictated tumor selectively. This bs-Ab-triggered cytolysis of tumor cells by CTL via CD3 is MHC unrestricted. Bs-MAb-targeted CTL can be used effectively for adoptive transfer of immunity. The "laboratory-engineered" immune lymphocytes are now used for clinical adoptive immunotherapy of ovarian carcinoma patients in a concerted action, with the Dr. Daniel den Hoed Cancer Center of Rotterdam, The Netherlands, the Academic Hospital, Leiden, The Netherlands, the Instituto di Ricerche Farmacologigiche Mario Negri, Milan, Italy, and the Instituto Nazionale per la Ricerca sul Cancro, Genova, Italy, as participating centers for a phase I and II clinical trial. The use of combinations of bs-MAb directed at distinct activation and/or adhesion sites on the lymphocytes and against TAA structures, respectively, will further increase the effectiveness of bs-MAb-retargeted CTL lymphocytes, as described earlier. Moreover, the use of bs-MAb directed against costimulatory molecules on the lymphocytes may provide the lymphocyte function-enhancing signal, which is not provided by (part of the) tumor cells because of the lack of expression of the relevant molecules. Employing such combinations of bs-MAb, we may be able to break tolerance or abrogate lymphocyte unresponsiveness. We previously proposed the hypothesis that multiple receptors are involved in MHC-unrestricted natural killer and lymphokine-activated killer cytolysis (10–12).

It was then predicted that the target cell specificity range of MHC-unrestricted lytic lymphocytes would be dictated by the combination of receptors that are functionally involved in effector-target cell interaction. The use of combinations of bs-MAb against such activation and/or adhesion sites can mimic this physiologic activation and trigger a cascade of (regulatory) immune functions. These combined molecular interactions of activation site, adhesion and triggering molecules, and tumor-associated antigens contribute to the activation program of the lymphocyte. The activation program comprises modulation of the lymphocyte migration capacity, proliferation, differentiation, and maturation, but also the target cell specificity repertoire of the lymphocyte. Addition of BRM to the proposed bs-MAb/CTL combinations for immunotherapy will further increase their antitumor efficacy.

REFERENCES

1. Canevari S, Ménard S, Mezzanzanica D, et al. Anti-ovarian carcinoma anti-T3 heteroconjugates or hybrid antibodies induce tumor cell lysis by cytotoxic T cells. Int J Cancer 1988; 2:18.
2. Van Dijk J, Warnaar SO, van Eendenburg JDN, et al. Induction of tumor-cell lysis by bi-specific monoclonal antibodies recognizing renal-cell carcinoma and CD3 antigen. Int J Cancer 1989; 43:344.

3. Bolhuis RLH, Gravekamp C, Van de Griend RJ. Cell-cell interactions. Clin Immunol Allergy 1986; 6:29.

4. Bolhuis RLH, van de Griend RJ. Phytohemagglutinin-induced proliferation and cytolytic activity in T3$^+$ but not in T3$^-$ cloned T lymphocytes requires the involvement of the T3 antigen for signal transmission. Cell Immunol 1985; 93:46.

5. Spits H, Yssel H, Leeuwenberg J, de Vries JE. Antigen-specific cytotoxic T cell and antigen-specific proliferating T cell clones can be induced to cytolytic activity by monoclonal antibodies against T3. Eur J Immunol 1985; 15:88.

6. Tax WJM, Reekers HW, Reekers PPM, Capel PJA, Koene RH. Polymorphism in mitogenic effect of IgG monoclonal antibodies against T3 antigen on human T cells. Nature 1983; 304:445.

7. Mentzer SJ, Barbosa JA, Burakoff SJ. T3 monoclonal antibody activation of nonspecific cytolysis: a mechanism of CTL inhibition. J Immunol 1985; 135:34.

8. Braakman E, Goedegebuure PS, Vreugdenhil RJ, Segal DM, Shaw S, Bolhuis RLH. ICAM$^-$ melanoma cells are relatively resistant to CD3-mediated T-cell lysis. Int J Cancer 1990; 46:475.

9. Springer TA, Dustin ML, Kishimotot TK, Marlin SD. The lymphocyte function-associated LFA-1, CD2 and LFA-3 molecules: cell adhesion receptors of the immune system. Annu Rev Immunol 1987; 5:223.

10. Hersey P, Bolhuis RLH. Non-specific MHC-unrestricted killer cells and their receptors. Immunol Today 1987; 8:233.

11. Bolhuis RLH, Braakman E. Lymphocyte-mediated responses: activation of and lysis by cytotoxic lymphocytes. Curr Opin Immunol 1988; 1:236.

12. Bolhuis RLH, Braakman E, Van de Griend RJ. Are cognitive receptors involved in ''non-specific'' MHC-unrestricted lytic activity? Res Immunol 1988; 139:460.

8

Gene Therapy in the Treatment of Murine Renal Cell Cancer

Drew M. Pardoll, Paul Golumbek, Hyam I. Levitsky, and Elizabeth M. Jaffee

Johns Hopkins University School of Medicine, Baltimore, Maryland

I. INTRODUCTION

The specificity of the immune response is orchestrated by two arms of the immune system (B cells and T cells), each possessing vast arrays of clonally distributed antigen receptors. It is the tremendous diversity of T and B cell receptors that endows the system with the ability to recognize foreign antigens and to discriminate self from nonself. For the generation of an antitumor response, two criteria must be fulfilled. First, the tumor must present novel antigens (neoepitopes) not found on normal cells. Second, the immune system must distinguish these neoantigens as distinct from self. It is this latter issue that determines the outcome of a potential response.

Despite the similarities in their receptor structure, B cells and T cells differ in the mechanisms by which they recognize antigen. To be recognized by antibodies, the tumor must present neoepitopes on the surface. In contrast, T cells recognize, via their T cell receptor (TCR), a complex of processed peptide antigens associated with major histocompatibility complex (MHC) proteins expressed on the cell surface.

It is now clear that at least two distinct pathways exist for the processing of antigens recognized by T cells. T helper (T_H) cells tend to recognize exogenously derived antigens endocytosed by antigen-presenting cells (APC) and degraded in low-pH endosomal compartments. Peptide fragments of the antigen then associate with class II MHC, and this complex is displayed on the surface. Alternatively, classic cytotoxic T lymphocytes (CTL) recognize peptides derived from endogenously synthesized proteins that are probably transported from the cytoplasm into the endoplasmic reticulum, where they associate with MHC class I molecules (1). These complexes then move through the Golgi and finally to the cell surface, where they are available for recognition by T cells. This scheme has critical implications for immunotherapy approaches utilizing T cells because the potential universe of tumor-specific antigens that can be recognized by the T cell arm is not confined to molecules expressed only on the surface of the tumor cell, but rather extends throughout the whole cell. Consequently, any point mutation, deletion, or recombination event that leads to the generation of a novel protein product can potentially provide a neoepitope recognizable by a CTL.

Recently, Boon and colleagues (2) demonstrated that mutagen treatment of tumor cells produced immunogenic variants that expressed novel peptides recognized by antigen-specific CTL. The gene that encoded this intracellular antigen, although expressed by both normal and tumor cells, was found to have a single point mutation in the tumors. This point mutation, which coded for an amino acid change from arginine to histidine, generated a new peptide capable of binding to class I MHC and being presented on the cell surface. These results established that neoepitopes generated by point mutations in tumor cells can be recognized by CTL. Probably all human tumor cells contain multiple specific genetic alterations responsible for their tumorigenicity. Mutations have been detected in all the common human tumors in oncogenes, such as $p21^{ras}$ (3), and in tumor suppressor genes, such as p53, Rb, DCC, MCC, NF, and WT1 (4).

A second type of tumor antigen was recently discovered by van der Bruggen et al. (5) in human melanomas. This antigen, called Mage-1, was the target for HLA-A1-restricted, melanoma-reactive T cells. The gene present in the tumors was not mutated. However, it was not found to be expressed in any normal tissues. It is thus likely that this gene is expressed only in early embryonic development, not in the adult. Hence, the immune system need not be tolerant to it and the unmutated form could serve as a tumor-specific antigen.

Although these tumors are considered immunogenic, it is still unclear whether the failure of an immune response to nonimmunogenic or poorly immunogenic tumors is due to an absence of neoepitopes or a defect in CTL regulation. The events leading to the activation of CTL are tightly regulated to protect against the development of inappropriate immune responses to self antigens or exaggerated responses to foreign antigens. This regulation is mediated by lymphokines produced by T_H cells (6–8). Most CTL express CD8 molecules on the surface, and most T_H express CD4. In general, CTL activation requires at least two signals. The first signal is generated by the cross-linking of TCR and CD8 by engagement of the peptide-class I MHC complex on the surface of the target cell. This first step induces the transcription of a number of genes, including interleukin-2 (IL-2) receptor (IL-2R). The second signal required for CTL activation involves binding of IL-2 by IL-2R (and probably other lymphokines as well), ultimately leading to killing of the target cell. Because most unprimed CTL are poor producers of IL-2, they must depend upon activated T_H cells to provide the second signal required for activation. Likewise, the activation of T_H cells also requires at least two signals. TCR and CD4 must be cross-linked by the engagement of the peptide-class II MHC complex. The second signal is delivered through an as yet undefined interaction between T_H cells and APC. One candidate for this second signal is the engagement of the T cell membrane receptor CD28 by its ligand, BB1 (9). Once activated, T_H cells begin to express surface IL-2R and secrete IL-2, along with other lymphokines, which leads to autocrine T_H proliferation and activation of CTL.

II. INTRODUCING LYMPHOKINE GENES INTO TUMOR CELLS: A NEW APPROACH TO GENERATING TUMOR-SPECIFIC IMMUNE RESPONSES

Our own group has been developing approaches to determine whether the failure of the immune system to reject nonimmunogenic tumors was due to an absence of tumor-specific CTL or a failure to generate adequate T cell help. We hypothesized that if T cell help was deficient, then tumors engineered to produce helper lymphokines normally made by T_H cells could effectively bypass the requirement for T_H cells in vivo. If tumor-specific CTL were indeed present, then the tumor cell could simultaneously engage TCR/CD8 by neopeptide plus class I MHC (signal I) and elaborate lymphokines needed for CTL activation (signal II). To experimentally address this question, we designed a system in which IL-2 is provided locally by the tumor cell target. This strategy addressed the critical principle in lymphokine biology that lymphokines act, not as hormones, but rather in a paracrine fashion. The novel feature of this system was that the tumor cell produced both the antigen and the helper lymphokine. Using a poorly immunogenic colon tumor model, CT26, we found that injection of tumor cells transfected with the gene for

IL-2 stimulated a CD8-dependent, MHC class I-restricted CTL response against the parental tumor (10). Most importantly, animals immunized with the engineered cells were able to reject a subsequent challenge at a distant site with the parental tumor cell line. In vivo elimination of CD8$^+$ (but not CD4$^+$) cells from syngeneic mice by monoclonal antibody injections and subsequent challenge with CT26 IL-2 resulted in growth of the transfectant. In addition, the IL-2-producing tumor grew in athymic (nude) mice.

These data established the role of a CD8$^+$ cytolytic T cell as an important effector cell responsible for this antitumor response and outlined two important principles. First, the immune response to a tumor may be primarily due to a helper arm deficiency of the immune system rather than an absence of CTL capable of recognizing tumor-specific antigens. A second principle illustrated by these studies was the effectiveness of providing "local help" to activate endogenous CTL. This strategy may have certain advantages over high-dose systemic lymphokine injections, because the tumor cell can deliver high concentrations of lymphokines where it is most needed—at the site of TCR/CD8 cross-linking on the CTL. Finally, the ability of these immunized animals also to reject a challenge with the parental tumor demonstrates that CTL activated locally can circulate and provide systemic antitumor immunity.

A number of potential mechanisms can account for a failure of help: (1) low precursor frequency of tumor-specific T_H cells, (2) lack of neoepitopes capable of being presented with class II MHC to T_H cells, (3) deletion of tumor-specific T_H cells, and (4) functional inactivation of tumor-specific T_H cells by the tumor. An in vitro model for T_H cell unresponsiveness has been developed in which engagement of the TCR with peptide plus class II MHC in the absence of second signal leads to inactivation of the lymphocyte (11,12). In this unresponsive state, there is no IL-2 gene transcription even if second signal is subsequently provided. This state of unresponsiveness can also be induced in T_H clones when antigen is presented by "nonprofessional" APC, such as MHC class II$^+$ keratinocytes (13). A number of transgeneic mouse models have provided evidence that a similar form of T cell anergy can be induced in vivo. For example, when the MHC class II I-Eα gene was introduced into the germ line of an I-E$^-$ strain under insulin promotor control, I-E was expressed exclusively on pancreatic islet cells. In these mice, I-E-specific T cells were functionally anergic, presumably as a result of engagement of I-E on the islet cells (14,15). Thus, an MHC class II$^+$ tumor that did not provide second signal could render responding T_H cells anergic, thereby leading to an absence of helper lymphokines needed to trigger the lytic mechanisms of tumor-specific CTL.

III. ENGINEERING RENAL TUMOR CELLS TO SECRETE IL-4

The encouraging results derived from IL-2 gene-transfected tumors prompted us to extend this paradigm to other lymphokines known to be important in immune response regulation. We therefore examined the immunologic consequences of introducing tumor cells engineered to secrete the helper lympholine IL-4. In addition to its role in the growth and differentiation of B cells, IL-4 has been shown to be important as a T cell growth factor and in the generation of CTL (16–19). Furthermore, IL-4 induces a different genetic program in activated CTL than IL-2, which correlates with increased lytic function (20).

Because of questions regarding the antigenic status of chemically or virally induced tumors, we chose to study a spontaneously arising renal cell carcinoma (RENCA) derived from a BALB/c mouse. When small numbers of RENCA cells (e.g., 1×10^3) are injected into BALB/c mice, they fail to be rejected and display a metastatic pattern quite similar to that of human renal cell carcinomas. RENCA tumor cells were transfected with a murine IL-4 cDNA in a bovine papillomavirus expression vector, and transfectants were selected in hygromycin. Clones were assayed for their ability to secrete bioactive IL-4. In vitro, RENCA-IL-4C has morphology, growth kinetics, and MHC expression identical to that of parental RENCA, indicating that IL-4 does not have direct cytotoxic or cytostatic effects on the tumor.

When RENCA-IL-4C cells were injected subcutaneously into BALB/c mice, they were completely rejected no matter how large the dose of cells. When RENCA-IL-4C cells were injected into BALB/c mice carrying either the *nude* (few T cells) or *scid* (no T cells or B cells) mutation, no growth was seen for the first 2 months, demonstrating that a major local antitumor response to RENCA-IL-4C could occur in the absence of T and B cells. Histologic examination of the injection site of RENCA-IL-4C in BALB/c mice demonstrated a tremendous influx of macrophages as well as some eosinophils. The predominant macrophage infiltrate in RENCA-IL-4C contrasts markedly with that of RENCA-IL-2 transfectants, which as previously reported for the IL-2-transfected CT26 colon tumor line, are predominantly infiltrated with T lymphocytes.

BALB/c mice immunized with RENCA-IL-4C rejected parental RENCA challenges at a distant site very efficiently. In contrast, CB17 *scid/scid* mice immunized with RENCA-IL-4C were completely incapable of rejecting contralateral parental RENCA challenges. In fact, the in vivo growth kinetics of wild-type RENCA in CB17 *scid/scid* mice were absolutely identical between unimmunized and RENCA-IL-4C–immunized groups. Taken together, these experiments implied that although the local rejection of RENCA-IL-4C was predominantly mediated by non-T cells, systemic immunity against the wild-type challenge was dependent on T cells. Furthermore, IL-4 was completely undetectable in the serum of these mice, indicating that the systemic immunity was not due to circulating IL-4. Histologic analysis of the rejecting challenge tumors revealed that, in contrast to the immunization site, lymphocytes were a major component of the infiltrating population early during the rejection. Immunoperoxidase staining showed that these lymphocytes were CD3$^+$, indicating that they were T cells.

The influx of macrophages seen at the immunization site, together with the CTL experiments, suggested a scenario in which tumor-infiltrating macrophages process tumor antigens and present them on MHC class II molecules to CD4$^+$ helper T cells, which in turn produce lymphokines that provide help for tumor-specific CD8$^+$ CTL. This model was tested in BALB/c mice that were selectively depleted of either CD4$^+$ or CD8$^+$ cells before immunization with RENCA-IL-4C and subsequently challenged with wild-type tumor. CD8 elimination completely abrogated the animals' ability to reject wild-type tumor challenges, but CD4 elimination had much less effect. Elimination of CD8$^+$ cells after RENCA-IL-4C immunization but before challenge also abrogated the animals' ability to reject wild-type tumor. These experiments demonstrate that CD8$^+$ effector cells are critical for producing the systemic immunity in vivo; the production of IL-4 locally appears to largely bypass the need for the CD4$^+$ helper T cell arm. The late recurrences in a few of the CD4-depleted mice are intriguing and suggest a role for CD4$^+$ cells in the augmentation of long-term ''memory'' CD8 responses.

A concern that is frequently raised about active immunotherapy strategies for human cancer treatment is that although immunity generated by tumor vaccines in animal models is sufficient to protect against challenges with limited numbers of tumor cells, they have never in the past been strong enough to cure animals of tumors. We therefore determined whether RENCA-IL-4C injections were capable of curing BALB/c mice that were injected with wild-type tumor cells at a distant site before inoculation with the engineered vaccine. Long-term cures could indeed be obtained when mice were treated with RENCA-IL-4C beginning at 6 or 9 days after introducing wild-type RENCA tumor cells. Histologic examination of RENCA wild-type challenge sites confirmed that by 6 days after injection, the tumor had indeed invaded surrounding tissues and therefore met the standard pathologic criterion for an established tumor at the time that RENCA-IL-4C therapy was started. Also, when the cured mice were reinjected with parental RENCA after 100 days, most rejected the challenge, indicating that a significant immune memory had been generated.

In conclusion, it appears that there are indeed antigens specific to tumors against which tolerance can be broken to generate beneficial responses. Without question, the major theoretical barrier to the sorts of approaches described here is the generation of autoreactivity. Are there additional layers of self tolerance against normal self antigens that are present from birth that will allow the immune system to effectively distinguish them from the neoantigens that have arisen within tumors? This critical issue will ultimately determine the limits of antigen-specific immunotherapy.

REFERENCES

1. Germain RN. Nature 1986; 322:687.
2. Lurquin C, Van Pel A, Mariame B, et al. Cell 1989; 58:293.
3. Hunter T. Cell 1991; 64:249.
4. Marshall CJ. Cell 1991; 64:313.
5. van der Bruggen P, Traversari C, Chomez P. Science 1991; 254:1643–1647.
6. Zinkernagel RM, Callahan GN, Althage A, Cooper S, Streilein JW, Klein J. J Exp Med 1978; 147:897.
7. von Boehmer H, Haas W. J Exp Med 1979; 150:1134.
8. Keene J, Forman J. J Exp Med 1982; 155:768.
9. Lindsey PS, Clark EA, Ledbetter J. Proc Natl Acad Sci U S A 1990; 87:5031.
10. Fearon ER, Pardoll DM, Itaya T, et al. Cell 1990; 60:397.
11. Jenkins MK, Pardoll DM, Mizuguchi J, Chused TM, Schwartz RH. Proc Natl Acad Sci U S A 1987; 84:5409.
12. Jenkins MK, Pardoll DM, Mizuguchi J, Quill H, Schwartz RH. Immunol Rev 1987; 95:113.
13. Gaspari A, Jenkins M, Katz SJ. Immunology 1988; 141:2216.
14. Lo D, Burkly L, Widera G, et al. Cell 1988; 53:159.
15. Markmann J, Lo D, Naji A, Palmiter R, Brinster R, Heber-Katz E. Nature 1988; 336:476.
16. Fernandez-Botran R, Sanders V, Oliver K. Proc Natl Acad Sci U S A 1986; 83:9689.
17. Hu-Li J, Shevach E, Mizuguchi J. J Exp Med 1987; 165:157.
18. Widmer M, Grabstein K. Nature 1987; 326:795.
19. Trenn G, Takayama H, Hu-Li J, Paul WE, Sitkovsky MV. J Immunol 1988; 140:1101.
20. Grusby MJ, et al. Cell 1990; 60:451.

9

Antiproliferative and Antitumor Effect of Interferon-α in Renal Cell Carcinoma

Correlation with the Expression of a Kidney-Associated Differentiation Glycoprotein

Neil H. Bander

New York Hospital–Cornell Medical Center, New York, New York

Guenther A. Gastl, David M. Nanus, Connie L. Finstad, and Anthony P. Albino

Memorial Sloan-Kettering Cancer Center, New York, New York

Lawrence M. Pfeffer

University of Tennessee Health Science Center, Memphis, Tennessee

I. INTRODUCTION

Approximately 20,000 cases of renal cell carcinoma (RCC) are diagnosed annually in the United States. About 25% of these patients have overt metastatic disease at the time of presentation. The median duration of survival in these patients has been reported as approximately 10 months. Among the balance of patients with cancers apparently localized to the kidney, the sole effective therapy is surgical excision of the cancer, typically by radical nephrectomy. About one-third of these patients with apparently localized disease (i.e., 25% of the total) later manifest metastatic disease and ultimately succumb to the cancer. The annual mortality rate for renal cancer in the United States is approximately 10,000.

Metastatic renal cancer has proven to be resistant to chemotherapeutic agents, both hormonal and nonhormonal (1). Immunotherapeutic strategies seem to be demonstrating greater promise, however. Currently, the two most active agents are interleukin-2 (IL-2) and interferon-α (IFN-α). IL-2, with or without lymphokine-activated killer cells, has produced response rates in the range of 0–35% (2–5). The treatment is intense, and the toxicity is substantial. Trials of IFN have produced objective response rates of 5–29% (6–10) with fewer side effects than seen in IL-2 trials. There has been no randomized trial comparing response rates of these two modalities in patients with renal cancer. Nevertheless, the reported response rates of IL-2- and IFN-based studies are quite comparable despite the generally better performance status, lower tumor burden, and more favorable distribution of metastatic sites (pulmonary lesions respond better than bone) of patients entering the IL-2-based studies. The lower morbidity of IFN and its general availability make IFN a very reasonable choice relative to IL-2.

IFN therapy, however, is not without problems of its own. It is expensive, and it is not without side effects. The problems of expense and toxicity are compounded by the long interval required to demonstrate response [median 3 months (6)] plus the fact that only about one in five patients who endure these problems derive an objective response.

II. RESULTS AND DISCUSSION

In the course of studies characterizing human renal cancer cell lines for cell surface antigen expression and biologic properties (e.g., growth factor production, growth on soft agar, and tumorigenicity in nude mice), we noted an antiproliferative and antitumor response in a subset of established human renal cancer cell lines when incubated with recombinant IFN-α (r-met-HuIFN-ConI, a consensus analog of the most frequent amino acid residues known to occur in subspecies of IFN-α; provided by Amgen, Inc.). This appeared to be a direct effect, occurring in the absence of any immune effector cells. Furthermore, the observed antitumor effect was noted at concentrations of IFN that could be achieved in vivo. When both the IFN-sensitive and IFN-resistant cell lines were molecularly phenotyped with six monoclonal antibodies (MAb) defining kidney-restricted differentiation antigens (Table 1), the binding pattern of one MAb (F33) demonstrated a 95% concordance with response to IFN (Table 2).

MAb F33 detects a 160,000 kD glycoprotein expressed by normal glo-

Table 1 Monoclonal Antibodies

Designation (Ig Subclass)	Antigen M_r	Site of expression[a]
MAb F33 (γ_1)	160,000	G, PT
MAb S22 (γ_1)	115,000	RC only
MAb S23 (γ_1)	120,000	PT, LH
MAb T43 (γ_1)	85,000	PT_c
MAb F23 (γ_{2a})	140,000	PT
MAb F31 (μ)	Glycolipid	PT_s

[a] G = glomerulus; PT = proximal tubule; LH = loop of Henle; RC = renal cancer; PT_c = proximal tubule, convoluted; PT_s = proximal tubule, straight.

merular and proximal tubular epithelial cells and by a subset of renal cancers in vivo and in vitro. All nine cell lines tested that expressed gp160 (gp160$^+$) were resistant to the antiproliferative effect of IFN, and eight of nine gp160$^-$ cell lines were IFN sensitive. This observation becomes even more provocative when juxtaposed with the results in another study of about 200 renal cancer specimens in which the incidence of gp160$^-$ renal cancers (the putative IFN-sensitive phenotype) accounted for approximately 20% of all renal cancers (Bander et al., unpublished observations), or approximately the incidence of responses seen in clinical trials of IFN.

We wanted to do a retrospective study of gp160 expression in patients previously entered in clinical trials of IFN to attempt to validate the in vitro findings. Unfortunately, this was not feasible because gp160 expression cannot be determined on routinely processed (i.e., formaldehyde-fixed and paraffin-embedded) tissue. Like most MAb to protein antigens, immunopathologic determination requires analysis on frozen sections. We therefore elected to study a nude mouse-human renal cancer xenograft model to determine if systemic in vivo administration of IFN would yield results similar to those we observed in vitro. Seven established human renal cancer cell lines (two gp 160$^+$ and five gp160$^-$) known to grow in nude mice were selected. Harvested cells from each line were injected subcutaneously into groups of 8–10 mice. Half of each group was treated with 1 million units IFN intraperitoneally three times weekly starting on the day of tumor inoculation. The remaining mice in each group served as untreated controls. Mice were monitored for tumor formation, which was defined as the time of initial presentation of a subcutaneous nodule $\geq$ 2 mm, which continued to enlarge. The results are shown

Table 2 Expression of Kidney Differentiation Antigens and Interferon-α Effect

Cell lines	S22	S23	T43	F23	F31	F33	IFN-α effect[a]
PT1	+	+ +	+ +	+ +	+	+ +	R
PT2	+	+ +	+ +	+ +	+	+ +	R
SK-RC-1	+ +	+ +	+ +	+ +	+	+ +	R
SK-RC-4	+ +	+ +	+	+	−	+ +	R
SK-RC-12		+ +	+ +	−	−	+ +	R
SK-RC-26	−	+ +	+ +	+	+	+ +	R
SK-RC-28	−	+ +	+ +	−	+	+ +	R
SK-RC-38		+ +	+ +	+ +	+ +	+ +	R
SK-RC-45	+ +	+ +	+ +	+ +	+	+ +	R
SK-RC-35		+ +	+ +	−	+	−	R
SK-RC-2	+ +	−	+ +	+ +	+	−	S
SK-RC-17		+ +	+ +	+ +	+ +	−	S
SK-RC-29	−	+ +	+ +	+ +	+	−	S
SK-RC-39		+ +	+ +	+ +	+	−	S
SK-RC-41		+ +	+ +	+	+	−	S
SK-RC-42	−	+ +	+ +	+ +	+	−	S
SK-RC-44		+ +	+ +	+	+ +	−	S
SK-RC-49		+ +	+ +	+ +	+ +	−	S

[a] IFN-α effect determined by growth inhibition assays (see Reference 11). S, >50% inhibition of cell growth compared to untreated control cultures at an IFN-α concentration of less than 1000 units/ml (except for SK-RC-29, where 50% inhibition occurred at 3000 units/ml). R, <20% inhibition of cell growth compared to untreated control cultures at an IFN-α concentration of up to 3000 units/ml. + +, indicates strong reactivity; +, weak reactivity; −, no reactivity by cell binding assays.

in Table 3. All the untreated mice developed tumors regardless of gp160 expression. Among the IFN-treated groups, mice inoculated with gp160[+] cell lines developed tumors just like their untreated counterparts; mice inoculated with gp160[−] tumors demonstrated significant delay or prevention of tumor take. The data were therefore entirely consistent with the in vitro data. We investigated the possibility that gp160 is related to the multidrug resistance (*mdr*) gene product (p170) because of their similar molecular weight, the known expression of *mdr* in renal tissue, and the role of *mdr* in resistance to chemotherapeutic agents. Our analysis indicates that p170 is different from gp160. Immunohistochemical analysis demonstrates different patterns of expression of these two molecules. For example, in normal kidney, gp160 is

Table 3   Antiproliferative Effect of Interferon-α on Renal Cancer Xenografts

Cell lines	gp160 expression	Median days to tumor formation[a]	
		− IFN-α	+ IFN-α[b]
SK-RC-01	+	14	15
SK-RC-45	+	10	10
SK-RC-17	−	6	>77
SK-RC-39	−	30	>73
SK-RC-42	−	40	NTF
SK-RC-44	−	7	NTF
SK-RC-49	−	5	NTF

[a] Tumor formation assessed as the initial presentation of a subcutaneous nodule > 2 mm, which continued to enlarge.
[b] IFN-α, treatment with 1 million units of recombinant DNA-derived α-IFN-Con1 intraperitoneally on a Monday-Wednesday-Friday schedule. See Reference 11. NTF, no tumor formation.

expressed by both glomerular and proximal tubular cells but p170 expression is limited to the proximal tubule. In addition, p170 is expressed by the adrenal, pancreas, and portions of the intestine but gp160 is not expressed by any of these tissues (12). RCC cell lines in vitro also do not cophenotype with MAb to gp160 and p170.

If gp160 mediates IFN resistance, its effect is likely limited to renal cancer because gp160 is a highly restricted renal differentiation antigen and is not expressed by other normal tissues or cancers (with the exception that some sarcomas appear to be gp160$^+$).

It is not yet clear whether gp160 directly mediates IFN resistance or if gp160 merely fortuitously cotypes with another gene product that is responsible for IFN resistance. However, we have found that there is a correlation between the apparent level of cell surface gp160 expression and IFN resistance. Of seven RCC lines which were gp160$^-$ by cell binding assay and by immunoprecipitation, all had an IC_{50} dose < 1000 U/ml. Cell lines with higher levels of expression required variously higher concentrations of IFN to reach the IC_{50}. These higher dose levels exceed those attainable in vivo.

We attempted to block IFN resistance in gp160$^+$ RCC lines in vitro using MAb to gp160. We could not demonstrate any change in resistance. This could indicate that gp160 does not directly mediate the resistance or that the MAb utilized do not block the active site.

III. SUMMARY

In conclusion, we observed an antiproliferative or antitumor effect among a subset of human renal cancers when incubated with IFN in vitro or when grown in an animal model and systemically treated with IFN. In neither setting does the response require the presence of immune effector cells. In 95% of the RCC lines tested (17 of 18), the response to IFN correlates with the expression of a kidney-restricted differentiation antigen, gp160. The sensitive phenotype (gp160⁻) occurs in approximately 20% of patients with renal cancer—approximately the response rate reported in numerous clinical trials. Recently, a prospective trial has begun to test the hypothesis that the gp160 phenotype is predictive of IFN response in patients. If confirmed, such a finding would be of obvious practical benefit.

Last, it is not currently known if gp160 directly mediates IFN resistance or merely cotypes with another gene product responsible for the phenomenon. Nor is the function of gp160 known. We are currently endeavoring to clone the gene to answer these questions. If gp160 mediates the resistance, it is tempting to contemplate the possibility of blocking its function. This could theoretically lead to higher response rates in patients with RCC treated with IFN.

REFERENCES

1. Yagoda A, Bander NH. Failure of cytotoxic chemotherapy, 1983–1988, and the emerging role of monoclonal antibodies for renal cancer. Urol Int 1989; 44: 338–45.
2. Rosenberg SA, Lotze MT, Muul LM, et al. A progress report on the treatment of 157 patients with advanced cancer using lymphokine-activated killer cells and interleukin-2 or high-dose interleukin-2 alone. N Engl J Med 1987; 316:889.
3. Parkinson DR, Fisher RI, Rayner AA, et al. Therapy of renal cell carcinoma with interleukin-2 and lymphokine-activated killer cells: phase II experience with a hybrid bolus and continuous infusion interleukin-2 regimen. J Clin Oncol 1990; 8:1630–6.
4. Abrams JS, Rayner AA, Wiernik PH, et al. High-dose recombinant interleukin-2 alone: a regimen with limited activity in the treatment of advanced renal cell carcinoma. J Natl Cancer Inst 1990; 82:1202–6.
5. Wang JCL, Walle A, Novogrodsky A, et al. A phase II clinical trial of adoptive immunotherapy for advanced renal cell carcinoma using mitogen-activated autologous leukocytes and continuous infusion interleukin-2. J Clin Oncol 1989; 7:1885–91.
6. Neidhart JA. Interferon therapy for the treatment of renal cancer. Cancer 1986; 57:1696–9.

7. Fossa SD, De Garis ST, Heier MS, et al. Recombinant interferon alfa-2a with or without vinblastine in metastatic renal cell carcinoma. Cancer 1986; 57:1700–4.

8. Sarna G, Figlin R, deKernion J. Interferon in renal cell carcinoma—the UCLA experience. Cancer 1987; 59:610–12.

9. Umeda T, Niijima T. Phase II study of alpha interferon on renal cell carcinoma—summary of three collaborative trials. Cancer 1986; 58:1231–5.

10. Krown SE. Interferon treatment of renal cell carcinoma—current status and future prospects. Cancer 1987; 59:647–51.

11. Nanus DM, Pfeffer LM, Bander NH, et al. Antiproliferative and antitumor effects of α-interferon in renal cell carcinomas: correlation with the expression of a kidney-associated differentiation glycoprotein. Cancer Res 1990; 50:4190–4.

12. Thiebaut F, Tsuruo T, Hamada H, et al. Proc Natl Acad Sci U S A 1987; 84:7735–8.

IV

Cell-Mediated Immune Responses and Adoptive Immunotherapy

10

Natural Killer Cells in Human Renal Cell Carcinoma

Kyogo Itoh

Kurume University School of Medicine, Kurume, Japan

Kazuhiro Hayakawa

Hirosaki University School of Medicine, Hirosaki, Japan

Andrew C. von Eschenbach

The University of Texas M. D. Anderson Cancer Center, Houston, Texas

Tatsuo Morita

Jichi Medical School, Tochigi-Ken, Japan

I. INTRODUCTION

Human renal cell carcinoma (RCC) is one of the few cancers responsive to various immunotherapies but relatively resistant to conventional chemo- or radiotherapies (1–4). There are uncommon but well-documented reports of spontaneous regression of RCC (5). The magnitude of lymphocyte infiltration in RCC was significantly higher than that of the other cancers (6). These results suggest that host immunity is largely involved in tumor regression. However, there has been very little evidence that either tumor-specific cytotoxic T lymphocytes (CTL) or T helper cells exist in tumor sites, peripheral compartments, or the other immune organs in patients with RCC (6–12). Instead of specific immunity, potent major histocompatibility complex

(MHC)-nonrestricted immunity primarily mediated by $CD3^-CD16^+$ natural killer (NK) or $CD3^-CD56^+$ NK cells predominated in lymphocytes residing in tumors (tumor-infiltrating lymphocytes, TIL) (10,11). This chapter addresses several key issues about the role of NK cells in human RCC.

II. IMMUNOLOGIC PROPERTIES OF RCC TIL: NK CELLS ARE A MAJOR EFFECTOR ARM FOR AUTOLOGOUS TUMOR CELL LYSIS

A. Surface Markers of RCC TIL Before and After Activation with IL-2

The vast majority (>70%) of RCC TIL in freshly isolated samples were T cells ($CD3^+$; Table 1). The percentage of $CD4^+$ T helper/inducer cells was slightly higher than that of $CD8^+$ T cytotoxic/suppressor cells. NK cells constituted only a small minority of RCC TIL ($\leq5\%$). This composition was not largely different from that of peripheral blood lymphocytes (6,10,12). These TIL were incubated in gas-permeable bags (duPont, Glasgow, PA) in AIM-V serum-free medium (GIBCO, Grand Island, NY) supplemented with 1000 U/ml of human rIL-2 for adoptive cellular therapy, as described previously (10). In all seven cases tested, RCC TIL proliferated well in culture with interleukin-2 (IL-2). Surface markers of IL-2-activated TIL 2–3 weeks after incubation were 50% of $CD3^+$ T cells, 32% of $CD4^+$ T cells, 19% of $CD8^+$ T cells, 8% of $CD3^-CD16^+$ NK cells, and 34% of $CD3^-CD56^+$ NK cells (Table 1). Thus, the percentages of $CD3^+$ T cells decreased, whereas those of NK cells, in particular $CD3^-CD56^+$ NK cells, significantly in-

Table 1 Surface Markers of RCC TIL Before and After Activation with IL-2[a]

Incubation with IL-2	T cells			NK cells	
	$CD3^+$	$CD4^+$	$CD8^+$	$CD26^+$	$CD3^-CD56^+$
Before culture	72 ± 17	38 ± 13	31 ± 11	5 ± 6	2 ± 2
Weeks 2–3	50 ± 32	32 ± 28	19 ± 15	8 ± 7	34 ± 25
Weeks 5–6	98 ± 1	64 ± 37	30 ± 31	<1	<1

[a] Single-cell suspensions of RCC from seven patients were incubated with AIM-V medium and 1000 U/ml of rIL-2 in the gas-permeable bags. Surface markers of TIL were analyzed using immunofluorescence techniques and flow cytometry before incubation and 2–3 and 5–6 weeks after incubation with IL-2. Values represent mean ± standard deviation of percentages of positive cells from six patients. Details of the methods and results are described elsewhere (6,10).

creased. Actual increase in the numbers of total TIL was 17.5-fold. Collectively, the mean n-fold increase in CD3$^+$ T cells and CD3$^-$CD56$^+$ NK cells was 10 and 651, respectively. In contrast to predominant proliferation of NK cells in the initial several weeks, T cells (in particular CD4$^+$ T cells) demonstrated overwhelming proliferation 5–6 weeks after the initiation of culture. They consisted of 98% CD3$^+$ T cells, 64% CD4$^+$ T cells, 30% CD8$^+$ T cells, <1% CD16$^+$ NK cells, and <1% CD3$^-$CD56$^+$ NK cells. The actual increase in the number of total TIL in those patients was 465-fold, and the mean n-fold increase in CD3$^-$ T cells and CD3$^-$CD56$^+$ NK cells was 743 and 31, respectively.

In summary, surface markers of freshly isolated RCC TIL, consisting mostly of T cells, were not significantly different from those found in peripheral blood lymphocytes. Predominant proliferation of CD3$^-$CD56$^+$ NK cells for several weeks in culture with IL-2 was of note, and it was different from TIL from either metastatic melanomas, where CD3$^+$ T cells predominated throughout the entire culture period (10), or the other human cancers (6).

B. Cytotoxicity of IL-2-Activated RCC TIL

IL-2-activated RCC TIL displayed potent cytotoxicity against freshly isolated autologous RCC cells as well as allogeneic RCC or melanoma cells (Table 2). They showed the highest cytotoxicity against K562 tumor cells (NK activity). CD3$^-$CD16$^+$ NK cells in RCC TIL were mostly responsible for the cytotoxicity, whereas CD3$^+$ T cells showed much lower MHC-nonrestricted cytotoxicity (Table 2). Kinetic study of autologous tumor cell lysis and NK cytotoxicity also revealed that the percentages of NK cells correlated well with the cytotoxicity (Figure 1). IL-2-activated RCC TIL during 2–3 weeks in culture possessed both higher levels of autologous tumor cell lysis and NK cytotox-

Table 2 Cytotoxicity in IL-2-Activated RCC TIL[a]

IL-2-activated RCC TIL	Cytotoxicity against (LU/10^6 cells)		
	Autologous RCC	Allogeneic melanoma	K562
Unseparated fractions	30	22	140
CD3$^-$CD16$^+$ NK cells	34	26	1670
CD3$^+$CD16$^-$ T cells	12	10	57

[a] RCC TIL were incubated with 200 U/ml of rIL-2 for 3 weeks followed by separation of CD3$^-$CD16$^+$ NK cells or CD3$^+$CD16$^-$ T cells using immunofluorescence techniques and a cell sorter. These cells were tested for cytotoxicity in a 4 h ^{51}Cr release assay.

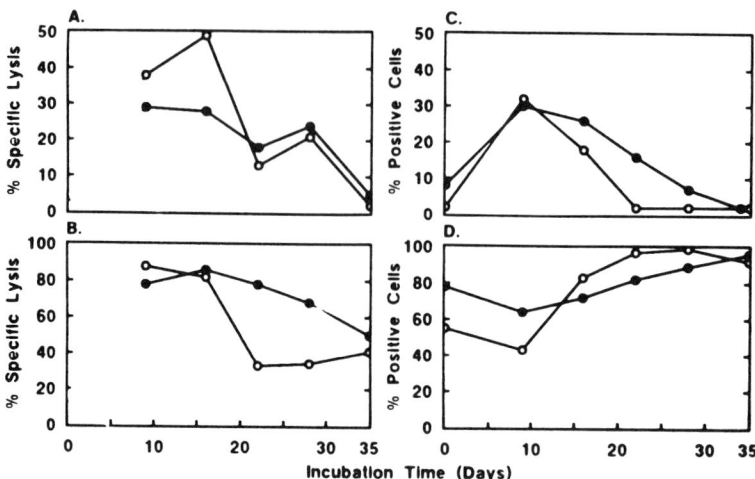

Figure 1 Comparison of phenotypes and cytotoxicity of RCC TIL from necrotic lesions to those from nonnecrotic lesions. Uncultured cells from necrotic or non-necrotic lesions of an RCC patient were separately isolated and incubated in an AIM-V/IL-2 bag. (A) A kinetic study of autologous tumor cell lysis at an effector-target cell (E/T) ratio of 40. (B) NK activity versus K562 cells at an E/T ratio of 40. (C) % CD3⁻CD56⁺ NK cells, and % CD3⁺ T cells (D) were investigated in IL-2-activated TIL from nonnecrotic lesions (filled circles) or necrotic lesions (open circles). (From Hayakawa et al., J Immunother 1991; 10:313.)

icity and higher percentages of NK cells. Those in the late stages of culture lost their cytotoxicity and also had lower percentages of NK cells. These results indicate that NK cells are a major arm for autologous tumor cell lysis in an MHC-nonrestricted fashion. T cells in RCC TIL have no or low levels of cytotoxicity. Indeed, T cell clones established from RCC TIL mostly demonstrated no cytotoxicity or lower levels of MHC-nonrestricted cytotoxicity (12).

C. Comparison of Immunologic Properties of RCC TIL from Necrotic Lesions to Those from Nonnecrotic Lesions

RCC usually consisted of both nonnecrotic and necrotic tumor lesions. Although TIL harvested from nonnecrotic lesions were primarily used for the study, necrotic tumor lesions also contained substantial numbers of TIL as well as live tumor cells. The immunologic properties of TIL harvested from necrotic lesions were compared with those from nonnecrotic lesions. Freshly isolated TIL from necrotic or nonnecrotic tumor lesions consisted of 55 or 77% CD3$^+$ T cells, 20 or 40% CD4$^+$ T cells, 30 or 40% CD8$^+$ T cells, and 2% or 0 CD16$^+$ cells. These cells were separately incubated with AIM-V medium and IL-2 in bags, and kinetic study was performed every 7–10 days for up to 35 days (Figure 1). Autologous tumor cell lysis (Figure 1A) and NK activity (Figure 1B) in IL-2-activated TIL from either necrotic or nonnecrotic lesions were high at both days 9 and 17 in culture and decreased thereafter. CD3$^-$CD56$^+$ NK cells increased from 2% (day 0) to 32% (day 9) in TIL from necrotic lesions and from 6% (day 0) to 29% (day 9) in TIL from nonnecrotic lesions (Figure 1C). Percentages of CD3$^-$CD56$^+$ NK cells in TIL from both lesions decreased thereafter and reached <1% at day 35 of incubation (Figure 1C). CD3$^+$ T cells in TIL from both lesions decreased a little from day 0 to day 9 and then increased, reaching nearly 100% at day 35 of incubation (Figure 1D). Thus, there was no significant difference between phenotypes and cytotoxicity of IL-2-activated TIL from necrotic lesions of RCC and those from nonnecrotic lesions, and NK cells are suggested as major effector cells to lyse autologous RCC cells.

D. Comparison of Different Culture Conditions for IL-2-Induced Activation of RCC TIL

Different culture conditions were compared with respect to IL-2-induced NK cell activation. TIL cultured with AIM-V medium and IL-2 in the bags consisted of 20% CD3$^+$ T cells and 69% CD3$^-$CD56$^+$ NK cells, whereas those cultured with RPMI medium, 10% fetal calf serum (FCS), and IL-2 (1000 U/ml) in microplates consisted of 85% CD3$^+$ T cells and 15% CD3$^-$CD56$^+$ NK cells (Table 3). The former TIL lysed autologous tumor cells, but the latter did not. In the second patient (RC11), TIL cultured with AIM-V and IL-2 in the bags had 28% CD3$^-$CD56$^+$ NK cells, whereas those with RPMI medium, 10% FCS, and IL-2 in microplates had only 5% CD3$^-$CD56$^+$ NK cells. TIL from the third case (RC6) cultured with AIM-V medium and IL-2 (1000 U/ml) in bags consisted of 70% CD3$^+$ T cells and 30% CD3$^-$CD56$^+$ NK cells and had potent autologous tumor cell lysis. In contrast, those with microplates had 90% CD3$^+$ T cells and 10% CD3$^-$CD56$^+$ NK cells and showed only NK cytotoxicity. A lower dose of IL-2 (20 or 200 U/ml) in AIM-V medium in the bags also induced the proliferation of CD3$^-$CD56$^+$ NK cells (data not shown). These results suggest that TIL subsets varied with culture conditions, and culture of TIL with AIM-V serum-free medium and IL-2 in gas-permeable bags raised more CD3$^-$CD56$^+$ NK cells with higher cytotoxicity than any other culture conditions tested.

Table 3 IL-2-Induced Activation of RCC TIL by Different Culture Conditions[a]

Patient	Culture conditions	Surface antigens (%)				% Cytotoxicity (E/T)					
						Autotumor			K562		
		CD3+	CD16+	CD56+	CD3−CD56+	40	20	10	40	20	10
RC1	AIM-V/IL-2 bag (day 25)	20	3	89	69	27	0	0	66	68	60
	RPMI/FCS/IL-2 microplate (day 25)	85	6	37	14	0	0	0	60	61	38
RC11	AIM-V/IL-2 bag (day 28)	70	15	80	28	—	—	—	—	—	—
	RPMI/FCS/IL-2 microplate (day 28)	95	2	31	5	—	—	—	—	—	—
RC6	AIM-V/IL-2 bag (day 16)	70	5	60	30	28	22	13	88	84	67
	AIM-V/IL-2 microplate (day 16)	90	16	16	10	2	0	0	73	56	41

[a] Single-cell suspensions of RCC from three patients were incubated under various culture conditions at the various incubation periods shown. AIM-V/IL-2 bag: culture with AIM-V serum-free medium and 1000 U/ml of rIL-2 in 3 liter gas-permeable bags. RPMI/FCS/IL-2/microplate: culture with RPMI medium 1640, 10% FCS, and 1000 U/ml of rIL-2 in 24-well microplates. AIM-V/IL-2 microplates: culture with AIM-V medium and 1000 U/ml of rIL-2 in 24-well microplates. After incubation, TIL were tested for phenotypic expression and cytotoxicity. Details of the methods and results are described elsewhere (10).

III. INTERACTION BETWEEN RCC CELLS AND NK CELLS: RCC CELLS POSSESS THE CAPABILITY TO ACTIVATE NK CELLS

In the previous section we showed that NK cells residing in RCC vigorously proliferated in culture with IL-2 and accounted for autologous tumor cell lysis in an MHC-nonrestricted fashion. NK cells from either peripheral blood or the other tumors usually did not vigorously proliferate in culture with IL-2. The results suggest that either NK cells in RCC TIL are different from those of peripheral blood lymphocytes or other cancers, or that cells besides NK cells residing in RCC are able to stimulate NK cells for vigorous proliferation in culture with IL-2. We investigated whether RCC cells can activate NK cells using cells from primary culture of human RCC cells (pRCC cells) as stimulator cells and human NK3.3 clones as effector cells.

A. Susceptibility of RCC Cells to NK Cell-Mediated Lysis

Cells from primary culture of human RCC cells were significantly more susceptible to lysis by NK cells than cells from primary culture of human melanoma cells or the other human cancer cells besides K562 target cells (13). Representative results at three different effector-target cell (E/T) ratios in 4 and 16 hour assays were shown (Figure 2).

B. Induction of NK Cell Proliferation

The RCC cells from all five patients tested induced significant proliferation of NK cells (Table 4). In contrast, none of the other cancer cells tested induced NK cell proliferation. Induction of NK cell proliferation by culture with RCC cells (RC7 or RC37) became significant at an effector-stimulator (E/S) ratio of 8:1 and reached a maximum at a ratio of 2:1 or 1:1, respectively (Figure 3). In contrast, none of three different cultures (two from established RCC cell lines, A704 or CAKI 2, or one culture of melanoma cells, M100) induced NK cell proliferation at any of the ratios tested besides a 1:2 ratio for A704 cells. Culture supernatants from none of the stimulators induced proliferation of NK cells. Culture supernatants from NK3.3 clones with these stimulators also failed to induce proliferation of NK cells (data not shown).

C. Increase in CD16 and IL-2Rα Expression

NK3.3 clones cultured with RCC cells increased their CD16 (87% positive) and CD25 (IL-2 receptor α; IL-2Rα 45% positive) expression compared to

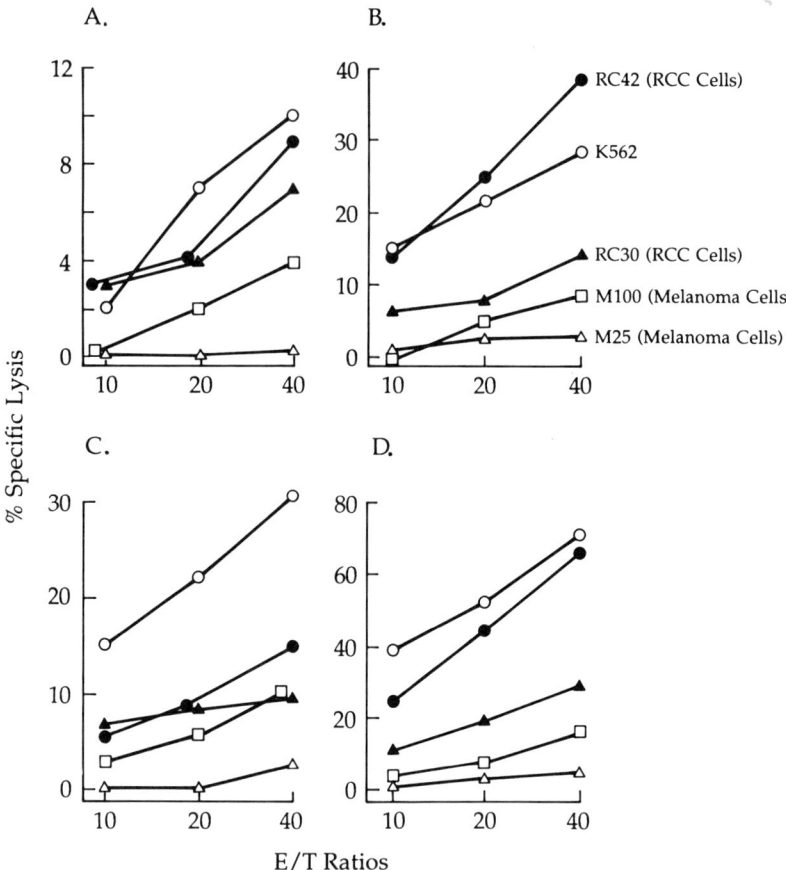

Figure 2 NK cell-mediated cytotoxicity against cells from primary cultures of RCC NK3.3 clones cultured with conditioned medium (CM; A and C) or 200 U/ml of rIL-2 (B and D) were used as effector cells. Target cells were RCC cells (RC30 and RC42) and cells from primary cultures of metastatic melanoma (M25, M100, and K562). Values represent mean percentage of specific lysis from triplicate determinations in 4 h (A and B) and 16 h (C and D) ^{51}Cr release assays at three different effector-target cell (E/T) ratios.

those with medium alone (64% CD16 or 14% CD25 positive) or with IL-2 (75% CD16 or 23% CD25 positive). There was no change in either the percentage of positive cells or the mean fluorescence intensity of CD56 antigen expression (data not shown). None of the T cell antigens (CD3, CD4, CD8, or TCR-δ-1) was induced in NK3.3 clones cultured with RCC cells.

Table 4 Induction of NK Cell Proliferation by Culture with RCC Cells[a]

		Proliferation of NK3.3 clones		
Stimulators	Patients	NK cell clone	NK cell clone plus tumor cells	SI
RCC	1	3255	13,802[b]	4.2
	2	380	6,487[b]	17.1
	3	4369	32,527[b]	7.4
	4	210	5,694[b]	27.1
	5	294	14,670[b]	49.9
Metastatic melanoma	1	4369	1,592	0.4
	2	4369	3,875	0.9
	3	174	268	1.5
K562		2410	2,610	1.1

[a] NK3.3 clones were incubated with irradiated tumor cells as shown in the absence of IL-2. [³H]TdR (thymidine) uptake of irradiated tumor cells alone were <1000 cpm. Values shown reflect subtraction of background. SI, stimulation index.
[b] At least $p < 0.05$ versus by NK cell alone (Student's two-tailed t-test).

D. Increase in Cytotoxicity

After incubation with RCC cells and IL-2 cells, NK3.3 cells demonstrated significantly higher ($p < 0.01$) cytotoxicity against RCC cells than that of those cultured with IL-2 alone (80% lysis versus 40% lysis), whereas in analogous IL-2 cultures with or without melanoma cells, no such difference in NK cytotoxicity was found. NK3.3 clones cultured with RCC cells also showed higher NK activity against K562 cells than those cultured with melanoma cells (data not shown).

In summary, human RCC cells (which are more susceptible to NK cytotoxicity than other cancer cells) possess the capability to induce proliferation of NK cells, increase CD16 and CD25 markers, and augment cytotoxicity in NK cells. These studies will be important for a better understanding of the immunobiology of RCC.

IV. CONCLUSION

NK cells residing in human renal cell carcinomas vigorously proliferated in culture with interleukin-2 and accounted for autologous tumor cell lysis in an MHC-nonrestricted fashion. In contrast, T cells residing in RCC had no or

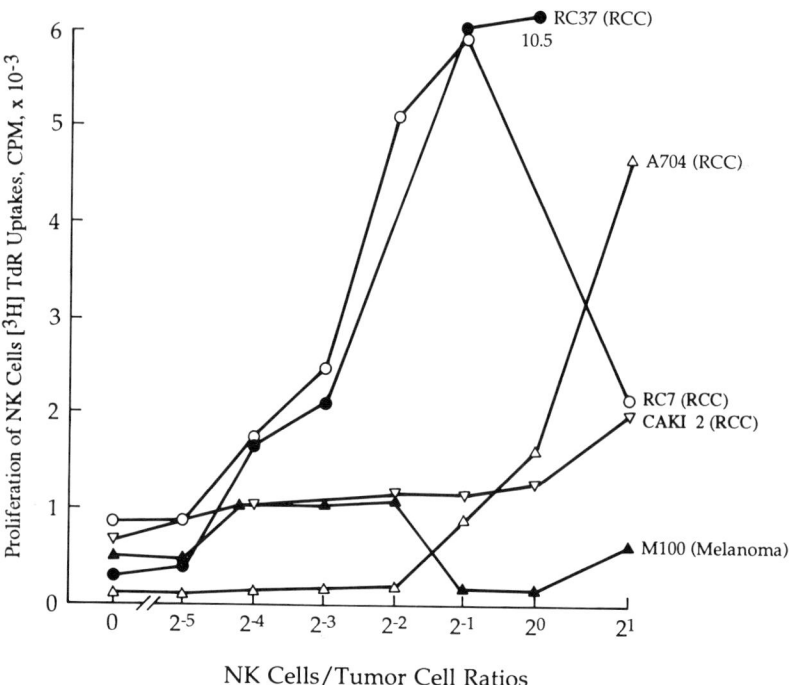

Figure 3 Stimulation of NK cell proliferation by incubation with RCC cells at different ratios. NK3.3 clones (4×10^4 cells per 0.2 ml per well) were incubated for 4 days in the absence of rIL-2 but in the presence of cells from primary culture of RCC (RC7 or RC37) or melanoma (M100) or cells from established RCC cell lines (A704 or CAKI 2) at various effector-stimulator (E/S) ratios. [^{3}H]TdR uptake of irradiated tumor cells was <1000 cpm and was subtracted from the values shown here.

very low cytotoxicity against autologous tumor cells, although they proliferated in the late stage of culture with IL-2. To address the mechanisms of the vigorous proliferation of natural killer cells residing in RCC, the interaction between RCC cells and NK cells was studied. Human RCC cells were more susceptible to lysis by NK cells than were melanoma cells or the other solid cancer cells tested. Incubation of NK cell clones with RCC cells in the absence of IL-2 resulted in (1) NK cell proliferation, (2) increased expression of CD16 and IL-2Rα antigens, and (3) augmentation of NK cell cytotoxicity. These results suggest that human RCC cells possess the capability of activating NK cells.

ACKNOWLEDGMENTS

This research was supported in part by Grant CA47891 from the National Cancer Institute and a grant from the University Cancer Foundation. We thank Ms. M. D. Young for manuscript preparation.

REFERENCES

1. Rosenberg SA, Lotze MT, Muul LM, et al. A progress report on the treatment of 157 patients with advanced cancer using lymphokine-activated killer cells and interleukin 2 or high-dose interleukin 2 alone. N Engl J Med 1987; 316:889–97.

2. Tallberg T, Tykka H. Specific activity immunotherapy in advanced renal cell carcinoma: a clinical long term followup study. World J Urol 1986; 3:234–44.

3. Poster DS, Bruno S, Ponta JS, Pinna K, Vilk P, MacDonald P. Current status of chemotherapy, hormonal therapy and immunotherapy in the treatment of renal cell carcinoma. Am J Clin Oncol 1982; 5:53–60.

4. Foon KA. Biological response modifiers: the new immunotherapy. Cancer Res 1989; 49:1621–39.

5. DeKernion J, Ramming K, Smith R. The natural history of metastatic renal cell carcinoma: a computer analysis. J Urol 1978; 120:148–52.

6. Balch CM, Riley LB, Bae Y-J, et al. Patterns of human tumor-infiltrating lymphocytes in 120 human cancers. Arch Surg 1990; 125:200–5.

7. Alexander J, Rayman P, Edinger M, et al. TILs from renal cell carcinoma: restimulation with tumor influences proliferation and cytotoxic activity. Int J Cancer 1990; 45:119–24.

8. Belldegrun A, Muul LM, Rosenberg SA. Interleukin 2 expanded tumor-infiltrating lymphocytes in human renal cell cancer: isolation, characterization, and antitumor activity. Cancer Res 1988; 48:206–14.

9. Finke JH, Rayman P, Alexander J, et al. Characterization of the cytotoxic activity of CD4$^+$ and CD8$^+$ tumor-infiltrating lymphocytes in human renal cell carcinoma. Cancer Res 1990; 50:2363–70.

10. Hayakawa K, Salmeron MA, Parkinson DR, et al. Study of tumor-infiltrating lymphocytes for adoptive therapy of renal cell carcinoma (RCC) and metastatic melanoma. Seqential proliferation of cytotoxic natural killer and noncytotoxic T cells in RCC. J Immunother 1991; 10:313–25.

11. Itoh K, Platsoucas CD, Balch CM. Autologous tumor-specific cytotoxic T lymphocytes in the infiltrate of human metastatic melanomas. Activation by interleukin 2 and autologous tumor cells, and involvement of the T cell receptor. J Exp Med 1988; 168:1419–41.

12. Kim T-Y, von Eschenbach AC, Filaccio MD, et al. Clonal analysis of lymphocytes from tumor, peripheral blood, and nontumorous kidney in primary renal cell carcinoma. Cancer Res 1990; 50:5263–8.

13. Hayakawa K, Morita T, Augustus LB, von Eschenbach AC, Itoh K. Human renal cell carcinoma cells possess the capability to activate natural killer cells. Int J Cancer 1992; 51:290–295.

11

Overview of Specific T Cell Therapy

Martin A. Cheever, Mary L. Disis, and Wei Chen

University of Washington, Seattle, Washington

David J. Peace

Loyola University, Maywood, Illinois

I. INTRODUCTION

The goal of developing specific T cell therapy for human malignancy is predicated in part on animal studies that show that T cell therapy can be effective and curative. In animal models, T cell therapy has been shown to be quantitative, with larger doses of immune T cells inducing longer survival times and greater percentages of cures. Therefore, effective specific T cell therapy in humans is dependent on being able to obtain adequate numbers of immune effector T cells.

In animal models it has been shown that small numbers of tumor-reactive T cells with limited therapeutic efficacy can be rendered curative by growing the T cells in vitro and treating with the increased numbers (1,2). [For a review of published works of others, see Reference 3.] The process of vaccination or immunization in vivo essentially involves induction of growth of the small subset of T cells recognizing the immunizing antigen via stimulation of specific T cell receptors with antigen. Stimulation of the T cell receptor with antigen induces T cell activation with upregulation of interleukin-2 (IL-2) receptors, secretion of IL-2, and induction of proliferation. Continued expansion of T cells in vitro can be mediated by either episodic restimulation with antigen or continued administration of exogenous IL-2.

T cells grown in vitro with exogenous IL-2 alone, as a major stimulus for proliferation, tend to become dependent upon IL-2, fail to synthesize endogenous IL-2 upon restimulation by antigen, and thereby become dependent upon IL-2. As a result, T cells grown in IL-2 alone often fail to survive long term in vivo to provide an optimal ongoing antitumor response and immunologic memory. In marked contrast, antigen-reactive T cells grown in vitro in response to intermittent restimulation with antigen, as the major stimulation for proliferation, can retain the ability to secrete IL-2 as well as other lymphokines and the ability to function normally in vivo (1). Normal function in vivo is defined in this circumstance as the ability to distribute widely, to proliferate in vivo in response to specific stimulation by tumor, to mediate specific tumor therapy, and to survive long-term in vivo to provide specific antitumor immunologic memory. Even the progeny of a single tumor-reactive T cell, if grown of large numbers in vitro under conditions that allow retention of the ability to respond to specific antigen, can provide all the necessary functions to eradicate tumor in vivo and can survive in vivo in large enough numbers to provide detectable specific antitumor immunologic memory long after adoptive transfer (2).

II. HIGH-DOSE IL-2 CAN CIRCUMVENT THE REQUIREMENT FOR HOST IMMUNOSUPPRESSION FOR OPTIMAL DONOR T CELL GROWTH AND LONG-TERM SURVIVAL IN VIVO

It has long been known that host "immunosuppression" with chemotherapy or radiation therapy greatly augments the adoptive transfer of T cell and B cell immunity. The most effective cancer therapy regimens employing the adoptive transfer of immune T cells have thus utilized either chemotherapy or total-body irradiation before adoptive cell transfer. Extrapolating from animal models, recent human cancer therapy trials with autologous tumor-infiltrating lymphocytes have employed both cyclophosphamide (CY) and IL-2. Similar interventions have been proposed as adjuncts to gene therapy regimens utilizing transfected autologous lymphocytes. However, very little is known about the interplay between chemotherapy and IL-2 for augmenting T cell transfer. Data from animal models (4) demonstrated that host pretreatment with CY increases both the short-term growth and the long-term survival of antigen-stimulated donor T cells in vivo. The administration of exogenous IL-2 for 7 days following T cell transfer also increases the growth and survival of donor T cells. The extent of growth induced by IL-2 correlates positively with the dose of IL-2. Pretreatment with CY increased donor T cell growth in vivo 2-fold. In comparison, IL-2 alone at doses of 2,500, 25,000, and 250,000 units per day increased the growth of antigen-stimulated donor T cells 6-, 14-, and 76-fold, respectively. Examination of the combination of CY and IL-2 revealed that the effects of low-dose IL-2 and CY were approximately additive. As the dose of IL-2 was increased, however, the advantage for CY pretreatment dissipated, and with the highest doses of IL-2 utilized, CY pretreatment was inhibitory and counterproductive.

III. CULTURED T CELLS CAN BE USED TO ACHIEVE A LEVEL OF IMMUNITY HERETOFORE IMPOSSIBLE

An essential observation supporting the concept of therapy with cultured T cells is that cultured T cells transferred in vivo can augment T cell responses substantially over those achievable by vaccination alone. For example, active immunization of mice with an antigenic tumor originally induced by the Friend leukemia virus (FBL-3) can increase the frequency of antigen-reactive T cells to approximately 1 in 150 T cells. In contrast, in representative experiments (4), a few tumor-reactive T cells (approximately 1×10^4) were expanded to 5×10^6 by stimulation in vitro with specific antigen followed by low-dose IL-2. The 5 million T cells were transferred in vivo followed by high-dose IL-2. Greater than 4×10^8 donor T cells were recovered in host ascites, spleen, and lymph nodes 1 week later. Therefore, the total increase in donor T cells in vivo was well over 80-fold. Moreover, the total number of T cells was increased 5- to 10-fold in regional lymph nodes and ascites, and thus the frequency of antigen-specific T cells in lymphoid organs was 9 of 10 versus the normal 1 of 150. Using transferred cultured T cells plus high-dose IL-2, hosts can essentially be "flooded" by antigen-reactive T cells, making the in vivo environment very inhospitable for any antigen-positive tumor cells. Importantly, the large numbers of donor T cells appeared to mediate no harm to the hosts.

IV. THE SURVIVAL AND FUNCTION OF DONOR T CELLS IN VIVO CAN BE GREATLY PROLONGED BY PERIODIC RESTIMULATION WITH ANTIGEN PLUS IL-2

The therapeutic efficacy of adoptively transferred T cells is related to both the number of T cells utilized and the time over which the donor T cells survive in vivo. Complete eradication of disseminated tumor often occurs over a prolonged period of time after T cell transfer. Thus, tumor elimination may be subject to both positive and negative influences over the same prolonged time. In unmanipulated hosts, transferred antigen-driven immune T cells diminish in number over time in a straight-line fashion on a semilogarithmic curve, implying that survival is predicated largely on factors intrinsic to the cells, as opposed to extrinsic factors, such as immune response to donor T cells (4). Studies have shown, however, that tumor-specific donor T cells surviving in vivo can be induced to regrow substantially at later points in time in response to repeated stimulation in vivo with tumor antigen plus exogenous IL-2 (5). Repeated courses of tumor plus IL-2 can induce repeated regrowth of donor T cells, with maintenance of donor T cell number at greater than the number input for more than 1 month. The increased donor T cell number can result in markedly increased immune function.

V. THE FUNCTION OF TUMOR-SPECIFIC T CELLS CAN BE MODIFIED BY RETROVIRAL TRANSDUCTION OF REGULATORY GENES

The requirement that T cells be intermittently restimulated with antigen for continual growth in response to IL-2 with maintenance of function makes it difficult to grow T cells. This problem is particularly relevant for human tumor immunology. Human T cells recognizing tumor-associated antigen often coexist with malignant cells at the sites of tumor. A major problem in developing such cells for therapy is that the antigens recognized have not been identified. Identification of antigens recognized by antibodies has been made easier by the use of B-B hybridomas to generate monoclonal antibodies. Similar T-T methodology has been difficult to establish for usage in antigen identification. T-T hybridomas are allogeneic to the host, and thus transplantation antigens are barriers for use in therapy. Therefore, recent experiments have begun to examine the use of transduction of autologous T cells with protein kinase C (PKC) and other genes to supercede T-T hybridoma technology and otherwise alter T cell function. Preliminary results have demonstrated that transduction of tumor-specific T cell clones with a retroviral vector containing the PKCγ gene upregulates IL-2 receptor expression and allows long-term growth in IL-2 alone with retention of specific function (6). In vivo therapy experiments revealed that the PKCγ-transduced T cell clones were as effective in curing mice of disseminated tumor as were the parental clones. The PKCγ-transduced T cell clones were not tumorigenic.

VI. THE PROTEIN PRODUCTS OF MUTATED ONCOGENES CAN BE IMMUNOGENIC BY VIRTUE OF UNIQUE AMINO ACID SEQUENCES

In humans, one ploy for generating large numbers of T cells immune to autologous tumor is to isolate T cells from tumor or regional lymph nodes and to grow the T cells with T cell growth factor (interleukin-2). This represents an attractive method for generating T cells immune to the unique display of antigens expressed by each individual's tumor. As a practical consideration, however, the use of autologous tumor cells as stimulators of T cell growth is limited by a number of factors, including the availability of autologous tumor and the secretion of tumor-derived suppressor factors.

An alternative approach for generating autologous tumor-reactive T cells is to stimulate the growth of T cells in response to defined antigens. In this circumstance the phenotype and function of the antigen-driven effector T cells generated can prospectively be chosen by the specific culture conditions utilized. For example, CD4$^+$ class II major histocompatibility complex (MHC)-restricted T cells can be enriched by the use of soluble tumor-associated antigens plus host antigen-presenting cells. Alternatively, CD8$^+$ class I MHC-restricted T cells can be generated by the use of antigen-presenting cells constructed to express the chosen antigen by use of transfection with DNA encoding tumor-associated antigens (7). Using established culture conditions, it is now possible to generate almost unlimited numbers of human T cells theoretically capable of functioning in vivo and reactive to virtually any antigen both expressed by tumor and within the host T cell repertoire.

A major remaining issue for prospectively testing antigen-specific T cell therapy for human malignancy is defining and characterizing which tumor-associated antigens on human tumors are within the host T cell repertoire and also appropriate for T cell attack. The antigens expressed by human malignancy have been extensively studied, characterized, and cataloged by many research groups. However, the majority of studies have focused on antigens recognized by antibody responses, and very little is known concerning which antigens are recognized or are potentially recognizable by autochthonous tumor-reactive T cells.

The primary event in the induction of malignancy is considered DNA mutation. Any protein expressed by a segment of mutated DNA is a potential tumor-specific antigen. Specific T cell therapy requires the existence of phenotypic differences between normal and malignant cells. A variety of cancer-related genes, including protooncogenes, have been shown to be mutated as an initiating event in the process of malignant transformation. Many activated protooncogenes and other cancer-related genes express predictable DNA mutations. Therefore, one focus of our studies is to evaluate whether the protein products of mutated cancer-related genes can be potential targets for T cell therapy (8,9).

The model system being studied is immunity to mutated *ras* protooncogene. Somatic mutations of the *ras* protooncogene are extremely common in human malignancy, occurring in approximately 20% of all patients. The mutations in general involve a single nucleotide substitution at codons 12 and 61, which results in the expression of a $p21^{ras}$ protein identical to a single substituted amino acid at residues 12 or 61. Only a limited number of possible amino acid substitutions can occur as the result of point mutations. Initial studies in mice (8,9) have shown that $p21^{ras}$ can be immunogenic to T cells by virtue of the expression of the single substituted amino acid. In these studies, mice were immunized with synthetic peptides corresponding to the mutated region of $p21^{ras}$ protein. Immune T cells were elicited that were specific for the peptide presented by class II MHC molecules. Importantly, aberrant $p21^{ras}$ protein could effectively stimulate specific T cells elicited with corresponding synthetic *ras* peptides. This demonstrated that $p21^{ras}$ protein could be processed by antigen-presenting cells (APC) so that the nominated segment of protein was bound to class II MHC molecules in a configuration similar to the immunizing peptide and in a concentration high enough to stimulate the specific antigen receptor on immune T cells.

More recent studies have shown that immunization of mice with whole mutated $p21^{ras}$ protein can similarly induce T cell responses and the T cell responses are directed against the mutated segment. This increases the likelihood that $p21^{ras}$ as released by patient tumor cells might be able to generate a detectable anti-*ras* response. Thus, $p21^{ras}$ protein represents a tumor-specific antigen related to the transforming events and shared by many individuals. Similar results have been obtained with proteins expressed by other cancer-related genes. Current studies are assessing various therapeutic ploys to determine how best T cells immune to *ras* can be used therapeutically.

REFERENCES

1. Cheever MA, Thompson DB, Klarnet JP, Greenberg PD. Antigen-driven long-term cultured T cells proliferate in vivo, distribute widely, mediate specific tumor therapy and persist long-term as functional memory T cells. J Exp Med 1986; 163:1100.
2. Klarnet JP, Matis LA, Kern DE, et al. Antigen-driven T cell clones can

proliferate in vivo, eradicate disseminated leukemia and provide specific immunologic memory. J Immunol 1987; 138:4012.

3. Greenberg PD. Adoptive T cell therapy of tumors: mechanisms operative in the recognition and elimination of tumor cells. Adv Immunol 1991; 49:281.

4. Chen W, Cheever MA. The requirement for host immunosuppression with chemotherapy for the optimal in vivo growth, function and long-term survival of adoptively transferred antigen-specific T cells can be circumvented by the administration of IL-2. Submitted.

5. Chen W, Reese VA, Cheever MA. Adoptively transferred antigen-specific T cells can be grown and maintained in large numbers in vivo for extended periods of time by intermittent restimulation with specific antigen plus IL-2. J Immunol 1990; 144:3659.

6. Chen W, Schweins L, Finn OJ, Cheever MA. Transduction of tumor-specific T cell clones with retroviral vector containing PKCr gene upregulates IL-2R expression and allows long-term growth in IL-2 alone with retention of functional specificity. Proc FASEB, 1991; abstract 5579.

7. Greenberg PD, Klarnet JP, Sugawara H, Schultz K, Cheever MA, Riddell SR. Requirements for antigen-specific induction and expression of CD4 [+] and CD8 [+] T cell responses to tumors. In: Lotze MT, Finn OJ, eds. Cellular immunity and immunotherapy of cancer, UCLA Symposia on Molecular and Cellular Biology, New Series. New York: Wiley-Liss, 1990; 235.

8. Cheever MA, Chen W, Nelson H, et al. T cell immunity to the oncogenic form of *ras* protein can be induced by immunization with synthetic peptides. In: Lotze MT, Finn OJ, eds. Cellular immunity and immunotherapy of cancer, UCLA Symposia on Molecular and Cellular Biology, New Series. New York: Wiley-Liss, 1990; 295.

9. Peace DJ, Chen W, Nelson H, Cheever MA. T cell recognition of transforming proteins encoded by mutated *ras* proto-oncogenes. J Immunol 1991; 146:2059.

12

Characterization of Tumor-Infiltrating Lymphocyte Lines Derived from Renal Cell Carcinoma

Demonstration of T Cells That Display Either Specific or Selective Response to Tumor

James H. Finke, Patricia Rayman, Mark Edinger, Raymond R. Tubbs, Eric A. Klein, and Ronald M. Bukowski

The Cleveland Clinic Foundation, Cleveland, Ohio

I. INTRODUCTION

T cells represent an important component of the host immune response to tumors. Animal studies have documented that T cells are involved in the antitumor immunity induced by cytokine therapy (1–7). Adoptive transfer studies have shown that specific T cells derived from tumor-bearing mice have the ability to inhibit metastatic disease (8–10). Evidence that T cells are part of the host defense against human tumors is suggested by the fact that most tumors are infiltrated with T cells (11–18) and some of these cells have specificity for the autologous tumor (11,13,14,16). During IL-2-based therapy regressing lesions exhibit an increase in T cell infiltration, suggesting an association between infiltrating T cells and response (19). In addition, antitumor activity has been observed in renal cell carcinoma and melanoma patients treated with tumor-infiltrating lymphocytes (TIL) combined with interleukin-2 (IL-2) therapy (20,21).

Characterization of the T cell response to human tumors is under investigation, and much of the work is focused on the cytotoxic activity of TIL. Specific T cells with lytic activity are readily detected in melanoma-derived TIL (14,16,22). In approximately one-third of the melanoma TIL cultures, the lytic response is due to major histocompatibility complex (MHC) class I-restricted cytotoxic T lymphocytes (CTL) (14,16,22). This high level of specific CTL activity has not been detected in TIL from other types of solid tumors (17,18,23–27). However, T cells with specific cytotoxicity for renal cell carcinoma (RCC) and ovarian carcinoma have been identified (28–31). Here we report on several TIL lines that display either specificity or selectivity for RCC in terms of proliferation, cytotoxic activity, and production of interferon-γ (IFN-γ).

II. MATERIALS AND METHODS

A. Isolation and In Vitro Growth of TIL from Human Renal Cell Carcinoma

Primary and metastatic renal cell carcinomas were processed as previously described (29,32). Briefly, tumor tissue was minced, weighed, and digested with the following enzymes for 2 h at 37°C; 20 ml of collagenase type III (1 mg/ml; Cooper Biomedical, Malvern, PA) and 1 ml of DNase type IV solution (2 mg/ml; Sigma Chemical Co., St. Louis, MO) for every 10 g tissue. The resulting cells were washed twice and counted.

TIL were expanded in vitro by culturing cells (5×10^5 per ml) in AIM-V medium supplemented with either 1000 U/ml of human recombinant IL-2, (Hoffmann-La Roche, Nutley, NJ) or 1000 U/ml of IL-2 plus 1000 U/ml of human recombinant IL-4 (Sterling Drug, Inc., Malvern, PA).

After 3 weeks in culture, TIL were separated into CD4$^+$ and CD8$^+$ subsets using anti-CD4-coated and anti-CD8-coated beads (AMAC, Inc., Westbrook, ME). This procedure included an initial negative selection followed by a positive selection as previously detailed (29). All the bioassays were conducted by culturing TIL in RPMI 1640 supplemented with 10% fetal calf serum (FCS).

B. Isolation of Tumor Targets

Short-term cultured autologous and allogeneic RCC were established by culturing tumor cells in complete RPMI (10% FCS, 200 mM L-glutamine, 25 mM HEPES, 100 mM sodium pyruvate, and 10 mM nonessential amino acids) for a minimum of 3–4 weeks (29,32). Cells that had been through two to three passages were characterized by immunostaining with antibodies to RCC (Monosan, Inc.), Uro 2 (Signet), and AE1/3 (Boehringer Mannheim). Positive staining with these antibodies demonstrated that the cultured cells were nonfibroblastic epithelial cells of renal origin and that the phenotype of the cultured cells was comparable to that of fresh tumor. In some cases freshly isolated tumor cells were used as either targets or stimulators, and the results obtained were comparable to those generated with the cultured tumor.

C. Bioassays

Lytic activity was detected using a 4 h ^{51}Cr release assay as previously described (32). Supernatant fluid from the 4 h assay was harvested with a Skatron system, and the amount of released ^{51}Cr was determined in a LKB gamma counter. In all the experiments the spontaneous release from tumor targets was never greater than 30%. For each effector-target cell (E/T) ratio, the percentage of specific lysis was calculated as previously reported (32).

The proliferation of TIL was measured by the uptake of [^{3}H]thymidine. TIL (5 × 10^4 cells per well) were incubated with one of the following for 3 days: medium, 5 U/ml of IL-2, autologous tumor cells (7000 R), various allogeneic tumor cells (7000 R), and tumor cells with 5 U/ml of IL-2. During the last 18 h of culture the cells were pulsed with [^{3}H]thymidine. Thereafter, cells were harvested and counted by a beta counter.

IFN-γ production was detected by culturing TIL (5 × 10^4 cells per well) under the same conditions described for measuring proliferation. After 3 days the supernatant fluid was tested for IFN-γ using a radioimmunoassay kit (Centocor, Malvern, PA).

D. Immunocytometry

FITC-, phycoerythrin-, and biotin-conjugated monoclonal antibodies were employed to phenotypically identify and quantitate lymphocyte subsets as previously described (29,32,33). Isotypic controls for each particular subclass of immunoglobulin and system employed were utilized to allow delineation of positive and autofluorescent populations and to control for nonspecific binding by a particular subclass of immunoglobulin. Analysis of TIL subsets was performed using the FACScan (Becton Dickinson).

III. RESULTS AND DISCUSSION

T cell lines were established from TIL that were grown in either IL-2 (1000 U/ml) or IL-2/IL-4 (1000 U/ml) for 3 weeks. CD4$^+$ and CD8$^+$ subsets were

isolated using anti-CD4- and anti-CD8-coated beads (29). The positively
selected cells were further expanded and, when tested, were greater than 95%
pure based on immunostaining. Subsets isolated from the IL-2-grown TIL (4
CD4$^+$ and 5 CD8$^+$ subsets) and the IL-2/IL-4-grown TIL (13 CD4$^+$ and 12
CD8$^+$ subsets) were tested for one or more of the following functions:
proliferation, cytotoxicity, or IFN-γ secretion. From these studies we established four different lines that consistently displayed either specificity or
selectivity for RCC (Table 1). One line was derived from the IL-2-grown TIL
and three from the IL-2/IL-4-grown cells. All these lines grew for 2–6 months
in vitro following subset isolation, and all maintained the original phenotype.
Flow analysis of two lines (RC-TIL1 and 2) also demonstrated their expression of the $\alpha\beta$ heterodimer of the T cell receptor (TCR) as defined by staining
with the WT31 antibody. Functional studies revealed that two CD8$^+$ lines
(RC-TIL1 and RC-TIL4) appeared to be specific in that they lysed the
autologous RCC but not four allogeneic RCC, autologous lymphoblasts,
Daudi, K562, Sk-Mel28, or HT29 (29). RC-TIL1 also proliferated and
produced IFN-γ specifically in response to the autologous tumor. Anti-CD3
antibody (OKT3) blocked all the functional activities, suggesting that recognition was through the TCR/CD3 complex (29). As shown in Table 2, RC-
TIL1 was MHC class I restricted. Preincubation of the targets cells with

Table 1   Activity of RCC-TIL Lines[a]

Line	Cytolytic[b] activity	Proliferation[c]	IFN-γ[d] secretion	MHC[e] restricted
RC-TIL 1	+	+	+	Class I
RC-TIL 2	−	+	+	ND
RC-TIL 3	+	−	−	ND
RC-TIL 4	+	ND	ND	ND

[a] Lines were tested for their ability to respond to autologous tumor and to allogeneic targets. Lines were tested three to five times to assess specificity.
[b] Tested for lysis against multiple targets in a 4 h ^{51}Cr release assay.
[c] TIL were rested for 2 days and then stimulated with various tumor targets in the presence and absence of IL-2 (5 U/ml). After 3 days in culture, proliferation of TIL was assessed by the uptake of [^{3}H]thymidine.
[d] Rested TIL were cultured with tumor cells in the presence or absence of IL-2 for 72 h. Thereafter, supernatant fluid was obtained and tested for IFN-γ using a RIA kit (Centocor, Malvern, PA).
[e] MHC restriction was determined by adding anti-HLA-ABC or anti-HLA-DR antibodies to the following bioassays: cytotoxic, proliferation, and cytokine production. As a control, nonimmune serum was added to bioassays.

Table 2 RCC-Specific TIL Line MHC Class I Restricted

Culture conditions[a] RC-TIL1		% Specific lysis[b] (E/T 12.5:1)	Proliferation[c]	
Antibody	Tumor		cpm ($\times 10^{-3}$ ± SD)	SI
Media	−	NA[d]	0.5 ± 0.1	NA
Media	+	21.8	9.4 ± 0.7	19.4
Anti-class I Ab	+	4.1	2.6 ± 0.3	5.3
Anti-class II Ab	+	14.6	8.8 ± 0.6	18.1
IgG control Ab	+	19.7	9.3 ± 0.7	19.1

[a] The following antibodies were added at a 1:5 dilution to various assays to determine if the RCC-specific CD8[+] TIL line (RC-TIL1) was MHC restricted: anti-HLA-ABC (IOT 2; AMAC, Inc., Westbrook, ME), anti-HLA-DR (IOT 2a; AMAC, Inc., Westbrook, ME), and IgG control (Jackson ImmunoResearch).

[b] ^{51}Cr-labeled autologous RCC were preincubated with the antibodies for 30 minutes before adding the effector cells to targets at an E/T ratio of 12.5:1 for 4 h. The spontaneous release for the targets were as follows: anti-class I, 12.2%; anti-class II, 21.4%; IgG control, 19.5%; and medium alone, 14.0%.

[c] The TIL line was rested in medium alone for 2 days and then added to 96-well plates containing medium alone, autologous RCC (7000 R), or autologous RCC (7000 R) pretreated for 30 minutes at 4°C with one of the antibodies at a dilution of 1:5. Cultures were incubated for 3 days and pulsed with [^{3}H]thymidine for the last 24 h. Cells were harvested and assessed for the uptake of [^{3}H]thymidine. SD, standard deviation; SI, stimulation index.

[d] NA, not applicable.

anti-HLA-ABC antibody reduced lysis of the autologous tumor by 80%. Proliferation to the autologous tumor was reduced by 72% following exposure of tumor cells to anti-MHC class I antibody (Table 2). Preincubation of RCC with a control antibody or an antibody to MHC class II antigens had a minimal effect on the functional activity of the RC-TIL1 cells. Also, production of IFN-γ in response to the autologous tumor was partially blocked by anti-MHC class I antibody (data not shown).

One CD4[+] culture (RC-TIL2) proliferated (Figure 1) and produced IFN-γ (Figure 2) when stimulated with autologous tumor but did not respond to three different allogeneic RCC. Moreover, this CD4[+] line was not cytotoxic for the autologous RCC, several allogeneic RCC, or K562 (data not shown). Although RC-TIL2 proliferated and produced IFN-γ in the absence of exogenous IL-2, the addition of IL-2 (<10 U/ml) potentiated both responses to the autologous tumor. The responses to exogenous IL-2 plus autologous tumor were synergistic compared to the responses generated by either stimulus alone (Figures 1 and 2). In addition, greater proliferation and IFN-γ production was observed when the responder-tumor ratio was reduced from 20:1 to 5:1. The

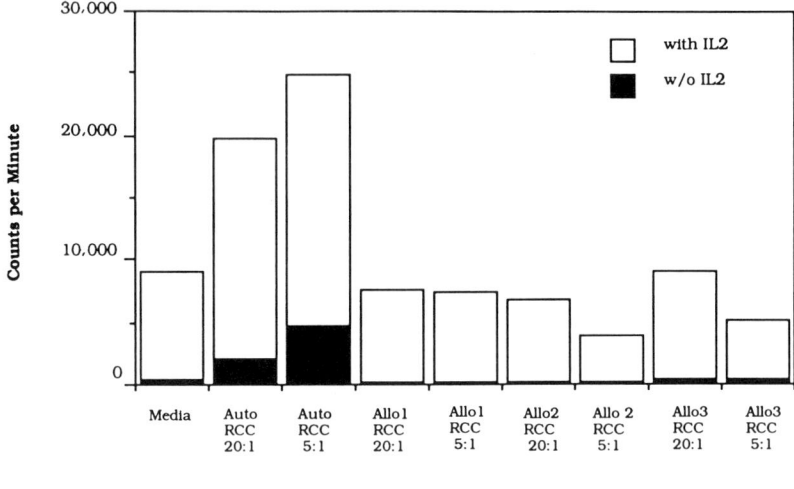

Figure 1 Proliferative response of RC-TIL2 (CD4[+]) cells following stimulation with medium, autologous RCC with or without IL-2 (5 U/ml), allogeneic RCC with and without IL-2 (5 U/ml), or IL-2 alone. Tumor cells were irradiated (7000 R) to prevent their replication. The ratios of TIL to tumor cells in these cultures were 20:1 and 5:1. The uptake of [^{3}H]thymidine was measured after 3 days of culture.

TIL was responsible for the IFN-γ detected in the cultures since tumor cells cultured alone or with IL-2 did not secrete detectable IFN-γ.

CD8[+] line from one additional patient displayed selective lysis for RCC upon repeated testing. RC-TIL3 was cytotoxic for the autologous tumor and two allogeneic RCC. However, this line was only minimally lytic for two other allogeneic RCC and did not lyse K562, Daudi, or Sk-Mel28. This line did not secrete IFN-γ in response to the autologous tumor; however, it was capable of producing IFN-γ in response to anti-CD3 antibody and IL-2. That RC-TIL3 can recognize the autologous tumor and mediate lysis but cannot secrete IFN-γ in response to tumor suggests that the stimulus provided by the tumor may be distinct for the induction of lysis and IFN-γ production. From the patient from whom the RC-TIL3 was derived we were also able to obtain TIL from a metastatic bone lesion. After expansion and separation, both the CD4[+] and CD8[+] T cell subsets from the bone lesion displayed a pattern of lysis comparable to that of the CD8[+] TIL (RC-TIL3) isolated from the primary renal tumor. A CD4[+] line (RC-TIL5) also showed selectivity for

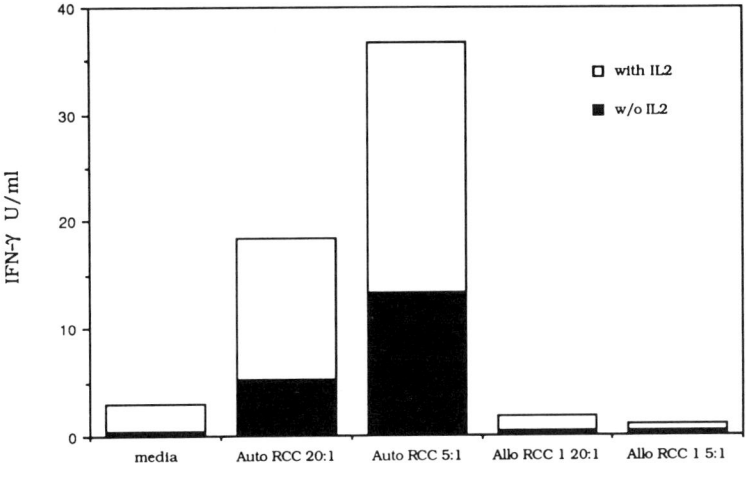

Figure 2 IFN-γ secretion by RC-TIL2 (CD4$^+$) cells was determined after culturing TIL with medium alone, IL-2 (5 U/ml), or autologous or allogeneic tumor with and without IL-2. The ratios of TIL to tumor cells (7000 R) were 5:1 and 20:1. After 3 days, supernatant fluid was tested for IFN-γ using a radioimmunoassay kit. Tumor cells (7000 R) cultured alone or with IL-2 did not secrete IFN-γ.

RCC in that it was lytic for autologous tumor and one allogeneic RCC but did not lyse three other allogeneic RCC or K562 (unpublished data).

The work presented here is in agreement with other work demonstrating that specific cytotoxic T cells are present in renal cell carcinoma TIL (28,29). Our results also illustrate that both CD4$^+$ and CD8$^+$ TIL can secrete IFN-γ specifically in response to autologous RCC. Similar findings were reported for melanoma and breast carcinoma TIL, in which IFN-γ as well as granulocyte-macrophage colony-stimulating factor (GM-CSF) and tumor necrosis factor α (TNF-α) were produced following stimulation with the autologous but not allogeneic tumor cells (34). The specific secretion of IFN-γ by T cells in response to syngeneic tumor has been reported for several murine models (35,36). Animal studies have also shown that IFN-γ secretion in response to tumor was involved in the antitumor activity mediated by T cells. The therapeutic activity of adoptively transferred T cells known to secrete IFN-γ in response to tumor was eliminated by the administration of antibodies to IFN-γ (35). The secretion of IFN-γ by tumor-specific T cells may enhance the host immune response to tumor cells through a number of different mechanisms. One possibility is that IFN-γ produced by TIL may serve to augment the cytolytic response by altering the sensitivity of tumor targets to lysis. Pretreatment with low concentrations (10 U/ml) of IFN-γ alone or in combination with TNF-α is known to make RCC and melanoma cells more susceptible to lysis by TIL but not to lysis by lymphokine-activated killer (LAK) cells (37) (Finke et al., manuscript in preparation). The reason for the increased susceptibility of IFN-γ-treated tumor cells to T cell lysis in not known but is being investigated.

Our studies have also identified non–MHC-restricted TIL that show selective lysis for RCC. These cultured TIL were not lytic for nonrenal tumor targets but lysed autologous RCC plus one or more allogeneic RCC. CTL that display selective lysis have been reported for other tumors. T cells derived from tumor-draining lymph nodes of patients with breast adenocarcinoma recognize breast and pancreatic tumors in a MHC-unrestricted fashion but not other tumors of epithelial origin. These cytotoxic T cells recognize a unique ductal epithelial mucin via the αβ TCR complex (38). In addition, CD8$^+$ T cells from the draining nodes of patients with squamous cell carcinoma of the head and neck (SCCHN) display MHC-unrestricted lysis that is selective for SCCHN (39).

The finding that anti-CD3 and anti-MHC class I antibodies can block the lysis and secretion of IFN-γ suggest that some TIL recognize RCC via TCR/CD3 complex and are MHC class I restricted. These results are similar to those reported for melanoma and ovarian TIL (31,40). It is not clear from our work if the TIL that display selective lysis for RCC recognize tumor via the TCR/CD3 complex.

The use of various separation procedures, including antibody-coated beads, has been important in defining the effector function of isolated T cell subsets (32,41). Previously we reported that the majority of lytic activity of RCC-derived TIL was nonspecific, non–MHC restricted, and mediated by CD3$^-$CD56$^+$ cells. We also reported that some positively selected CD4$^+$ and CD8$^+$ TIL had low levels of lytic activity for the autologous tumor and all had lytic activity in an 18 h assay (32). It is possible that the detection of TIL with specificity or selectivity for RCC reported here is related to a refinement in the positive selection procedure employed and in the use of IL-2/IL-4 for in vitro culture of TIL. Previous work in melanoma demonstrated that the growth of TIL in IL-2/IL-4 versus IL2 alone augmented the development of a specific CTL response (42). Continued efforts to modify the culture conditions for the expansion of TIL may improve the detection and maintenance of RCC-specific and RCC-selective T cells. These cells will be important in the further analysis of T cell immunity to human RCC and possibly in the development of new forms of immunotherapy for this disease.

ACKNOWLEDGMENTS

Supported by NO1-CM-97622 and a grant from Sterling Drug, Inc.

REFERENCES

1. Talmadge JE, Chirigos MA. Comparison of immunomodulating and immuno-therapeutic properties of biologic response modifiers. Springer Semin Immunopathol 1985; 8:429–43.
2. Rosenberg SA, Mulé JJ, Spiess PJ, Reichert CM, Schwarz SL. Regression of established pulmonary metastases and subcutaneous tumor mediated by the systemic administration of high-dose recombinant interleukin 2. J Exp Med 1985; 161:1169–88.
3. Mule JJ, Yang JC, Lafreniere RL, Shu S, Rosenberg SA. Identification of cellular mechanisms operational in vivo during the regression of established pulmonary metastases by the systemic administration of high-dose recombinant interleukin 2. J Immunol 1987; 139:285–94.
4. Rosenberg SA, Schwarz SL, Spiess PJ. Combination immunotherapy for cancer: synergistic antitumor interactions of interleukin-2, alfa interferon and tumor-infiltrating lymphocytes. J Natl Cancer Inst 1987; 80:1393–7.
5. Gansbacher B, Zier K, Daniels B, Cronin K, Bannergi R, Gilboa E. Interleukin 2 gene transfer into tumor cells abrogates tumorigenicity and induces protective immunity. J Exp Med 1990; 172:1217–24.
6. Watanabe Y, Kuribayashi S, Miyatake K, et al. Exogenous expression of mouse interferon-gamma cDNA in mouse neuroblastoma C1300 cells results in reduced tumorigenicity by augmented antitumor immunity. Proc Natl Acad Sci U S A 1989; 86:9456–61.
7. Golumbek PT, Lazenby AJ, Levitsky HJ, et al. Treatment of established renal cancer by tumor cells engineered to secrete interleukin 4. Science 1991; 254:713–6.
8. Cheever MA, Greenberg PD, Fefer A. Specificity of adoptive chemoimmunotherapy of established syngeneic tumors. J Immunol 1980; 125:711–6.
9. Rosenberg SA, Spiess P, Lafreniere R. A new approach to the adoptive immunotherapy of cancer with tumor-infiltrating lymphocytes. Science 1986; 233:1318–21.
10. Spiess PJ, Yang JC, Rosenberg SA. In vivo antitumor activity of tumor-infiltrating lymphocytes expanded in recombinant interleukin 2. J Natl Cancer Inst 1987; 75:1067–75.
11. Vose BM, Moore M. Human tumor-infiltrating lymphocytes: a marker of host response. Semin Hematol 1985; 22:27–35.
12. Whiteside TL, Miescher S, Hurlimann J, Moretta L, Von Fliedner V. Separation, phenotyping and limiting dilution analysis of T-lymphocytes infiltrating human solid tumors. Int J Cancer 1986; 37:803–11.
13. Whiteside TL, Miescher S, Hurlimann J, Moretta L, Von Fliedner V. Clonal

analysis and in situ characterization of lymphocytes infiltrating human breast carcinomas. Cancer Immunol Immunother 1986; 23:169–78.

14. Itoh K, Tilden AB, Balch CM. Interleukin 2 activation of cytotoxic T-lymphocytes infiltrating into human metastatic melanomas. Cancer Res 1986; 46:3011–7.

15. Kurnick JT, Kradin RL, Blumberg R, Schneeberger EE, Boyle LA. Functional characterization of T lymphocytes propagated from human lung carcinomas. Clin Immunol Immunother 1986; 38:367–80.

16. Muul LM, Spiess PJ, Director EP, Rosenberg SA. Identification of specific cytolytic immune responses against autologous tumor in humans bearing malignant melanoma. J Immunol 1987; 138:989–95.

17. Finke JH, Tubbs R, Connelly B, Pontes E, Montie J. Tumor-infiltrating lymphocytes in patients with renal-cell carcinoma. Ann N Y Acad Sci 1987; 532:387–94.

18. Belldegrun A, Muul LM, Rosenberg SA. Interleukin 2 expanded tumor-infiltrating lymphocytes in human renal cell cancer: isolation, characterization and antitumor activity. Cancer Res 1988; 48:206–14.

19. Rubin TT, Elwood LJ, Rosenberg SA, Lotze MT. Immunohistochemical correlates of response to recombinant interleukin-2 based immunotherapy in humans. Cancer Res 1989; 49:7089–92.

20. Topalian SL, Solomon D, Avis FF, et al. Immunotherapy of patients with advanced cancer using tumor-infiltrating lymphocytes and recombinant interleukin-2: A pilot study. J Clin Oncol 1988; 6:839–53.

21. Kradin RL, Lazarus DS, Dubinett SM, et al. Tumor-infiltrating lymphocytes and interleukin-2 in treatment of advanced cancer. Lancet 1989; 1:577–80.

22. Topalian SL, Solomon D, Rosenberg SA. Tumor specific cytolysis by lymphocytes infiltrating human melanomas. J Immunol 1989; 142:3714–25.

23. Alexander J, Rayman P, Edinger M, et al. TIL from renal cell carcinoma: restimulation with tumor influences proliferation and cytolytic activity. Int J Cancer 1990; 45:119–24.

24. Heo DS, Whiteside TL, Kanbour A, Herberman RB. Lymphocytes infiltrating human ovarian tumors. I. Role of Leu-19 (NKH1)-positive recombinant IL-2 activated cultures of lymphocytes infiltrating human ovarian tumors. J Immunol 1988; 140:4042–9.

25. Lotzova E. Ovarian-tumor-infiltrating-lymphocytes: phenotype and antitumor activity. Nat Immun Cell Growth Regul 1988; 7:226–9.

26. Whiteside TL, Heo DS, Takagi S, Johnson JT, Iwatsuki S, Herberman RB. Cytolytic antitumor effector cells in long-term cultures of human tumor-infiltrating lymphocytes in recombinant interleukin-2. Cancer Immunol Immunother 1988; 26:1–10.

27. Heo DS, Whiteside TL, Johnson JT, Chen K, Barnes EL, Herberman RB. Long-term interleukin 2-dependent growth and cytotoxic activity of tumor-infiltrating lymphocytes from human squamous cell carcinomas of the head and neck. Cancer Res 1987; 47:6353–62.

28. Koo AS, Tso C-L, Shimabukuro T, Peyret C, deKernion JB, Belldegrun A.

Autologous tumor-specific cytotoxicity of tumor-infiltrating lymphocytes derived from human renal cell carcinoma. J Immunother 1991; 10:347–54.

29. Finke JH, Rayman P, Edinger M, et al. Characterization of a human renal cell carcinomas specific cytotoxic CD8[+] T cell line. J Immunother 1992; 11:1–11.

30. Ferrini S, Biassoni R, Moretta A, Bruzonne M, Nicolin A, Morretta L. Clonal analysis of T lymphocytes isolated from ovarian carcinoma ascitic fluid. Phenotypic and functional characterization of T cell clones capable of lysing. Int J Cancer 1985; 36:337–40.

31. Ioannides CG, Freedman RS, Platsoucas CD, Rashad S, Kim YP. Cytotoxic T cell clones isolated from ovarian tumor-infiltrating lymphocytes recognize multiple antigenic epitopes on autologous tumor cells. J Immunol 1991; 146:1700–7.

32. Finke JH, Rayman P, Alexander J, et al. Characterization of the cytolytic activity of CD4[+] and CD8[+] TIL subsets in human renal cell carcinoma. Cancer Res 1990; 50:2363–70.

33. Lanier LL, Le AM, Civin CJ, Loken MR, Phillips JH. The relationship of CD16 (Leu 11) and Leu 19 (NKH-1) antigen expression on human peripheral blood NK cells and cytotoxic T lymphocytes. J Immunol 1986; 136:4480–6.

34. Schwartzentruber DJ, Topalian SL, Mancini M, Rosenberg SA. Specific release of granulocyte-macrophage colony-stimulating factor, tumor necrosis factor-α and IFN-γ by human tumor-infiltrating lymphocytes after autologous tumor stimulation. J Immunol 1991; 146:3674–81.

35. Barth RJ, Mule JJ, Spiess PJ, Rosenberg SA. Interferon γ and tumor necrosis factor have a role in tumor regressions mediated by murine CD8 tumor-infiltrating lymphocytes. J Exp Med 1991; 173:647–58.

36. Yamasaki T, Handa H, Yamashita J, Watanabe Y, Namba Y, Hamaoka M. Specific adoptive immunotherapy with tumor specific CTL clone for murine malignant gliomas. Cancer Res 1984; 44:1776–82.

37. Stotter H, Wiebke EA, Shorken T, et al. Cytokines alter target cell susceptibility to lysis. II. Evaluation of tumor infiltrating lymphocytes. J Immunol 1989; 142:1767–73.

38. Jerome KR, Barnd DL, Bendt KM, et al. Cytotoxic T-lymphocytes derived from patients with breast adenocarcinoma recognize an epitope present on the protein core of a mucin molecule preferentially expressed by malignant cells. Cancer Res 1991; 51:2908–16.

39. Letessier EM, Heo DS, Okarma T, Johnson JT, Herberman RB, Whiteside TL. Enrichment in tumor-reactive CD8[+] T-lymphocytes by positive selection from the blood and lymph nodes of patients with head and neck cancer. Cancer Res 1991; 51:3891–9.

40. Itoh K, Platsoucas CD, Balch CM. Autologous tumor-specific cytotoxic T lymphocytes in the infiltrate of human metastatic melanomas. Activation of interleukin 2 and autologous tumor cells, and involvement of the T cell receptor. J Exp Med 1988; 168:1419–41.

41. Wong JT, Pinto CE, Gifford JD, Kurnick JT, Kradin RL. Characterization of the

CD4$^+$ and CD8$^+$ tumor infiltrating lymphocytes propagated with bispecific monoclonal antibodies. J Immunol 1989; 143:3404–11.

42. Kawakami Y, Rosenberg SA, Lotze MT. Interleukin 4 promotes the growth of tumor-infiltrating lymphocytes cytotoxic for human autologous melanoma. J Exp Med 1988; 168:2183–91.

13

Tumor-Infiltrating Lymphocytes in Metastatic Renal Cell Carcinoma

The Cleveland Clinic Experience

Ronald M. Bukowski, Siva R. Murthy, Eric A. Klein, Laurie Bauer, Raymond R. Tubbs, G. Thomas Budd, James S. Sergi, Vicki Gibson, Patricia Rayman, Jill Stanley, and James H. Finke

The Cleveland Clinic Foundation, Cleveland, Ohio

I. INTRODUCTION

Tumor-infiltrating lymphocytes (TIL) may represent part of the host immune response to human malignancy and contain an enriched population of cells having cytotoxic and helper functions (1). When TIL are expanded by recombinant interleukin-2 (rIL-2), a mixed population of $CD3^+CD4^+$ and $CD3^+CD8^+$ T cells (2–4) results. Importantly, TIL contain antigen-specific as well nonspecific cytotoxic lymphocytes (2–4). In view of preclinical studies demonstrating that rIL-2-activated TIL are 50–100 times more effective in their therapeutic potency than lymphokine-activated killer (LAK) cells (5) and several preliminary reports in which TIL were given to patients with metastatic malignant melanoma, renal cell carcinoma (RCC), and lung cancer (6,7), both phase I and phase II trials utilizing TIL in renal cancer patients were initiated at The Cleveland Clinic Foundation. This report summarizes the results of the initial phase I trial.

Interleukin-4 was originally termed B cell stimulating factor 1 and is a lymphokine with multiple biologic activities (8). One of these is its influence on the growth and cytolytic potential of T lymphocytes. Recent studies have shown IL-4 functions to augment the generation of specific cytotoxic T lymphocytes (CTL) in mixed lymphocyte cultures (9,10) and that it also abrogated the development of nonspecific cytotoxic activity (9,10). IL-4 is also a potent inhibitor of LAK activity induced by IL-2 (11,12). Finally, Kawakami et al. (13) demonstrated that IL-4 when combined with IL-2 may enhance the growth and lytic activity of melanoma-specific TIL and inhibit the nonspecific lytic activity. In view of these observations and the results of our first trial utilizing TIL, a second study utilizing rIL-2 and recombinant human IL-4 (rhIL-4) to expand TIL in vitro with periodic autologous tumor restimulation has been initiated. The preliminary results of this trial are also reported.

II. MATERIALS AND METHODS

A. Patient Population

Patients $\geq$ 18 years with metastatic RCC, which was surgically incurable, who had tumor tissue (primary tumor or metastatic lesion) accessible for surgical removal and from whose tumors produced adequate numbers of autologous TIL $\geq$ 1 $\times$ 10^9 were eligible. Objectively measurable (phase II trial) or evaluable disease (phase I trial) was required. Patients were also required to have a performance status (PS) $\leq$ 1 (Eastern Cooperative Oncology Group), a life expectancy $\geq$ 3 months, and to be fully recovered ($\geq$14 days) from any recent surgical procedures or any infection ($\geq$21 days). Minimal tumor burden was required and was defined as having had a previous nephrectomy, $\leq$30% liver involvement by tumor, absence of central nervous system metastases, and a normal serum calcium in the presence of osseous metastases. Prior radiotherapy ($\geq$28 days) was allowed for control of pain, but previous chemotherapy, immunotherapy, or hormonal therapy was not permitted. Adequate hematologic, biochemical, pulmonary, and cardiac function were required as previously described (14). Informed consent was obtained in accordance with the National Cancer Institute (NCI) and institutional guidelines.

Patients with a clinical or pathologic diagnosis of metastatic RCC who met the eligibility criteria underwent surgery for removal of their primary or metastatic tumor. Specimens were then processed for TIL preparation as previously described (14). When adequate TIL growth (generally 4–6 weeks) was seen, therapy was initiated. Biochemical and hematologic baseline studies were repeated and, if present, the status of measurable disease determined.

B. Treatment and Study Design

Two sequential studies have been performed, the first a phase I trial to determine the toxicity of TIL and the second a phase II trial to study efficacy. The characteristics of these two trials are outlined in Table 1.

The rIL-2 (NSC 60064) employed in these trials was produced by Hoffmann-LaRoche and supplied by the NCI. It was produced using a gene cloned from human DNA that was expressed in *Escherichia coli*. The rIL-2 had specific activity between 5 and 15 $\times$ 10^6 U/mg protein; it was reconstituted with sterile water and administered as a constant infusion via the Pharmacia CADD I ambulatory infusion pump in 100 ml of a 5% solution of dextrose in water. The TIL were administered without a filter via a central intravenous (IV) catheter on specified days (see Table 1) and the rIL-2 as a continuous IV infusion. No dose escalation within individual patients was permitted. Most patients received acetaminophen (650 mg orally every 6 h), ranitidine (150 mg orally every 12 h) as prophylaxis for gastrointestinal bleeding, and meperidine (25–50 mg IV) to control rigors throughout the course of treatment. Hydroxyzine hydrochloride (25 mg IV) was given to control pruritus, prochlorperazine (10 mg IV every 4–6 h) to treat nausea and vomiting, and diphenoxylate hydrochloride with atropine sulfate (2.5–5.0 mg orally) to control diarrhea. Hypotension was managed with fluid administration and/or phenylephrine hydrochloride at 0.3 μg/kg/minute titrated to maintain the systolic blood pressure between 90 and 100 mm Hg.

Table 1 Phase I and Phase II TIL Trials in Renal Cell Carcinoma

	Phase I	Phase II
TIL growth in vitro		
rIL-2	1000 U/ml	1000 U/ml
rhIL-4	–	1000 U/ml
Autologous tumor		
restimulation	–	+
Treatment schedules		
TIL $\geq 1 \times 10^9$		
cells infusion	Days 1, 8	Days 1, 2, 3, . . .
rIL-2 (CI)	0, 1.0, 3.0,	4.5 $\times$ 10^6 U/day,
	4.5 $\times$ 10^6 U/day,	days 1–5, 8–12,
	days 1–5, 8–12	15–19
Patients per dose		
level	3–6	Phase II trial

C. Study Monitoring

Within 14 days of the start of therapy, studies were performed in all patients to determine eligibility. All patients were treated on a regular oncology nursing floor. Vascular access was obtained with a triple-lumen central venous catheter. Vital signs were obtained every 15 minutes during and for 30 minutes after the TIL infusion and every 4 h during the administration of rIL-2. Weights were obtained on a daily basis, and tumor response was assessed using standardized criteria (Southwest Oncology Group) on day 28 and monthly thereafter. Laboratory evaluation during treatment included daily hematologic studies and biochemical studies three times weekly.

The NCI common toxicity criteria were utilized. The occurrence of grade III or IV toxicity, with the exceptions of fever and/or hematologic abnormalities, were considered dose limiting. Although the cardiovascular, hepatic, neurologic, and pulmonary toxicities of rIL-2 are significant, they are readily reversible. Therefore, the definitions of dose-limiting toxicity were modified to allow continued therapy within the limits of patient safety. Therapy was held in the presence of any of the following: serum creatinine or a total bilirubin ≥ 5.0 mg/dl, hypotension refractory to phenylephrine hydrochloride, altered mental status or coma, dyspnea at rest, or requirement for mechanical ventilatory support. In the presence of these adverse effects or other grade III or IV toxicity, therapy was withheld until there was a return to a grade I level. The rIL-2 was then restarted with a 50% dose reduction. Development of any grade IV nonhematologic toxicity required the discontinuation of therapy.

D. Human Renal Cell Carcinoma TIL Isolation and Expansion In Vitro

The kidneys obtained at nephrectomy were perfused with 50 ml Hanks' balanced salt solution (Whittaker Bioproducts, Walkersville, MD) to remove extraneous blood. In the phase I trial, the primary and metastatic tumors were minced, cultured with rIL-2 (1000 U/ml), and processed as previously described (14,15).

In the phase II trial (Table 1), TIL were cultured with rIL-2 (1000 U/ml) and rhIL-4 (1000 U/ml) and restimulated with fresh autologous tumor cells on days 22 and 29. The rhIL-4 (NSC 620211) was produced by Immunex Corporation, prepared by Sterling Drug (Kansas), and supplied by the NCI. It was produced using a gene cloned from human DNA and expressed in yeast cultures. The rhIL-4 had a specific activity of 1.8×10^6 U/mg. In both trials,

TIL used for adoptive therapy were harvested using the Stericell system (E. I. duPont de Nemours).

E. In Vitro Studies

Tumor targets were isolated and cytolytic assays were performed using a 4 h ^{51}Cr release assay as previously described (4,15). Phenotypic analysis of cultured TIL was performed utilizing three-color immunocytometry as described in our previous reports (8).

F. Statistical Analysis

Summary statistical values and data analysis were performed in a manner similar to that used in our previous publications (8).

III. RESULTS

A. Phase I Trial

A group of 26 patients were entered into this study, with one patient declared ineligible because of prior therapy with rIL-2 and interferon-α. A total of 25 patients were eligible, and 18 (72%) were eventually treated. Reasons for nontreatment included inadequate TIL growth in two patients, contamination of cultures in three, and rapid disease progression in two.

The toxicity in the 18 patients treated resembled that reported with continuous-infusion rIL-2 (16,17). There were no previously unrecognized or fatal toxic effects, and all side effects resolved completely when rIL-2 was discontinued. Because of toxicity, three patients failed to complete the two weeks of rIL-2 therapy. Fever and/or chills were the only toxic effects associated with TIL infusion. Moderate gastrointestinal toxicity (nausea and vomiting) was seen in all patients. Reversible serum creatinine elevation was also common (83% of patients). Dose-limiting toxicity occurred at a dose of rIL-2 4.5×10^6 U/m^2 and consisted of dyspnea and hypoxia in three patients. This developed on days 13, 15, and 17 of rIL-2, respectively, and was not related to TIL infusion. Ventilatory support was not required.

In the 18 patients evaluable for response, no objective tumor regression was seen. However, a single patient demonstrated a minor decrease in the size of pulmonary nodules. Of the 17 remaining patients, eight had stable disease and nine had progressive disease at the end of 4 weeks.

In the 18 patients who were treated with TIL, expansion to $\geq 1.0 \times 10^9$ cells was possible in all instances. The level of TIL expansion in vitro was not

Table 2 Phenotypes of TIL Infused During Phase I Trial

Phenotype	Number	Mean (%)	Median (%)	Range (%)
CD3$^+$	18	77.8	86.5	27.8–99.6
CD56$^+$	18	39.2	32.0	6.8–87.2
CD3$^+$CD25$^+$HLA-DR$^+$	18	16.2	3.0	0.0–64.0
CD8$^+$CD3$^+$CD4$^-$	18	42.8	37.0	0.0–97.1
CD4$^+$CD3$^+$CD8$^-$	18	23.6	13.2	0.0–96.5

associated with tumor site (metastatic versus primary), the degree of initial lymphoid infiltrate, or the phenotype of cultured TIL. The total number of TIL infused per patient ranged from 1.2×10^9 to 2×10^{12}, and in 8 of 18 patients $> 1 \times 10^{11}$ cells were infused.

Phenotypes of the cultured TIL in the 18 eligible patients are summarized in Table 2. In 14 of 18 instances >70% of TIL were T cells with a CD3$^+$ phenotype. The number of CD3$^+$CD4$^+$ and CD3$^+$CD8$^+$ subsets within the cultured TIL varied considerably from one patient to the next. In 4 of 18 patients, TIL were predominantly CD56$^+$, and in two of these cases, cells with the phenotype of natural killer (NK) cells (CD3$^-$CD56$^+$CD8$^-$ or CD3-CD16a$^+$CD56$^+$) predominated. Therefore, analysis demonstrated that cultured TIL from renal tumors were mostly T cells but were extremely heterogenous in their phenotypes. Lymphocytes with the phenotype of NK cells

Table 3 Cytolytic Activity of TIL Cultures: Phase I Trial[a]

	Autologous tumor	Daudi	RCC-2[b]
Patients tested	14	16	7
LU per 10^6 cells			
Mean ± SEM[c]	44.6 ± 14.2	244.6 ± 103.3	21.8 ± 6.8
Median	28.9	95.2	17.1
Range	0.0–169.8	0.0–1549.3	0.0–102.7
Patient 11	44.2	0.0	0.0
Patient 15	148.3	141.7	32.9

[a] TIL infused on day 1.
[b] Renal cell carcinoma cell line (18).
[c] Standard error of the mean.

rarely predominated in culture, although some preparations contained a significant number of these cells.

The cytolytic activity of the cultured TIL is outlined in Table 3. The majority of cultures displayed non–major histocompatibility complex (MHC)-restricted lytic activity as illustrated by patient 15. In 12 of 14 instances, TIL were cytotoxic to autologous tumor targets, and in one of 14 instances cytotoxicity was detected against autologous tumor only (patient 11). Non–MHC-restricted cytotoxicity was found against the Daudi cell line in 14 of 17 TIL cultures and against the allogeneic renal carcinoma cell line RCC-2 (18) in 9 of 17 cultures.

B. Phase II Trial

A total of 14 patients have been entered into this trial, and all were eligible; three patients were never treated, and one is too early to assess. Reasons for nontreatment included inadequate TIL growth in two patients, and disease progression in one instance. The toxicity of TIL expanded with rIL-2 and rhIL-4 and administered with rIL-2 resembled that seen in the phase I trial. In 1 of 10 patients, rIL-2 toxicity resulted in dose modification.

The TIL expansion data are summarized in Table 4, and an apparent increase in proliferation compared with the first trial is evident. The phenotypes of the infused TIL and the cytotoxicity data are summarized in Tables 5 and 6, respectively. Most TIL cultures were >98% $CD3^+$, with both $CD4^+$ and $CD8^+$ subsets present. Cytotoxicity data, however, demonstrated minimal if any lytic activity in most cultures. In one instance (patient 10), lytic activity restricted to only autologous tumor was present.

In the 10 patients evaluable for response, one minor regression of a pulmonary metastasis and one partial response of a pulmonary lesion have been seen.

Table 4 TIL Expansion Data: Phase II Trial TIL Cultured with rIL-2/rhIL-4[a]

	Median	Range
TIL infused	2.52×10^{11}	3.4×10^9–5.29×10^{11}
Fold increase	3017	28.3–20179

[a] Data based on first eight patients.

Table 5 Phenotypes of TIL Cultured with rIL-2/rhIL-4: Phase II Trial[a]

Phenotype	Mean (%)	Range (%)
CD3[+]	98.6	96.7–99.6
CD4[+]	63.8	32.3–99.5
CD8[+]	34.0	4.1–88.9
CD56[+]	6.9	1.4–19.9
CD3[+]CD25[−]HLA-DR[+]	69.0	44.4–91.7
CD3[+]CD25[+]HLA-DR[−]	27.4	2.9–54.0
CD3[+]CD56[−]CD2[+]	91.6	77.4–98.3

[a] Data based on first eight patients.

Table 6 Cytotoxicity of TIL Cultured in rIL-2/rhIL-4: Phase II Trial[a]

	LU per 10[6] cells			
Patient	Autologous tumor	Daudi	RCC-2[b]	Nonrenal cell line[c]
1	0.0	0.0	0.0	ND
2	0.0	0.0	0.0	0.0
3	0.0	0.0	ND	0.0
4	ND[2]	0.0	ND	0.0
6	0.0	NE[3]	0.0	0.0
7	2.2	NE	0.0	NE
9	ND	5.5	0.0	0.0
10	21.1	0.0	0.0	ND

[a] Data based on first eight patients. ND, not done; NE, not evaluable.
[b] Renal cell carcinoma cell line (18).
[c] Included: SK-MEL 28.

IV. DISCUSSION

The two trials discussed in this report demonstrate the feasibility of large-scale culture of TIL from primary tumors and metastatic lesions obtained from patients with renal cell carcinoma. In both trials the toxicity of TIL administered with interleukin-2 was similar to that reported with continuous infusion of this cytokine (16,17). The toxicity of TIL alone in the phase I trial was minimal.

In the first study, 18 patients were treated and only one minor tumor regression was seen. The interesting feature noted during this trial was the extreme heterogeneity of the cultured TIL. This was demonstrated by detailed three-color flow cytometry. The heterogeneity of the TIL may be a major contributing factor in abrogating or diluting the activity of any particular subset in the population. Additionally, the phase I nature of this trial makes any conclusion preliminary regarding efficacy.

The definitive analysis of the TIL administered to patients in this first trial demonstrated that they were activated based on their expression of HLA-DR. The functional analysis of TIL from these renal tumors demonstrated that they displayed non-MHC cytolytic activity. In one patient there appeared to be some restricted lytic activity against autologous tumor, and recent reports (19,20) have demonstrated that specific CTL can be isolated from renal cell carcinoma tumors.

The phase II trial was initiated to determine if altering the culture conditions utilizing interleukin-4 and restimulating with autologous tumor would affect the clinical and laboratory results. Interleukin-4 is an immunoregulatory cytokine that has variable effects on cultured lymphocytes. Previous reports indicated it may facilitate the generation of specific CTL and inhibit the nonspecific cytolytic activity observed during the first TIL trial (9,10). The preliminary results of this trial demonstrate no differences in toxicity from the phase I trial, and again the major side effects are attributable to continuous-infusion interleukin-2. The in vitro data, however, show some different and interesting results. The inclusion of high-dose interleukin-4 in the cultures resulted in a change in TIL phenotypes, the majority being CD3$^+$ and either CD4$^+$ or CD8$^+$. Few CD56$^+$ cells were found. The expansion data demonstrate that proliferation of TIL may indeed be superior to that seen in the initial phase I trial, in which rIL-2 alone was used in vitro. In contrast, the cytolytic studies demonstrated that the majority of cultures exhibited little if any lytic activity against autologous tumor or other cell lines. This is in contrast to the TIL that were cultured in interleukin-2 alone, which were broadly cytolytic.

Further studies of these TIL have demonstrated that even though cytolytic activity is absent, interferon-γ production by some TIL cultures in response to autologous tumor is present (data not shown). This was demonstrated by isolating and testing the CD4 and CD subsets. Interestingly, in the two patients with objective tumor regression, the TIL demonstrated interferon-γ production when cultured in the presence of autologous tumor.

The two trials presented in this report represent the largest series of patients with metastatic RCC treated with TIL and rIL-2. Comparisons with other series (6,7,21) are difficult, since most investigators have utilized different culture methods, different schedules and/or doses of rIL-2, and in some instances concomitant chemotherapy with cyclophosphamide. To date 48 patients with metastatic RCC have been treated with TIL with or without rIL-2, and 4 major responses have been reported. These results, although disappointing, should be considered preliminary. In a similar manner our understanding of the biology of TIL, their mechanisms of action, and in vitro growth requirements are also preliminary.

In conclusion, we performed two trials utilizing TIL cultured from primary renal tumors or metastatic lesions in patients with renal cell carcinoma. The phase II trial is ongoing and demonstrates that the manipulation of in vitro culture conditions in terms of additional cytokines and restimulation with autologous tumor can result in a more homogeneous population of TIL than was noted in our phase I trial. The phase II trial is in progress, and clinical results are preliminary.

Additional investigations into the biology of TIL to further characterize the presence of specific CTL and the potential proliferative defect noted by Finke's group (22) are required. Future studies may involve genetically altered RCC cells to potentially enhance a selective CTL response.

ACKNOWLEDGMENTS

Supported by N01-CM-97622 and a grant from Sterling Drug, Inc.

REFERENCES

1. Vose BM, Moore M. Human tumor-infiltrating lymphocytes: a marker of host response. Semin Hematol 1985; 11:17.
2. Whiteside TL, Miescher S, Hurlimann J, Moretta L, Von Fliedner V. Separation, phenotyping and limiting dilution analysis of T-lymphocytes infiltrating human solid tumors. Int J Cancer 1986; 37:803.
3. Itoh K, Tilden AB, Balch CM. Interleukin-2 activation of cytotoxic T-lymphocytes infiltrating into human metastatic melanomas. Cancer Res 1986; 46:3011–7.
4. Muul LM, Spiess PJ, Director EP, Rosenberg SA. Identification of specific cytolytic immune response against autologous tumor in humans bearing malignant melanoma. J Immunol 1987; 138:989–95.
5. Rosenberg SA, Spiess P, Lafreniere R. A new approach to the adoptive immunotherapy of cancer with infiltrating lymphocytes. Science 1986; 233:1318.
6. Topalian SL, Solomon D, Avis FF, et al. Immunotherapy of patients with advanced cancer using tumor-infiltrating lymphocytes and recombinant interleukin-2: a pilot study. J Clin Oncol 1988; 6:839–53.
7. Kradin RL, Lazarus DS, Dubinett SM, et al. Tumor-infiltrating lymphocytes and interleukin-2 in treatment of advanced cancer. Lancet 1989; 1:577–80.
8. Yokota T, Arai N, et al. Molecular biology of interleukin-4 and interleukin-5

genes and biology of their products that stimulate B cells, T cells and hematopoietic cells. Immunol Rev 1988; 102:137.

9. Spits H, Yssel H, et al. Recombinant interleukin-4 promotes the growth of human T-cells. J Immunol 1987; 139:1142.

10. Widmer M, Acres RB, et al. Regulation of cytolytic cell populations from human peripheral blood by B cell stimulatory factor 1 (interleukin-4). J Exp Med 1987; 166:1447.

11. Spits H, Yssel H, et al. IL-4 inhibits IL-2 mediated induction of human lymphokine activated killer cells, but not the generation of antigen-specific cytotoxic T lymphocytes in mixed leukocyte cultures. J Immunol 1988; 141:29.

12. Nagler A, Lanier LL, Phillips JH. The effects of IL-4 on human natural killer cells. A potent regulator of IL-2 activation and proliferation. J Immunol 1988; 141:2349.

13. Kawakami Y, Rosenberg SA, Lotze MT. Interleukin-4 promotes the growth of tumor-infiltrating lymphocytes cytotoxic for human autologous melanoma. J Exp Med 1988; 168:2183.

14. Bukowski RM, Sharfman W, Murthy S, et al. Clinical results and characterization of tumor-infiltrating lymphocytes with or without recombinant interleukin-2 in human metastatic renal cell carcinoma. Cancer Res 1991; 51:4199–205.

15. Finke JH, Tubbs R, Connelly R, Pontes E, Montie J. Tumor-infiltrating lymphocytes in patients with renal cell carcinoma. New York Academy of Science. 1988; 387–94.

16. Sosman JA, Kohler PC, Hank JA, et al. Repetitive weekly cycles of interleukin-2. II. Clinical and Immunologic effects of dose, schedule, and addition of indomethacin. J Natl Cancer Inst 1988; 80:1451–61.

17. Thompson JA, Lee DJ, Lindgren CG, et al. Influence of dose and duration of infusion of interleukin-2 on toxicity and immunomodulation. J Clin Oncol 1988; 6:669–78.

18. Hasimura T, Tubbs R, Connelly R, et al. Characterization of two cell lines with distinct phenotypes and genotypes established from a patient from renal cell carcinoma. Cancer Res 1989; 49:7064–71.

19. Belldegrun A, Kasid A, Uppenkamp M, Rosenberg SA. Lymphokine mRNA profile and functional analysis of a human CD4[+] clone with unique anti-tumor specificity isolated from renal cell carcinoma ascitic fluid. Cancer Immunol Immunother 1990; 31:1–10.

20. Finke JH, Rayman P, Edinger M, et al. Characterization of a renal cell carcinoma specific cytotoxic CD8[+] T-cell line. J Immunother (in press).

21. Oldham RK, Dillman RO, Yanelli JR, et al. Continuous infusion interleukin-2 and tumor derived activated cells as treatment of advanced solid tumors: a National Biotherapy Study Group trial. Mol Biother 3:38–73.

22. Alexander J, Edinger M, Tubbs R, et al. Selective unresponsiveness of tumor derived T-lymphocytes. Proc FASEB 1992; (submitted).

14

Adoptive Immunotherapy of Disseminated Renal Cell Cancer

European Experience and Perspective

Gerrit Stoter, S. Hoo Goey, Diane Batchelor, Alexander M. M. Eggermont, Cor Lamers, Jan W. Gratama, and Reinder L. H. Bolhuis

Rotterdam Cancer Institute, Daniel den Hoed Cancer Center, Rotterdam, The Netherlands

I. INTRODUCTION

Interleukin-2 (IL-2) is a glycoprotein produced by activated T lymphocytes (1). In vitro activation of peripheral blood lymphocytes with IL-2 yields effector cells capable of lysing autologous as well as allogeneic tumor cell lines and fresh tumor preparations. This observation is designated the lymphokine-activated killer cell phenomenon (LAK) (2). DNA technology has made it possible to clone the gene for IL-2 and insert it into *Escherichia coli* to produce large amounts of recombinant human interleukin-2 (3).

Animal experiments have shown that there is a dose-effect relationship for IL-2 and that the combination of IL-2 with LAK is superior to either component when used alone. In addition, it appeared that divided daily doses were the most effective schedule for the administration of IL-2 in animal experiments (4,5).

These observations have led to clinical investigations with IL-2 and LAK. The first results were published by Rosenberg et al. (6,7). It was shown that renal cell cancer and melanoma were the most sensitive tumors. Response rates varied from 20 to 35%, and the median duration of response was 8 months (8). Of 35 responders 7 remain continuously free of disease for an observation period of 2.5 to more than 5 years (9). There was suggestive evidence for a survival advantage of the combination of IL-2 and LAK over that by IL-2 alone ($p = 0.07$).

The side effects of high-dose intermittent daily administration of IL-2 and LAK were substantial, including fever, chills, skin rash, anorexia, nausea, diarrhea, hypotension, oliguria, weight gain, lung edema, and cardiac rhythm disturbances (6–8).

In contrast to Rosenberg's high-dose intermittent scheme of bolus administration of 24×10^6 IU/m^2 of IL-2 three times daily for 5 days, West et al. introduced a schedule of continuous administration of IL-2 at 18×10^6 IU/m^2/day for 5 days (Cetus IL-2, 3×10^6 U = 18×10^6 IU) (10). The rationale for this schedule was based on theoretical considerations of efficacy and toxicity. Later, Thompson et al. performed a comparative clinical study of different dose levels of IL-2 given as a 2 or 24 h infusion or as three bolus injections over 24 h. It was shown that both toxicity and immunomodulation were dose dependent (11) and that immunomodulation was better with continuous infusion than with bolus administration (12).

More recently, it has been demonstrated that the combination of IL-2 and interferon-α (IFN-α) is synergistic in animal experiments (13–16). In addition, increasing doses of the combination of IL-2 and IFN-α have yielded increased response rates as high as 38% in a group of patients with renal cell cancer (17). This combination has now undergone extensive phase I trials and is currently explored in phase II studies with the use of various schedules. The compiled data of six published phase I and II studies show an overall response rate of 28% (13% complete response and 15% partial response) in a total of 85 treated patients (17–22).

These investigations have led to a series of adoptive immunotherapy studies in Europe, starting with IL-2 alone (23) and followed by IL-2 and LAK (24). At present, a single-institution study is being conducted at the Rotterdam Cancer Institute exploring the combination of IL-2 with LAK and IFN-α (25).

II. MULTICENTER STUDIES IN EUROPE

A. IL-2 Alone

From December 1987 to June 1989, a group of European investigators performed a phase II study of IL-2 alone for the treatment of patients with measurable metastases of renal cell cancer. Cetus IL-2 was given as a continuous infusion at a dose of 18×10^6 IU/m^2/day on days 1–5 (120 h) and on days 11–15 (108 h), with a repeat cycle starting on day 36. After these two induction cycles, patients with stable disease or response were scheduled to receive four maintenance cycles of continuous infusion of IL-2 at 18×10^6 IU/m^2/day on days 1–5, every 4 weeks. Response to treatment was evaluated every 2 months. Eligibility criteria required histologic proof of renal cell cancer, bidimensionally measurable metastases, performance status Karnofsky index > 80, normal organ functions of heart, lung, bone marrow, and kidney, and normal serum bilirubin and coagulation tests. Prior immunotherapy was not allowed. Patients with hypertension and a history of myocardial infarction or arrhythmias were excluded, and so were patients with infections and steroid medication.

A group of 57 patients were entered on study, with a median age of 53 years (range 21–80): 79% of patients had two or more metastatic organ sites, and 42 patients (67%) underwent prior nephrectomy. Although 37 patients (65%) received the two induction cycles, dose reductions or interruptions were applied in 50% of patients, mainly because of hypotension.

In the 51 patients who were evaluable, response was assessed according to World Health Organization (WHO) criteria (26). Two patients achieved a complete response (4%) and 6 a partial response (12%), for an overall response rate of 16%. Stable disease was seen in 10, and 33 developed progression. As of October 1991, progression-free survival for complete responders is 9 and 31$^+$ months and for partial responders, 5–19 months. The median progression-free survival for complete responders has not been reached and is 12 months for partial responders and 3 months (range 2–27$^+$) for patients with stable disease. The median overall survival for all patients is 8.5 months.

Common side effects were fever, skin rash, fatigue, anorexia, and diarrhea. Hypotension occurred frequently. Elevations of serum creatinine and bilirubin were transient and did not pose clinical problems. Culture-proven septicemia occurred in six patients. There were three treatment-related deaths. One patient died of *Staphylococcus epidermidis*-induced endocarditis, one of *Klebsiella* sepsis, and one of hypotension and anuria in combination with rapidly progressive disease.

B. IL-2 with LAK

The second multicenter phase II study used the combination of IL-2 and LAK. IL-2 was given as a continuous infusion of 18×10^6 IU/m^2/day on days 1–5. Leukapheresis was performed on days 8–11, and in vitro IL-2-cultured lymphocytes (LAK) were infused on days 12–15. IL-2 was given on days 12–16, that is, until 24 h after the fifth and last administration of LAK. This IL-2 and LAK cycle was repeated on day 36. Patients with stable disease or response were assigned to receive four monthly maintenance cycles with IL-2 at 18 × 10^6 IU/m²/day on days 1–5. The eligibility criteria for this protocol were similar to those just described.

A total of 56 eligible patients were entered on study; all were evaluable for toxicity and 53 for response, with a median age of 55 years (23–70): 90% developed metastases within 2 years from the diagnosis of the primary tumor, 71% had two or more metastatic organ sites, and 41 patients (73%) had previously undergone nephrectomy. Of 53 patients, 37 (70%) received two induction cycles. The median number of IL-2-cultured lymphocytes (LAK) per treatment cycle was 15 × 10^9 cells.

A complete response was achieved in 3 patients (6%) and in 7 a partial response was seen (13%), for an overall response rate of 19%. A total of 14 patients had stable disease, and 29 developed progression. As of August 1991, the time to progression-free survival for complete responders ranged from 16 to 32^+ months and for partial responders, from 4 to 25 months. The median progression-free survival for complete responders has not yet been reached. The median progression-free survival for partial responders is 11 months and for stable patients, 8 months (range 4–33^+). The median overall survival for all patients is 12 months.

Hypotension was the reason for treatment interruptions or dose reductions in 18 patients (32%). Side effects included fever, skin rash, nausea and vomiting, diarrhea, and hypotension. No toxic deaths were observed.

III. SINGLE-INSTITUTION STUDY OF IL-2 WITH LAK AND IFN-α

In March 1989 a phase II study of the combination of IL-2 with IFN-α and LAK was initiated at the Rotterdam Cancer Institute (25). The rationale for this combination is described in the introduction. The eligibility criteria in this protocol differ in one aspect from the studies already described; that is, patients must have nephrectomy to resect the primary tumor. The initial scheme consisted of Cetus IL-2, 18 × 10^6 IU/m²/day, as a continuous infusion on days 1–5. Leukapheresis was performed on days 7–9. IL-2-cultured lymphocytes (LAK) were reinfused on days 12–14, with IL-2 on days 12–16 (108 h). IFN-α was given intramuscularly on days 12–15 at a daily dose of 5 × 10^6 U/m². This cycle was repeated on day 36. Because of the moderate and manageable toxicity observed in the first 17 patients, we modified the protocol in that IFN-α was added on days 1–5. For logistic reasons Roche IL-2 was substituted for Cetus IL-2 (Cetus IL-2 3 × 10⁶ U = Roche IL-2 6.9 × 10⁶ U = 18 × 10⁶ IU). Patients with stable disease or response were scheduled for maintenance treatment with four monthly cycles of IL-2 at 18 × 10⁶ IU/m²/day on days 1–4 and IFN-α at 5 × 10⁶ U/m²/day on days 1–4.

Of the 17 patients in the first part of the study 16 were evaluable for response. The 17th patient died of myocardial infarction complicated by a ventricular septum defect 2 weeks after the completion of the second induction cycle. This complication was probably caused by this form of immunotherapy. A total of three patients (19%) achieved a complete response, and 1 (6%) a partial response. As of October 1991, progression-free survival is 6, 18, and 32⁺ months for complete responders and 6 months for the partial responder. Apart from the cardiac adverse event, the toxicity was manageable and all patients received 100% of the protocol regimen. This opened the possibility of adding IFN-α to the priming phase with IL-2, which carries the possible advantage of increased expression of major histocompatibility and tumor-associated antigens, which could enhance the cytolytic machinery.

A group of 28 patients have been entered: 60% had two or more metastatic organ sites. A total of 5 patients are too early yet for evaluation, and 1 has been lost to follow-up from the end of the second induction cycle; 3 patients received inadequate treatment because of grade 4 toxicity. Thus, 19 patients are evaluable for response: 3 (16%) have achieved a complete response and 6 (32%), a partial response. If one considers the 3 patients with inadequate therapy as treatment failures, the overall response rate is 41%. As of October 1991, progression-free survival for the complete responders is 4⁺, 10⁺, and 17⁺ months and, for partial responders, 2, 2⁺, 3⁺, 4, 10⁺, and 17 months.

The toxicity of the intensified regimen is considerable with WHO grades 3–4 hypotension in 50% of the patients, oliguria or anuria in 60%, diarrhea and metabolic acidosis in 40%, confusion in 30%, lung edema in 20%, and electrocardiographic (ECG) abnormalities in 15% of the patients. Only 28% of the patients received the full induction treatment. Dose reductions of 25–50% were applied in 30% of patients. Less than 50% of IL-2 and IFN-α was given to 42% of the patients. This illustrates that the maximum tolerated treatment intensity has been reached.

IV. CONCLUSIONS AND PERSPECTIVES

The results of these studies show that IL-2-based immunotherapy of disseminated renal cell cancer can be effective. The response rate in the first study of IL-2 alone is low (16%) but comparable to the average outcome of five other reported IL-2-alone studies, with 38 of 224 responses (17%, range 0–24%) (17,21,27–29).

The study of IL-2 and LAK has yielded a 19% overall response rate, which is again similar to the combined results of five other reports, with 49 responses in 187 patients (26%, range 3–50%) (8–10,29,30). In contrast to the findings of West et al. (10), we have not found clinical or immunologic correlates to predict treatment outcome.

The results of the ongoing study of IL-2 with LAK and IFN-α must await further patient recruitment and longer follow-up before conclusions can be drawn, but a relatively high response rate of approximately 40% with good durability has been observed thus far.

It is difficult to define the relative merits of LAK in combination with IL-2 and IFN-α. The literature now reports six phase I and II studies of the combination of IL-2 and IFN-α without adoptive cell transfer. An overall response rate of 24 of 85 patients (28%) has been observed (17–22). A randomized study is needed to demonstrate an additional therapeutic value of LAK in combination with IL-2 and IFN-α.

One of the drawbacks of current adoptive cellular immunotherapy is the lack of homing efficiency of the effector cells (31). It may be that the approach with tumor-infiltrating lymphocytes (TIL) offers a way to use effector T cells specific for the tumor cells of the host from whom they have been cultured. In mouse models TIL are at least much more effective than LAK (32).

In the human being the best perspectives for TIL may be in melanoma (33). In melanoma patients the use of TIL has yielded partial responses in about half of the patients (34). The results of TIL in renal cell cancer are disappointing, with 2 partial responses in 7 patients in one series (35) and no responses in another series of 18 patients (36).

Another way to improve the homing capacity of effector cells is the use of bifunctional antibodies with specificity for an activation antigen on the effector cell and for a tumor-associated antigen. Such bispecific antibodies can be constructed chemically (37) or by somatic hybridization of either two hybridomas (quadroma) or a hybridoma and a spleen lymphocyte (trioma), each producing one of the required specificities (38–40). It has been reported that effective triggering and activation of the lytic machinery of T and natural killer (NK) cells can be obtained with monoclonal antibodies for CD2, CD3, or CD16 (41–44). Only 3–5% of the lysis-promoting receptors need to be targeted for effective activation of the lymphocytes. Therefore, the required concentrations of bispecific antibody are very low, of the order of 1 mg per 10^9 cells. The tumor cell lysis mediated by these targeted lymphocytes is further enhanced by incubation of the effector cells with IL-2 (45). Bispecific antibodies are now available for several solid tumors, including renal cell cancer. As a model approach, a Dutch clinical investigation is now studying the role of activated T lymphocytes coated with a bispecific antibody (OC-TR) with specificity for the activation antigen CD3 and for a tumor-associated antigen of ovarian cancer (MOv-18) (39,40,46–48).

Centocor Europe B.V., Leiden, The Netherlands, produces the trioma-derived bispecific antibody OC-TR, of which one F(ab′) binding site is directed against the CD3 activation site on the T lymphocyte and the other to an ovarian cancer-associated membrane antigen (MOv-18) (39). In vitro experiments with the MOv-18 antibody showed a high affinity and specificity for several ovarian cancer cell lines. Fluorescein isothiocyanate-labeled antibody staining of frozen ovarian cancer sections and single-cell suspensions derived from ovarian carcinomas showed reactivity in virtually 100% of nonmucinous carcinoma specimens, almost all cells binding the MOv-18 antibody. There was cross-reactivity in only 3 of 141 sections (2%) with nonovarian tumors. No reactivity was seen in normal tissues, including kidney, spleen, bladder, ovary, uterus, prostate, pancreas, colon, stomach, liver, skin, parotid gland, thyroid, larynx, breast, testis, lung, bone marrow, and peripheral blood lymphocytes (46). OC-TR induced a 75% target cell lysis at a lymphocyte-target cell ratio of 100:1 in the 4 h ^{51}Cr release assay, in contrast to 16% when no OC-TR was added to the peripheral blood lymphocytes (39,40). The cytotoxicity appeared to be specific since no lysis occurred with normal and nonovarian cancer target cells (40).

In addition to the in vitro data, in vivo studies in a nude mouse model showed that OC-TR-targeted activated peripheral blood T cells could eliminate MOv-18-positive ovarian cancer (OVCAR3) growing in the peritoneal cavity of nude mice (49). Biolocalization studies with nude mice indicate that MOv-18 bound preferentially to human ovarian carcinomas. Moreover, it was shown in a clinical study with 18 ovarian cancer patients that ^{131}I-labeled MOv-18 gave positive images in 27 of 32 lesions detected at laparotomy (48).

In The Netherlands a clinical phase II study has been initiated for the intraperitoneal administration of OC-TR-labeled activated T lymphocytes. Ovarian cancer patients who relapse after first-line chemotherapy are selected. Laparoscopy is performed to obtain fresh tumor biopsies, which are examined for the presence of MOv-18. Patients with positive biopsy specimens are subject to debulking laparotomy, at which time the remaining measurable and evaluable indicator lesions are documented and a Tenckhoff catheter is inserted. Leukapheresis is performed 1 day before surgery to obtain 10^8 lymphocytes, which are cultured and activated with IL-2 and phytohemagglutinin (PHA). After 2–3 weeks of culture there is an approximately 50-fold proliferation of cells. These activated lymphocytes are then coated with OC-TR and infused with IL-2 at 600,000 IU daily for 5 days at 10^9 cells per day via the Tenckhoff catheter. This treatment cycle is repeated 3 weeks later, and a second-look laparotomy is scheduled at 8 weeks after the last cell transfer.

A total of six patients have completed therapy. Toxicity was much less than with systemic high-dose IL-2 therapies. Fever, anorexia, and abdominal bloating were the most important side effects. Ascitic fluid cytology became negative in two patients within 5 days of therapy, and ascites became infiltrated with lymphocytes, eosinophils and granulocytes. These observations suggest that the anticipated inflammatory immune response is indeed evoked by this treatment, resulting in tumor cell death.

Before exploratory laparotomy was performed, three patients showed progression of disease outside the peritoneal cavity. The three remaining patients were operated upon. Two showed complete and partial tumor regression at accessible sites on the peritoneal surface. These results are encouraging and indicate that this treatment strategy should be further developed in the treatment of cancer. Bispecific antibodies are now also available for renal cell cancer.

REFERENCES

1. Taniguchi T, Matsui H, Fujita T, et al. Structure and expression of a cloned cDNA for human interleukin-2. Nature 1983; 302:305–7.
2. Grimm EA, Mazumder A, Zhang HZ, Rosenberg SA. Lymphokine activated killer cell phenomenon: lysis of NK resistant fresh solid tumor cells by IL2 activated autologous human peripheral blood lymphocytes. J Exp Med 1982; 155:1823–41.
3. Rosenberg SA, Grimm EA, McGrogan M, et al. Biological activity of recombinant human interleukin-2 produced in *Escherichia coli*. Science 1984; 223:1412–15.
4. Mulé JJ, Shu S, Schwarz SL, Rosenberg SA. Adoptive immunotherapy of established pulmonary melanoma by the intravenous adoptive transfer of syngeneic lymphocytes activated in vitro by interleukin-2. Science 1984; 225:1487–92.
5. Lafreniere R, Rosenberg SA. Adoptive immunotherapy of murine hepatic metastases with lymphokine activated killer (LAK) cells and recombinant interleukin-2 (rIL2) can mediate the regression of both immunogenic and nonimmunogenic sarcomas and an adenocarcinoma. J Immunol 1985; 135:4273–80.
6. Rosenberg SA, Lotze MT, Muul LM, et al. Special report: observations on the

systemic administration of autologous lymphokine-activated killer cells and recombinant interleukin-2 to patients with metastatic cancer. N Engl J Med 1985; 313:1485–92.

7. Rosenberg SA, Lotze MT, Muul LM, et al. A progress report on the treatment of 157 patients with advanced cancer using lymphokine-activated killer cells and interleukin-2 or high-dose interleukin-2 alone. N Engl J Med 1987; 316:889–97.

8. Rosenberg SA, Lotze MT, Yang JC, et al. Experience with the use of high-dose interleukin-2 in the treatment of 652 cancer patients. Ann Surg 1989; 210:474–84.

9. Rosenberg SA. Adoptive cellular therapy in patients with advanced cancer; an update. Biol Ther Cancer Updates 1991; 1:1–15.

10. West WH, Tauer KW, Yanelli JR, et al. Constant-infusion recombinant interleukin-2 in adoptive immunotherapy of advanced cancer. N Engl J Med 1987; 316:898–905.

11. Thompson JA, Lee DJ, Lindgren CG, et al. Influence of dose and duration of infusion of interleukin-2 on toxicity and immunomodulation. J Clin Oncol 1988; 6:669–78.

12. Thompson JA, Lee DJ, Lindgren CG, et al. Influence of schedule of interleukin-2 administration on therapy with interleukin-2 and lymphokine activated killer cells. Cancer Res 1989; 49:235–40.

13. Brunda MJ, Bellantoni D, Sulich V. In vivo antitumor activity of combinations of interferon-α and interleukin-2 in a murine model. Correlation of efficacy with the induction of cytotoxic cells resembling natural killer cells. Int J Cancer 1987; 40:365–71.

14. Cameron RB, McIntosh JK, Rosenberg SA. Synergistic antitumor effects of combination immunotherapy with recombinant interleukin-2 and a recombinant hybrid alpha interferon in the treatment of established murine hepatic metastases. Cancer Res 1988; 48:5810–17.

15. Iigo M, Sakurai J, Tamura T, et al. In vivo antitumor activity of multiple injections of recombinant interleukin-2 alone and in combination with three different types of recombinant interferon on various syngeneic murine tumors. Cancer Res 1988; 48:260–4.

16. Rosenberg SA. The development of new immunotherapies for the treatment of cancer using interleukin-2. Ann Surg 1988; 208:121–35.

17. Rosenberg SA, Lotze MT, Yang JC, et al. Combination therapy with interleukin-2 and alpha interferon for the treatment of patients with advanced cancer. J Clin Oncol 1989; 7:1863–74.

18. Lee KH, Talpaz M, Rothberg JL, et al. Concomitant administration of recombinant human interleukin-2 and recombinant interferon α-2a in cancer patients: a phase I study. J Clin Oncol 1989; 7:1726–32.

19. Budd GT, Osgood B, Barna B, et al. Phase I clinical trial of interleukin-2 and α-interferon: toxicity and immunologic effects. Cancer Res 1989; 49:6432–6.

20. Sznol M, Mier JW, Sparano J, et al. A phase I study of high-dose interleukin-2 in combination with interferon-α2b. J Biol Response Mod 1990; 9:529–37.

21. Bukowski RM, Murthy S, Sergi J, et al. Phase I trial of continuous infusion

recombinant interleukin-2 and intermittent recombinant interferon-α2a: clinical effects. J Biol Response Mod 1990; 9:538–45.

22. Hirsh M, Lipton A, Harvey H, et al. Phase I study of interleukin-2 and interferon-α2a as outpatient therapy for patients with advanced malignancy. J Clin Oncol 1990; 8:1657–63.

23. Von der Maase H, Geertsen P, Thatcher N, et al. Recombinant interleukin-2 in metastatic renal cell carcinoma—a European multicenter phase II study. Eur J Cancer 1991; 27:1583–1589.

24. Negrier S, Philip T, Stoter G, et al. Interleukin-2 with or without LAK cells in metastatic renal cell carcinoma: a report of a European mulitcentre study. Eur J Cancer Clin Oncol 1989; 25:S21–8.

25. Stoter G, Goey SH, Punt CJA, et al. Recombinant human interleukin-2 (IL2) + IL2 activated lymphocytes (LAK) + alpha-interferon (αIFN) in metastatic renal cell carcinoma. Proc Am Soc Clin Oncol 1990; 9:187.

26. WHO. Handbook for reporting results of cancer treatment. Geneva, 1979.

27. Abrams JS, Rayner AA, Wiernik PH, et al. High-dose recombinant interleukin-2 alone: a regimen with limited activity in the treatment of advanced renal cell carcinoma. J Natl Cancer Inst 1990; 82:1202–6.

28. Sosman JA, Kohler PC, Hank JA, et al. Repetitive weekly cycles of interleukin-2: responses of renal carcinoma with acceptable toxicity. J Natl Cancer Inst 1988; 80:60–3.

29. Dillman RO, Oldham RK, Tauer KW, et al. Continuous interleukin-2 and lymphokine-activated killer cells for advanced cancer: a national biotherapy study group trial. J Clin Oncol 1991; 9:1233–40.

30. Fisher RI, Coltman CA Jr, Doroshow JH, et al. Metastatic renal cell cancer treated with interleukin-2 and lymphokine-activated killer cells. Ann Intern Med 1988; 108:518–23.

31. Ortaldo JR, Longo DL. Human natural lymphocyte effector cells: definition, analysis of activity, and clinical effectiveness. J Natl Cancer Inst 1988; 80:999–1010.

32. Spiess P, Yang J, Rosenberg SA. In vivo activity of murine tumor-infiltrating lymphocytes. J Natl Cancer Inst 1987; 79:1067–75.

33. Belldegrunm A, Muul LM, Rosenberg SA. Interleukin-2 expanded tumor-infiltrating lymphocytes in human renal cell cancer: isolation, characterization and antitumor activity. Cancer Res 1988; 48:206–14.

34. Rosenberg SA, Packard BS, Aebersold PM, et al. Use of tumor-infiltrating lymphocytes and interleukin-2 in the immunotherapy of patients with metastatic melanoma. N Engl J Med 1988; 319:1676–80.

35. Kradin RL, Kurnick JT, Lazarus DS, et al. Tumour-infiltrating lymphocytes and interleukin-2 in treatment of advanced cancer. Lancet 1989; 577–80.

36. Bukowski RM, Sharfman W, Murthy S, et al. Clinical results and characterization of tumor-infiltrating lymphocytes with or without recombinant interleukin-2 in human metastatic renal cell carcinoma. Cancer Res 1991; 51:4199–05.

37. Titus JA, Perez P, Kaubisch A, et al. Human natural killer cells targeted with hetero-cross-linked antibodies specifically lyse tumor cells in vitro and prevent tumor growth in vivo. J Immunol 1987; 139:3153–8.

38. Van Dijk J, Warnaar SO, van Eendenburg JDH, et al. Induction of tumor cell lysis by bispecific monoclonal antibodies recognizing renal cell carcinoma and CD3 antigen. Int J Cancer 1989; 43:344–9.

39. Mezzanzanica D, Canevari S, Ménard S, et al. Human ovarian carcinoma lysis by cytotoxic T-cells targeted by bispecific monoclonal antibodies: analysis of the antibody components. Int J Cancer 1988; 41:609–15.

40. Pupa SM, Canevari S, Fontanelli R, et al. Activation of mononuclear cells to be used for hybrid monoclonal antibody-induced lysis of human ovarian carcinoma cells. Int J Cancer 1988; 42:455–9.

41. Van de Griend RJ, Bolhuis RLH, Stoter G, et al. Regulation of cytolytic activity in CD3$^-$ and CD3$^+$ killer cell clones by monoclonal antibodies (anti-CD16, anti-CD2, anti-CD3) depends on subclass specificity of target cell IgG-FcR. J Immunol 1987; 138:3137–44.

42. Bolhuis RLH, Roozemond RC, van de Griend RJ. Induction and blocking of cytolysis in CD2$^+$CD3$^-$ NK and CD2$^+$, CD3$^+$ cytotoxic T-lymphocytes via CD2 50 kD sheep erythrocyte receptor. J Immunol 1986; 136:3939–44.

43. Lanzavecchia A, Scheidegger D. The use of hybrid hybridomas to target human cytotoxic T-lymphocytes. Eur J Immunol 1987; 17:105–11.

44. Van de Griend RJ, Tax WJM, van Krimpen BA, et al. Lysis of tumor cells by CD3$^+$4$^-$8$^-$16$^+$ T cell receptor $\alpha\beta^-$ clones, regulated via CD3 and CD16 activation sites, recombinant interleukin-2 and interfon-β. J Immunol 1987; 138:1627–33.

45. Perez P, Hoffman RW, Titus JA, et al. Specific targeting of human peripheral blood T-cells by heteroaggregates containing anti-T3 cross-linked to anti-target cell antibodies. J Exp Med 1986; 163:166–78.

46. Miotti S, Canevari S, Ménard S, et al. Characterization of human ovarian carcinoma-associated antigens defined by novel monoclonal antibodies with tumor-restricted specificity. Int J Cancer 1987; 39:297–303.

47. Colnaghi MI, Buraggi GL, Canevari S, et al. Evaluation of the suitability of a monoclonal antibody raised against human ovarian carcinoma for therapeutic approaches. Nucl Med Biol 1989; 16:633–6.

48. Crippa F, Buraggi GL, Di Re E, et al. Radioimmunoscintigraphy of ovarian cancer with the MOv18 monoclonal antibody. Eur J Cancer 1991; 27:724–9.

49. Mezzanzanica D, Garrido MA, Neblock DS, et al. Human T-lymphocytes targeted against an established human ovarian carcinoma with a bispecific F(ab')$_2$ antibody prolong host survival in a murine xenograft model. Cancer Res 1991; 57:5716–5721.

15

Adoptive Immunotherapy for Renal Cell Carcinoma Using Cytokine-Modulated Tumor-Infiltrating Lymphocytes

The UCLA Experience

Arie Belldegrun, Gunther Steger, Cho-Lea Tso, Randhir Kaboo, Thomas Duckett, Robert A. Figlin, and Jean B. deKernion

UCLA School of Medicine, Los Angeles, California

I. INTRODUCTION

Immunotherapy using combination of immune lymphoid cells and cytokines, such as interleukin-2 (IL-2), is a new approach to the therapy for human cancers. Modern recombinant DNA technology has overcome the problem of supplying high quantities of purified cytokines, and laboratory methods have been established for ex vivo large-scale production of lymphoid cell populations for use in adoptive therapy programs.

Murine models of cellular therapy using tumor-infiltrating lymphocytes (TIL) have demonstrated a protective antitumor activity against intravenous challenge (1). The injected TIL not only provides tumor protection but are also capable of surviving in vivo for periods of up to 6 weeks even in the absence of exogenously supplied IL-2 (2,3). Furthermore, additional work using murine models has established that T cell subpopulations, such as cytolytic CD8$^+$ clones and CD8$^+$ lymphocyte cultures, can be effective against established tumors (4–6). Regardless of the dominant phenotype, adoptively transferred TIL can be substantially more reactive to the autologous tumor than lymphokine-activated (LAK) cells (7).

Thus far, only IL-2 and, on some occasions, IL-4 have been used for in vitro expansion and generation of TIL for clinical use. Several other cytokines with T cell stimulatory properties, however, are now available and are awaiting further testings. Modifications in culture conditions, use of specific lymphoid cell populations, and restimulation with autologous tumor are all important concepts currently being investigated. This chapter summarizes some of our experience with adoptive cellular therapy and the approaches we have taken to enhance the potency of TIL therapy.

II. STUDIES WITH INTERLEUKIN-4

IL-4, initially termed B cell stimulatory factor 1, is a B cell-derived lymphokine originally characterized as a costimulator for B cell proliferation. More recently it was shown that IL-4 can also induce the proliferation of some activated T cells and augment allogeneic generation of cytotoxic T lymphocytes (CTL) (8–11). In addition, IL-4 is an important regulator of natural killer (NK) cell activity in humans (12,13). In the mouse, IL-4 generates LAK activity from murine splenocytes independently, as well as in combination with IL-2 (14,15). Conversely, human IL-4 inhibits LAK activity generated in human peripheral blood leukocytes (PBL) from IL-2 (16). Thus recently we studied the in vitro effects of IL-4 cocultured with various doses of IL-2 on the proliferation, phenotypic expression, and cytotoxicity of human renal cell carcinoma TIL. Specifically, we were interested in determining whether IL-4 is capable of suppressing the growth of nonspecific NK cells and LAK cells while expanding a more pure population of specific, major histocompatibility complex (MHC)-restricted cytotoxic T cells with more potent in vivo activity. Compared to culture in IL-2 alone, the addition of IL-4 improved overall expansion in both high-dose (1000 units/ml) IL-2, with a mean fold expansion of 2061 versus 1087, and low-dose IL-2 (20 units/ml), with a mean fold expansion of 1904 versus 262. Enhancement of TIL proliferation was dependent on the timing of IL-4 addition to the culture. Augmented growth of TIL from renal cell carcinoma occurred only when IL-4 was added with or following activation by IL-2. The phenotype consisted primarily of $CD3^+$ $CD4^+$ lymphocytes, with a reciprocal reduction in $CD56^+CD16^+$ cells. Importantly, there was a significant reduction in nonspecific cytotoxicity against K562, M14, and allogeneic tumor targets but no significant change against autologous tumor. It thus appears that IL-4 has an important regulatory effect on the expansion of IL-2-stimulated TIL by promoting the growth of $CD3^+CD4^+$ lymphocytes and inhibiting the growth and nonspecific cytotoxicity associated with LAK-like $CD16^+CD56^+$ cells (17).

We also evaluated the effects of irradiated autologous tumor restimulation on TIL cultures. The greatest total fold expansion was seen in those cultures containing the combination of IL-4, low-dose IL-2, and irradiated autologous tumor cells, which exhibited a 5.2- $\pm$ 2.4-fold greater expansion of TIL cultures than those grown with the standard 1000 units/ml of IL-2 alone (1992, in press). These results suggest that IL-4 and irradiated autologous tumor cells can be effective growth stimulators when used in combination with a low-dose IL-2 regimen and may be of significant benefit for growing activated TIL from patients with renal cell carcinoma.

III. STUDIES WITH INTERLEUKIN-6 AND INTERLEUKIN-7

IL-6 and IL-7 are two cytokines that were recently shown to stimulate T cells (18–22). We investigated the effects of varying doses of IL-6 (0, 25, and 100 units/ml) together with IL-2 (400 units/ml) on the in vitro expansion, proliferation, cytotoxicity, and cell surface phenotype of long-term renal TIL cultures from patients with renal cell carcinoma (23). TIL cultures grown in IL-6 alone showed no growth. No consistent effect on proliferation could be demonstrated when high-dose IL-6 was added to the cultures. At an early stage of the culture (days 22–27), there was no significant influence on TIL growth, and when tested at a later stage (days 56–71), two of three cultures demonstrated enhanced proliferative response. No major advantages of IL-6-treated TIL compared to those grown in IL-2 alone were noted. Typically, IL-6-treated cultures had a higher $CD8^+$ percentage of cells and fewer $CD4^+$ cells. It thus appears that IL-6 can enhance the growth of some TIL from renal cell carcinoma, although these effects are not consistent in all cultures and can alter the functional characteristics of these TIL. The impact of these data on the immunotherapy of renal cell carcinoma needs further investigation.

We recently analyzed the effect of IL-7 on the growth of TIL. Of 10 TIL cultures 5 proliferated in response to IL-7 alone, but this proliferation response was significantly lower (70–90%) than that with IL-2 alone. Combination of IL-2 and IL-7 showed a synergistic effect on TIL proliferation measured by thymidine incorporation. IL-7-driven proliferation could be partly blocked by anti-IL-2 and anti-IL-2 receptor antibodies, suggesting a partial dependence of the proliferation in response to IL-7 on the activation of the IL-2 pathway. These data are in accordance with previous reports that IL-7 stimulation of concanavalin A (ConA)-activated T cells is associated with the production of IL-2 and the IL-2 receptor expression. Phenotypically, a significant increase in the number of CD3$^+$ cells with a decrease in CD56$^+$ was observed, with a predominance of CD4$^+$ cells. When IL-7 was combined with IL-2 to stimulate TIL, these phenotypic changes were not observed. Our studies with IL-7 demonstrated a synergistic effect with IL-2 on the proliferation of TIL derived from renal cell carcinoma but no enhancement or influence on the cytolytic activity against autologous tumor killing.

IV. TUMOR-SPECIFIC TIL

TIL currently in use for clinical trials are expanded in relatively high doses of interleukin-2, which may not select the small proportion of lymphocytes dedicated to autologous tumor. Variabilities in the tumor, the host, and culture conditions all contribute to TIL specificity and may result in a nonspecific population of effectors (24). We recently showed that by varying culture conditions, tumor-specific TIL clones from renal cell carcinoma can be selected (25). In these studies we used a modified technique for growing TIL from renal cell carcinoma with a low (20 units/ml) dose of IL-2 and continuous stimulation with the autologous tumor cells (TIL-tumor ratio, 10:1). Tumor-stimulated TIL grown in low-dose IL-2 expanded significantly better than TIL growing in high-dose IL-2 alone (586,744- versus 35,464-fold) and exhibited absolute specific lysis between 50 and 190 days in culture. Killing was MHC restricted and could be blocked by W6-32 but not by HLA-DR. Fluorescence-activated cell sorting (FACS) analysis revealed a CD3$^+$ CD8$^+$CD16$^-$ phenotype. These studies demonstrated that CTL with specific antitumor activity can be selectively grown from bulk culture TIL derived from human renal cell carcinoma by using a low dose of IL-2 and continuous stimulation with irradiated autologous tumor cells. The generation and maintenance of persistent autologous tumor-specific cytotoxicity in long-term and expandable bulk cultures of TIL may improve the efficacy and potency of adoptive immunotherapy.

Unlike some malignant melanomas, renal cell carcinoma presents a special problem with respect to TIL therapy because of the original cellular heterogeneity. The proportion of CD8$^+$ TIL from renal cell carcinoma can often be lower than 30% and ranges between 7 and 75% (26,27). Furthermore, with time in culture the percentage of CD4$^+$ cells can be significantly increased (28). If the CD8$^+$ T cell is indeed the principal antitumor effector cell, current processes using bulk cultures are less than optimal in efficiency, with a high degree of individual variability. At present, no practical techniques are available for generating therapeutically useful numbers of tumor antigen-specific TIL. In an attempt to make the process more efficient by isolating CD8$^+$ TIL before the initiation of large-scale production of effector T cells, we developed a single-step selection process for the large-scale ex vivo production of CD8$^+$ TIL. Enzymatic digestions were performed on resected from renal cell carcinoma to produce bulk TIL culture. The tumor digests were cultured for 10–20 days ex vivo using high-dose recombinant IL-2. Isolations of lymphocyte subsets were performed using the CD8$^+$ AIS-Cellector (Applied Immune Sciences, Menlo Park, CA) device. The cultures were greater than 90% CD8$^+$ at the time of culture termination. Phenotypic analysis after isolation revealed 99% CD8$^+$ and $\alpha\beta$ T cell receptor positivity, whereas only partial CD56 and virtually no CD16 surface expression were observed. Lytic activity from these cultures at an early time point was high in both natural killer (NK cell activity, as measured against K562) and T cell type killing measured against a variety of fresh tumor targets. Late-culture cytotoxicity testing of the CD8$^+$ cultures showed a dramatic reduction in NK-like killing, with generally sustained levels of T cell-like killing. The propagated CD8$^+$ cells expressed lytic activity against autologous renal cell carcinoma that ranged from approximately 1 to 18 lytic units per 10^6 cells. Kinetic analysis of the lytic activity from two of the cultured CD8$^+$ TIL showed that natural and LAK cell against K562 and Dandi cell lines dropped steadily. Comparison of bulk, complementary CD4$^+$ TIL and CD8$^+$ TIL from the same patient showed that the majority of the proliferative and lytic activity against autologous tumor was contained within the CD8$^+$ fraction (1992, submitted for publication). These observations formed the basis for current studies using highly purified CD8$^+$ immune T cells as part of an adoptive immunotherapy protocol in patients with metastatic renal cell carcinoma.

V. IN VIVO CYTOKINE PRIMING

To improve the efficacy of TIL immunotherapy, 10 patients with advanced renal cell carcinoma were primed with interferon-α before nephrectomy and then treated with a combination of primed TIL (pTIL) (up to 2.8 $\times$ 10^{11} cells per patient), interleukin-2, and interferon-α (29). A total of 0.2–2.5 $\times$ 10^9 cells (20–72% lymphocytes) extracted from 35–100 g tumor were propagated in AIM-V medium in the presence of 400 units IL-2 (Hoffman-LaRoche). All TIL cultures were successfully expanded to greater than 1 $\times$ 10^{11} cells. By FACS analysis, most pTIL were CD3$^+$, with 15–91% CD8$^+$ cells. All pTIL exhibited enhanced antiautologous killing of 2.0–4.9 lytic units (30%). Patients were evaluated for clinical response after 4–8 weeks of treatment: 3

patients are currently free of cancer; 2 patients are complete responders with a follow-up of 22^+ and 21^+ months. The third patient is a surgical complete responder. His pulmonary metastasis regressed, and upon further exploration, he was rendered a complete responder. Further studies are currently underway to optimize the priming conditions before radical nephrectomy. We are analyzing the effect of tumor necrosis factor, interferon-γ, interferon-α, and interleukin-2 as possible priming agents.

Genetic engineering is largely responsible for our progress in cytokine and cell therapy and will determine the future course of biologic response modifier therapy. Cells can now be tailored to produce specific cytokines. The insertion of cytokine genes into the tumor or the TIL has initiated the new field of "gene therapy." TIL can be modified to produce specific cytokines, and cytokine genes can be directly inserted into the tumor, delivering high levels of local cytokine production. Alternatively, the tumor cell can be modified to produce a vaccine. Successful transfections of such cells have been accomplished in our laboratory as well as in others. Based on these studies, we have obtained permission from the U.S. Food and Drug Administration Human Gene Therapy Subcommittee and the Human Recombinant Advisory Committee to treat patients with metastatic malignant melanoma and renal cell carcinoma using in vitro expanded and genetically engineered (neomycin phosphotransferase) bulk, $CD8^+$, and/or $CD4^+$ TIL and bulk, $CD8^+$, and/or $CD4^+$ peripheral blood leukocytes (PBL) in combination with recombinant interleukin-2 alone or with recombinant IL-2 and recombinant interferon-α. The novel feature of this protocol is that two cell populations from the same patient, TIL and PBL, will each be transfected with a different retroviral vector containing the neomycin phosphotransferase (neo-R) gene (30). The ability to "genetically mark" two different cell populations will permit us to address the important questions of TIL trafficking, tumor localization, and in vivo life span.

In summary, some patients respond to the new strategies of immunotherapy, and combinations of cytokines or cytokine-stimulated cells show great promise. Imaginative techniques to modify cells and segregate cell subpopulation for therapy must be explored.

ACKNOWLEDGMENTS

Supported by Grants 52 499-01 and CA-09120 from the National Institutes of Health.

REFERENCES

1. Speiss PJ, Yang JC, Rosenberg SA. In vivo antitumor activity of tumor infiltrating lymphocytes expanded in recombinant interleukin-2. J Natl Cancer Inst 1987; 79:1067–72.

2. Alexander RB, Rosenberg SA. Long term survival of adoptively transferred tumor-infiltrating lymphocytes in mice. J Immunol 1990; 145:1615–20.

3. Wong RA, Alexander RB, Puri RK, Rosenberg SA. In vivo proliferation of adoptively transferred tumor-infiltrating lymphocytes in mice. J Immunother 1991; 10:120–30.

4. Yamasaki T, Handa H, Yamashita J, Watanabe Y, Namba Y, Hamaoka M. Specific adoptive immunotherapy with tumor specific CTL clone for murine malignant gliomas. Cancer Res 1984; 44:1776–82.

5. Greenberg PD, Cheever MA. Effector mechanisms operative in adoptive therapy of tumor-bearing animals: implications for the use of interleukin-2. J Biol Response Mod 1984; 3:455–62.

6. Barth RJ, Mule JJ, Spiess PJ, Rosenberg SA. Interferon gamma and tumor necrosis factor have a role in tumor regressions mediated by murine CD8$^+$ tumor-infiltrating lymphocytes. J Exp Med 1991; 173:647–52.

7. Rosenberg SA, Speiss P, Lafreniere R. A new approach to the adoptive immunotherapy of cancer with tumor-infiltrating lymphocytes. Science 1986; 233:1318–21.

8. Paul WE, Ohara J. B-cell stimulatory factor 1/interleukin 4. Annu Rev Immunol 1987; 5:429.

9. Widmer MB, Acres RB, Sassenfeld HM, Grabstein KM. Regulation of cytolytic cells populations from human peripheral blood by B cell stimulating factor 1 (interleukin 4). J Exp Med 1987; 166:1447.

10. Spits H, Yssel H, Takebe Y, et al. Recombinant interleukin 4 promotes the growth of human T cells. J Immunol 1987; 139:1142.

11. Mitchell LC, Davis LS, Lipsky PE. Promotion of human T lymphocyte proliferation by IL-4. J Immunol 1989; 142:1548.

12. Spits H, Yssel H, Paliard X, Kastelein R, Figdor C, de Vries JE. IL-4 inhibits IL-2 mediated induction of human lymphokine activated killer cells, but not the generation of antigen-specific cytotoxic T lymphocytes in mixed leukocyte culture. J Immunol 1988; 141:29.

13. Han X, Itoh K, Balch CM, Pellis NR. Recombinant interleukin-4 (rIL-4) inhibits interleukin-2 induced activation of peripheral blood lymphocytes. Lymphokine Res 1988; 7(3):227.

14. Mulé JJ, Smith CA, Rosenberg SA. Interleukin-4 (B-cell stimulatory factor-1) can mediate the induction of LAK activity directed against fresh tumor cells. J Exp Med 1987; 166:792–7.

15. Peace DJ, Kern DE, Schultz KR, Greenberg PD, Cheever MA. IL-4 induced lymphokine-activated killer cells: lytic activity is mediated by phenotypically

distinct natural killer like and T cell like large granular lymphocytes. J Immunol 1988; 140:3679–85.

16. Kawakami Y, Custer M, Rosenberg SA, Lotze MT. Interleukin-4 regulates interleukin-2 induction of lymphokine activated killer activity from human lymphocytes. (Submitted for publication.)

17. Koo A, Lee T, Peyret C, et al. Regulatory effects of combination lymphokines on tumor infiltrating lymphocytes (TIL) from renal cell cancer. Cancer Res 1990; 31:296, A1758.

18. Lotze M, Jirik F, Kabouridis P, et al. B cell stimulating factor 2/interleukin-6 is a co-stimulant for human thymocytes and T lymphocytes. J Exp Med 1988; 167:1253–6.

19. Takai Y, Wong GG, Clark SC, Burakoff SJ, Herrmann SH. B cell stimulatory factor 2 is involved in the differentiation of cytotoxic lymphocytes. J Immunol 1988; 140:508–12.

20. Uyttenhove C, Coulie PG, Van Snick J. T cell growth and differentiation induced by interleukin-HP 1/IL-6, the murine hybridoma/plasmacytoma growth factor. J Exp Med 1988; 167:1417–22.

21. Lynch DH, Namen AE, Miller RE. In vivo evaluation of the effects of interleukins 2, 4 and 7 on enhancing the immunotherapeutic efficacy of anti-tumor cytotoxic T lymphocytes. Eur J Immunol 1991; 21:2977–85.

22. Jicha DL, Mulé JJ, Rosenberg SA. Interleukin 7 generates antitumor cytotoxic T lymphocytes against murine sarcomas with efficacy in cellular adoptive therapy. J Exp Med 1991; 174:1511–15.

23. Lee T, Koo A, Peyret C, Shimabukuro T, deKernion J, Belldegrun A. The effects of interleukin-6 on tumor-infiltrating lymphocytes derived from human renal cell cancer. J Urol 1991; 145:663–7.

24. Kim T-Y, von Eschenback AC, Filaccio MD, et al. Clonal analysis of lymphocytes from tumor, peripheral blood and nontumorous kidney in primary renal cell carcinoma. Cancer Res 1990; 50:5263–8.

25. Koo A, Tso CL, Shimabukuro T, Peyret C, deKernion JB, Belldegrun A. Autologous-tumor-specific cytotoxicity of tumor infiltrating lymphocytes derived from human renal cell carcinoma. J Immunother 1991; 10:347–354.

26. Finke JN, Rayman P, Alexander J, et al. Characterization of the cytolytic activity of CD4[+] and CD8[+] tumor-infiltrating lymphocytes in human renal cell carcinoma. Cancer Res 1990; 50:2363–71.

27. Belldegrun A, Muul LM, Rosenberg AR. Interleukin-2 expanded tumor infiltrating lymphocytes in human renal cell cancer: isolation, characterization and antitumor activity. Cancer Res. 1988; 48:206–14.

28. Belldegrun A, Kasid A, Uppenkamp M, Rosenberg SA. Lymphokine mRNA profile and functional analysis of a human CD4[+] clone with unique antitumor specificity isolated from renal cell carcinoma ascitic fluid. Cancer Immunol Immunother 1990; 31:1–10.

29. Belldegrun A, Tso CL, Sakata T, et al. Characterization of tumor infiltrating lymphocytes (TIL) primed in-vivo with interferon-alpha as part of a combined immunotherapy protocol for advanced renal cell carcinoma (proceedings). Cancer Res 1991; 32:251, A1495.

30. Chandler CF, Skotzko M, Lee JD, et al. Retroviral-mediated gene transfer of interleukin-6 and interleukin-7 into human tumor infiltrating lymphocytes. Surg Forum 1991; 42:470–7.

V

Interleukin-2 and Other Cytokines

16

T Cell Growth Factors in the Treatment of Renal Cancer

Michael T. Lotze

University of Pittsburgh, Pittsburgh, Pennsylvania

I. INTRODUCTION

That T cells are central to the immune response to many murine and some human tumors is now well established (1). Regressing lesions on a variety of immunotherapy protocols demonstrate infiltrating T cells within responding lesions (2). This includes both metastatic melanoma as well as renal cell carcinoma. The rapid progress in defining the prototypic T cell growth factor, interleukin-2 (IL-2), and subsequent factors acting either alone or synergistically with IL-2 in promoting T cell growth has allowed the opportunity to test these reagents in clinical trials (3). The operational strategy employed in the development of these imunotherapies is constantly undergoing alteration as we learn more about these factors and the regulation of the immune response. Our current premise is that antigenic differences recognizable by T cells exist within tumors and that in a progressively growing tumor an inadequate host response is observed. Operationally this is defined as immunologic tolerance (4–6). We know from experimental studies in murine models that recognition and rejection of a mutagenized P815 mastocytoma can be mediated by T cell recognition of a single amino acid substitution dictated by a single base change within a variety of different genes (7). The role of therapies employing T cell growth factors is to either enhance the number and range of specificities of thymic emigrants or to break peripheral tolerance. Studies of both progressing and regressing tumors can instruct us in some of the requisite factors and cells important in an antitumor response. For example, when P815 is placed in the subconjunctival space in animals, it is rejected (8,9). This same tumor placed in the anterior chamber grows progressively. Both tumors have cytolytically specific precursor T cells and produce IL-2 upon specific stimulation. Only the regressing tumor in the subconjunctival space, however, produces IL-4. These types of studies in murine models can help us further refine our approaches to applying cytokines in the treatment of patients with cancer.

T cell precursors migrate from the bone marrow, where they are produced, to the thymus, where they undergo maturational events involving a variety of different cytokines. T cells, which are capable of binding to autologous antigens presented within the thymus, are eliminated through a process of negative selection. Those T cells with "allowed" T cell receptors emigrate from the thymus to peripheral sites. So-called naive T cells circulate until they encounter antigen. At this time they can either be tolerized (4–6) through poorly understood events or similarly expanded into mature effector cells. Although it has widely been believed that the thymus is no longer necessary after fetal and early childhood development, it is clear that thymic emigrants can be detected into adult life. Indeed, the function of the thymus may also be assumed by other sites within the host. Recently it was also suggested that thymic reentry of T cells occurs and that this is restricted to activated T cells (10). This may explain the seeming paradox that IL-7, a novel T cell growth factor, has profound effects on mature T cells and yet thus far has been found to be produced only by bone marrow and thymic stromal cells (11). The circulation of T cells is a dynamic process. At least 50% of peripheral T cells are replaced every 2–3 days (reviewed in Ref. 12). In addition to IL-1, IL-6, tumor necrosis factor (TNF), and transforming growth factor β (TGF-β) also regulate the reactivity of T cells. At least five separate factors profoundly regulate T cell growth.

The best studied factors are IL-2, IL-4, and IL-7. Only limited studies have been performed for IL-10 and IL-12, more recently described factors (13–16). Their role in the maturation of the immune response to tumors is discussed in relationship to their use in clinical trials.

II. INTERLEUKIN-2

The first studies of IL-2 were based on its ability to activate large granular lymphocytes to develop lymphokine-activated killer (LAK) activity and its ability to serve as the major T cell growth factor (12). It has been widely applied in clinical trials, and in a recent update of the National Cancer Institute (NCI) Surgery Branch experience, 1023 patients were reported to have been treated on IL-2-based regimens with an overall mortality of 1.3%. In the NCI/IL-2 Working Group, a total of 515 patients were treated on IL-2-based trials, with a 3.5% mortality. Approximately one-third of the patients required a portion of their care in the intensive care unit, predominantly because of the hemodynamic effects related to IL-2 therapy. In 60 patients with renal cell cancer treated with IL-2 alone in the NCI Surgery Branch, an 18% complete and partial response (CR and PR) rate were noted compared to a 35% partial and complete response in 72 patients receiving combinations of IL-2 and lymphokine-activated killer cells. In an as yet unreported prospective randomized trial of IL-2 compared to IL-2 and LAK in which 91 and 90 patients were treated, respectively (79 and 85 evaluable), a total of 16 PR were noted with IL-2 alone and with LAK and IL-2, a total of 24. The p2 value for this comparison was 0.098. A subsequent escalating dose protocol utilizing combinations of IL-2 and interferon-α for the treatment of patients with advanced cancer was performed in 94 patients (17). Interferon-α was administered either once or three times daily and IL-2 given three times daily as an intravenous bolus. The highest response rate (41%) overall was observed in patients receiving interferon-α at 10^6 U/m^2 intravenously three times daily and 4.5 million Cetus units/m^2 three times daily of IL-2. In renal cell carcinoma at this dose a total of 13 patients were treated, with 3 PR and 2 CR, for an overall 30% response rate. These responses tend to be less durable than those observed with IL-2 alone, and subsequent studies using lower doses of IL-2 and interferon-α have not shown substantive improvement (17). This may be because of the lower overall dosage employed. Similarly, combination of IL-2 and TNF have not appeared to be substantively better than IL-2 alone (18). Combinations of interferon-α and interferon-γ administered to patients with metastatic renal cell cancer at the University of Pittsburgh Medical Center revealed a maximum tolerated dose of 10 million U/m^2 of recombinant interferon-α given subcutaneously daily in the evening or late afternoon for 5 days at the beginning of each of 3 week cycles (19). Interferon-α was given at a maximum tolerated dose of 1000 μg/m^2 intravenously in a phase IA trial. Objective responses were observed in 8 of 30 evaluable patients. In a total of 30 patients treated in a subsequent phase IB trial (20) with doses of interferon-α ranging from 2.5 to 20 billion/U/m^2 and interferon-γ 30–1000 μg/m^2, a total of eight partial and complete responses were noted. No combinations of these agents with IL-2 have yet to be reported and represent high-priority clinical trials. They raise the possibility that sequential administration of cytokines may be important in obtaining overall responses.

Our future studies with IL-2 alone are designed to decrease toxicity and improve ease of administration.

III. INTERLEUKIN-4

We first evaluated the role of IL-4, a potent immunomodulatory agent acting on B cells, T cells, and macrophages, in a total of 48 patients in a phase I trial. Patients were administered IL-4 either once or three times daily over two weekly cycles of therapy interrupted by 10–14 days of rest. Toxicities were usually mild and observed at the highest doses administered (10–30 μg/kg three times daily). IL-4 induces a vascular leak syndrome similar to what we have previously seen with IL-2 and is associated with oliguria and rare postural hypertension. Interestingly, a remarkable sensation of nasal congestion, as well as gastritis and frank gastric ulceration, has been noted. IL-4 has a rapid clearance, with an α distribution phase of approximately 8 minutes and a β clearance phase of approximately 48 minutes (21). We treated a total of 48 patients on an escalating dose protocol of IL-2 and IL-4 given three times daily. A total of 18 patients with renal cell carcinoma were treated, with 3 partial and complete responses. The first of these (a complete response) was observed in a patient at the lowest dose administered (2 μg/kg of IL-4) given three times daily and IL-2 at 216,000 IU/kg, also given three times daily. Toxicity was similar to that observed with IL-2 alone. We believe the maximum tolerated dose of this combination is 20 μg/kg of IL-4 given three times daily and 720,000 IU/kg of IL-2. Our future studies of IL-4 involve administering gene-marked tumor-infiltrating lymphocytes (22) expanded with IL-2 and IL-4 given with combinations of these agents. In addition we are performing studies with direct IL-4 gene transfer into fibroblasts as a tumor vaccine that was suggested by studies in murine models (23–25).

IV. OTHER T CELL GROWTH FACTORS

Similarly to IL-4, IL-7 was initially identified as a factor that enhanced B cell precursor maturation (26). Cloned stromal cells produced a pre-B cell growth factor of 30,000–40,000 daltons using a precursor B cell line sensitive to its presence. Initially the murine and subsequently the human factor (27) was identified and cloned. IL-7 promotes the growth of early thymic T cells (28) as well as mitogen-stimulated peripheral T cells. In addition it induces lymphokine-activated killer cell activity alone in both mouse (29) and human (30) and synergizes with IL-2. Interestingly, IL-4 also inhibits both the IL-2- and IL-7-mediated activity in stimulating lymphokine-activated killing. Human studies of IL-7 in vivo have not yet been performed, but administration to normal mice stimulates B lymphopoiesis, peripheral lymphadenopathy, and increased numbers of CD8$^+$ and CD4$^+$ T cells in the lymph node and spleen (11). IL-7 administered alone or in combination with IL-2 and/or IL-4 may have a role in further expanding T cells in the host.

IL-10 was originally identified as a cytokine synthesis inhibitory factor as well as a T cell growth factor (31,32). It inhibits the production of interferon-γ and IL-2 by so-called TH1 cells in the mouse and appear to be a significant cell growth factor cofactor for thymocyte, spleen, and lymph node cells with IL-2, IL-4, and IL-7. In addition it was recently identified as a novel cytotoxic T cell differentiation factor (13) that appears not to have intrinsic LAK-inducing activity. Human studies have not yet been extensively reported, but less profound effects on T cell growth have been noted.

Finally, IL-12 was initially identified as a cytotoxic lymphocyte maturation factor derived from a human B lymphoblastoid cell line (14). Similar studies demonstrated that it is also a natural killer (NK) cell stimulatory factor (15) and exists as a 70 kD disulfide-linked heterodimer consisting of a 35 kD and a 40 kD chain (16). IL-12 appears to be a major inducer of interferon-γ production by T cells and NK cells. It may mediate many of its activities through induction of this important cytokine. Its precise role in regulating immune reactivity in humans remains to be determined but again, like IL-7 and IL-10, may be found to have a role, both in the early development of an immune response and in promoting the final maturation of precursor cytolytic T cells.

REFERENCES

1. Lotze MT, Finn OJ. Preface. Current paradigms in cellular immunology: Implications for immunity to cancer. In: Lotze MT, Finn OJ, eds. Cellular immunology and the immunotherapy of cancer. New York: Wiley-Liss, 1990.

2. Rubin JT, Elwood L, Rosenberg SA, Lotze MT. Immunohistochemical correlates of response to recombinant interleukin-2 based immunotherapy. Cancer Res 1989; 49:7086-92.

3. Lotze MT, Custer MC, Kawakami Y, et al. T cell growth factors and the expansion of lymphoid cells with antitumor activity in vitro and in vivo. In: Lotze MT, Finn OJ, eds. Cellular immunity and the immunotherapy of cancer. New York: Wiley-Liss, 1990.

4. Jenkins MK, Pardoll DM, Mizuguchi J, Chused, Schwartz RH. Molecular events in the induction of a nonresponsive state in interleukin-2 producing helper T-lymphocyte clones. Proc Natl Acad Sci U S A 1987; 84:5409.

5. Nossal GJV. Immunological tolerance: collaboration between antigen and lympokines. Science 1989; 245:147.

6. Dallman MJ, Shiho O, Page TH, Wood KJ, Morris PJ. Peripheral tolerance to alloantigen results from altered regulation of the interleukin 2 pathway. J Exp Med 1991; 173:79-87.

7. Lurquin C, Van Pel A, Marianne B, et al. Structure of the gene of tum transplantation antigen P91A: the mutated exon encodes a peptide recognized with L^d by cytotoxic T cells. Cell 1989; 58:293-303.

8. Ksander BR, Mammolenti MM, Streilein JW. Termination of immune privilege in the anterior chamber of the eye when tumor-infiltrating lymphocytes acquire cytolytic function. Transplantation 1991; 52:128-33.

9. Bando Y, Ksander BR, Streilein JW. Characterization of specific T helper cell activity in mice bearing alloantigenic tumors in the anterior chamber of the eye. Eur J Immunol in press.

10. Agus DB, Surh CD, Sprent J. Reentry of T cells to the adult thymus is restricted to activated T cells. J Exp Med 1991; 173:1039-46.

11. Morrissey PJ, Conlon P, Charrier K, et al. Administration of IL-7 to normal mice stimulates B-lymphophoiesis and peripheral lymphadenopathy. J Immunol 1991; 147:561-8.

12. Lotze MT. Interleukin-2 basic principals. In Devita V, Hellman S, Rosenberg SA, eds. Principles and practice of biologic therapy. Philadelphia: Lippincott, 1991; 123–41.

13. Chen W-F, Zlotnik A. IL-10: a novel cytotoxic T cell differentiation factor. J Immunol 1991; 147:528-34.

14. Stern AS, Podlaski FJ, Hulmes JD, et al. Purification to homogeneity and partial characterization of cytotoxic lymphocyte maturation factor from human B-lymphoblastoid cells. Proc Natl Acad Sci U S A 87:6808-12.

15. Chan SH, Perussia B, Gupta JW, et al. Induction of interferon γ production by natural killer cell stimulatory factor: characterization of responder cells and synergy with other inducers. J Exp Med 1991; 173:869-79.

16. Gately MK, Desal BB, Wolitzky AG, et al. Regulation of human lymphocyte proliferation by a heterodimeric cytokine, IL-12 (cytotoxic lymphocyte maturation factor). J Immunol 1991; 147:874-82.

17. Sznol M, Mier JW, Sparano J, et al. A phase I study of high-dose interleukin-2 in combination with interferon-alpha 2b. J Bio Res Mod 1990; 9:529-37.

18. Rosenberg SA. Lotze MT, Yang JC, et al. Experience with the use of high dose interleukin-2 in the treatment of 652 patients with cancer. Ann Surg 1989; 210:474-85.

19. Ernstoff MS, Nair S, Bahnson RR, et al. A phase IA trial of sequential administration recombinant DNA produced interferons: combinations rIFN gamma and rIFM alpha in patients with metastatic renal cell carcinoma. J Clin Oncol 1990; 8:1637-1649.

20. Ernstoff MS, Gooding W, Nair S, et al. A phase IB of the combination of

recombinant interferons gamma and alpha in patients with metastatic renal cell carcinoma. Cancer Res 1992; 52:851-856.

21. Custer MC, Lotze MT. A biologic assay specific for interleukin-4: rapid fluorescence assay for IL-4 detection in supernatants and serum. J Immunol Methods 1990; 128:109-17.

22. Rosenberg SA, Sebersold P, Cornetta K, et al. Gene transfer into humans: immunotherapy of patients with advanced melanoma using tumor infiltrating lymphocytes modified by retroviral gene transduction. N Engl J Med 1990; 323:570-8.

23. Oliff A, Defeo-Jones D, Boyer M, et al. Tumors secreating human TNF/cachectin induce cachexia in mice. Cell 1987; 50:555-63.

24. Tepper RI, Pattengale PK, Leder P. Murine interleukin-4 displays potent antitumor activity in vivo. Cell 1989; 57:503-12.

25. Fearon ER, Pardoll DM, Itaya T, et al. Interleukin-2 production by tumor cells bypasses T helper function in the genration of an antitumor response. Cell 1990; 60:397-403.

26. Namen AE, Lupton S, Hjerrild K, et al. Stimulation of B-cell progenitors by cloned murine interleukin-7. Nature 1988; 333:571-3.

27. Goodwin RG, Lupton S, Schmierer AN, et al. Human interleukin 7: molecular coloning and growth factor activity on human and murine B-lineage cells. Proc Natl Acad Sci U S A 1989; 86:302-6.

28. Watson JD, Morrissey PH, Namen AE, Conlon PJ, Widmer MB. Effect of IL-7 on the growth of fetal thymocytes in culture. J Immunol 1989; 143:1214-22.

29. Alderson MR, Sassenfeld HM, Widmer MB. Interleukin-7 enhances cytolytic T lymphocyte generation and induces lymphokine-activated killer cells from human peripheral blood. J Exp Med 1990; 172:577-87.

30. Stotter H, Custer MC, Bolton ES, Guedez L, Lotze MT. Interleukin-7 induces human lymphokine activated killer (LAK) cells and is regulated by interleukin-4. J Immunol 1991; 146:144-50.

31. Fiorentino DF, Bond MW, Mosmann TR. Two types of mouse T helper cell. IV: Th2 clones secrete a factor that inhibits cytokine production by Th1 clones. J Exp Med 1989; 170:2081-95.

32. MacNeil IA, Suda T, Moore KW, Mosmann TR, Zlotnik A. IL-10, a novel growth cofactor for mature and immature T cells. J Immunol 1990; 145:4167-73.

17

Overview of Interleukin-2 Trials in Patients with Renal Cell Carcinoma

Mario Sznol, Anne Thurn, and David R. Parkinson

National Cancer Institute, National Institutes of Health, Bethesda, Maryland

I. INTRODUCTION

In articles published in the *New England Journal of Medicine* in December 1985 and April 1987, Rosenberg et al. reported 4 complete and 8 partial responses in 36 patients with renal cell carcinoma (RCC) treated with a novel regimen of interleukin-2 (IL-2) and lymphokine-activated killer (LAK) cells (1,2). These data were remarkable for a variety of reasons: RCC was considered refractory to standard therapeutic agents, complete and durable responses were seen, and regression of tumor was induced by an agent that presumably activated the host immune system and had no direct antiproliferative effects. Subsequently, IL-2 has been administered in various doses and schedules, both as a single agent and combined with adoptive immunotherapy or other biologic agents to confirm and improve upon the activity first demonstrated in the National Cancer Institute (NCI) Surgery Branch trials. The results of the studies published to date and many of the unresolved issues related to IL-2 treatment of RCC are discussed in this review.

II. PATIENTS SELECTED FOR IL-2 STUDIES

Before the introduction of IL-2 into the clinic, animal tumor models in the NCI Surgery Branch showed that its efficacy was dose related and was enhanced by the adoptive transfer of LAK cells (3). Therefore, the initial clinical trials sought to give IL-2 alone or in combination with LAK at the maximum tolerated dose (MTD). The most serious common toxicities seen at the MTD were hypotension and a vascular leak syndrome (VLS), which developed in the majority of patients. IL-2 could continue to be given for a limited time despite these toxicities by administering vasopressors and supplemental oxygen in an intensive care unit or its equivalent. The hypotension and VLS, as well as the other renal, hematologic, hepatic, and gastrointestinal toxicities, were found to be rapidly reversible in most patients after IL-2 was discontinued.

During the course of these early studies, it was observed that the severe acute cardiovascular and pulmonary stresses induced by treatment posed a more serious risk for myocardial infarction or pulmonary failure in those patients with underlying coronary artery disease or pulmonary insufficiency. As a result, patients entered in most IL-2 trials, particularly those placed on aggressive regimens that produced intensive care unit (ICU)-level toxicity, were required to meet rigorous eligibility criteria. IL-2 treatment was limited to those with an Eastern Cooperative Oncology Group (ECOG) performance status (PS) of 0 or 1, normal stress treadmill examinations, forced expiratory volume in one second on pulmonary function tests greater than 70% of predicted, and normal renal, liver, and hematologic parameters. In this population, most patients had undergone previous nephrectomy and otherwise had minimal or no pretreatment with chemotherapy or other biologic or hormonal agents. The selection of patients in this manner allowed investigators to give as much IL-2 as possible for determination of the maximum therapeutic benefit while minimizing the possibility of serious permanent toxicity. When comparing the results of high-dose IL-2 to that of other cytotoxic or biologic agents, however, it is important to note that IL-2 trials contain a uniquely screened and selected population of RCC patients.

III. STUDIES OF IL-2 ALONE

The initial objective clinical responses in patients with metastatic RCC treated with IL-2 were noted in trials administering both IL-2 and LAK cells (1,2); subsequently, considerable experience has been obtained with IL-2 alone. Based on the therapeutic experiments in animal models, a three times daily intravenous (IV) bolus schedule has been the predominant regimen tested in clinical trials. The results of the major studies of high-dose intravenous bolus Cetus IL-2 (600,000–720,000 IU/kg every 8 h, days 1–5 and 11–15 or 15–19) are listed in Table 1 (4–8). Patients received a median of 15–20 doses of IL-2

Table 1 High-Dose Bolus IL-2 in Patients with RCC

Study	IL-2 supplier	Reference	Dose and schedule[a]	Patients: total no. entered (no. evaluable)	CR	PR	Response rate: (CR + PR)/N (%)	Duration (months)[b]
Rosenberg	Cetus	4	720,000 IU/kg, every 8 h, days 1–5, 11–15	54	4	8	22	CR: 34^+, 28^+, 27^+, 25^+ PR: 27^+, 27^+, 25^+, 21^+, 21^+, 19^+, 15^+, 3^+
ILWG	Cetus	5	600,000 IU/kg, every 8 h, days 1–5, 15–19	30	1	7	27	CR: 7^+ PR: 11^+, 10^+, 6^+, 4^+, 4^+, 3^+, 2
Abrams	Cetus	6	600,000 IU/kg, every 8 h, days 1–5, 12–16	16	0	0	0	
Modified Group C	Cetus	7	600,000 IU/kg, every 8 h, days 1–5, 11–15	37	1	2	8	10^+, 20^c, 5^c
Poo	Cetus	8	600,000 IU/kg, every 8 h, days 1–5, 11–15	20 (15)	0	4	27	NA

[a] Cetus IL-2 1 mg = 3 million Cetus units = 18 million International Units (IU).
[b] CR, complete response; PR, partial response; NA, not applicable.
[c] Surgical resection to NED status.

over the 3-week treatment period. In 152 evaluable patients, 6 complete and 21 partial responses were seen, for an overall response rate of 17.8%. Although the response rates were low, responses were durable in all but 1 patient listed in Table 1, with a range of 3^+–34^+ months.

Cetus Corporation has carefully analyzed a series of 166 patients treated with the every 8 h bolus IV regimen of IL-2. The data base includes almost all patients listed in Table 1, as well as patients treated in other trials, and was updated to include follow-up information for the patients past the publication date (Arthur Louie, Cetus Corporation, personal communication, 1991). In the Cetus Series, 7 complete and 21 partial responses were observed, for an overall response rate of 17%. Of the 28 responses, 18 were ongoing (measured from on-study date) at the date of last analysis, with a range of 6^+–51^+ months. Of all responding patients, 41% were projected to have response durations of 24 months or more, with a median duration of response of 20.7 months. When subset analyses were done, ECOG performance status 0 patients (n = 108) had a 21% response rate, including all the complete responses. Although 16 of 28 responding patients had disease limited to lung and/or lymph nodes and there was a trend toward a higher response rate in patients with lung-only disease, responses occurred at most sites, including recurrent renal bed masses, adrenal, and spleen. Of these patients 4% died of treatment-related toxicity, but otherwise toxicity was completely reversible in most patients. The toxicity profile was similar to that seen in patients treated with IL-2/LAK, which has been reviewed in great detail by others (9–11).

Several trials were conducted with a continuous-infusion schedule of single-agent IL-2 (Table 2) (12,13). Those trials using Cetus IL-2 were initiated primarily in Europe and used 18 million IU/m^2/day for 120 h separated by 1 week of rest (12). In the single published trial, no toxic deaths were reported and only 3% of patients developed dyspnea. Hypotension was managed by dose reduction rather than by instituting pressors, so that few patients actually required dopamine and ICU-level monitoring to continue treatment. A response rate of 19% was seen, comparable to that obtained with the every 8 h IV bolus regimen. A separate multicenter randomized trial compared Hoffmann-LaRoche IL-2 at a dose of 9 million IU/m^2/day for 96 h for 4 weeks with the same dose and schedule of IL-2 administered together with LAK cells (13). Among 24 patients in the IL-2-alone arm there was a 13% response rate, including 1 complete response in lung metastases. A more intensive continuous-infusion regimen of Hoffmann-LaRoche IL-2 alone is currently being evaluated by the Southwest Oncology Group (SWOG).

Other investigators are exploring regimens administering IL-2 by continuous infusion for 24 h once or twice weekly and have reported responses in

Table 2 Continuous-Infusion IL-2 Alone in Patients with RCC

Study	IL-2 supplier	Reference	Dose and schedule[a]	Patients: total no. entered (no. evaluable)	CR	PR	Response rate: (CR + PR)/N (%)	Duration (months)
Negrier	Cetus	12	18 MIU/m²/day, days 1–5, 11–15	42 (32)	2	4	19	Median progression-free survival > 7.8
Bajorin	Hoffmann-LaRoche	13	9 MIU/m²/day, days 1–4, × 4 weeks	24	1	2	13	CR: 16⁺

[a] Cetus IL-2 1 mg = 3 million Cetus units = 18 million International Units (IU). Hoffmann-LaRoche IL-2 units were arbitrarily converted to IU as 1 Hoffmann-LaRoche unit = 3 IU.

patients with RCC, but full phase II studies have not been completed. In the latter schedules much higher total cumulative doses of IL-2 can be administered over a short period of time without significantly increasing toxicity (14,15).

IL-2 alone has also been tested in doses and schedules designed for outpatient administration (Table 3). Bukowski et al. administered 60 MIU/m^2 (Cetus IL-2) by IV bolus three times per week to 41 evaluable patients with RCC (16). It is important to note that only 56% of the patients had undergone a previous nephrectomy and over 50% were ECOG performance status 1 or 2. Most patients were unable to tolerate the starting dose of IL-2 and required a dose reduction after a median of four doses. Nevertheless, an overall response rate of 12% was observed, including a durable complete response lasting 20$^+$ months. Among ECOG PS 0 patients the response rate was 21% (4 of 19), similar to that with the most intense IL-2 regimens, although the partial responses were of short duration. Another outpatient regimen of IL-2, in this case administered by the subcutaneous route (SC) daily for 5 days each week at a dose of 18 MIU/day, produced a 29% response rate in 21 patients (17). Although the results of the latter study are promising and suggest low-dose outpatient IL-2 may have similar efficacy to the ICU-level inpatient regimens, the study is small and requires confirmation and others have reported a high rate of neutralizing antibodies in patients receiving SC Cetus IL-2 (18).

IV. STUDIES OF IL-2 ALONE IN COMBINATION WITH LAK

The major trials of IL-2 administered in combination with LAK are listed in Table 4 (4,13,19–24). As noted, most of the early studies of IL-2 in patients with RCC included LAK because animal models predicted that adoptive transfer of LAK with IL-2 resulted in optimum antitumor activity in vivo (4). Therefore, the greatest number of RCC patients who have received IL-2, particularly at the highest dose levels, have been treated with IL-2/LAK regimens. As a result, follow-up for the purpose of determining durability of response or persistence of toxicities is longer for patients entered on IL-2/ LAK protocols than for those receiving IL-2 alone or IL-2 combined with other biologic agents.

To date, the combined response rate of published trials administering IV bolus IL-2 every 8 h with LAK is 23.5% (43 of 183, Table 4) (4,7,19,22). In these trials there were 12 (6.5%) complete responses, and the median duration of all responses was approximately 11 months. The responses of 16 of 43 patients (37%) achieving partial or complete remission and followed for

Table 3 Outpatient IL-2-Alone Studies in Patients with RCC

Study	IL-2 supplier	Reference	Dose and schedule[a]	Patients: total no. entered (no. evaluable)	CR	PR	Response rate: (CR + PR)/N (%)	Duration (months)
SWOG	Cetus	16	60 MIU/m^2, IV, 3 times per week	44 (41)	1	4	12	CR: 20$^+$ PR: 12, 4, 3, 2
Sleijfer	Cetus	17	9–18 MIU/day, SC, days 1–5 × 6 weeks	27 (21)	2	4	29	NA

[a] Cetus IL-2 1 mg = 3 million Cetus units = 18 million International Units (IU).

Table 4 Studies of IL-2/LAK in Patients with RCC

Study	IL-2 supplier	Reference	Dose and schedule[a]	Patients: total no. entered (no. evaluable)	CR	PR	Response rate: (CR + PR)/N (%)	Duration (months)
Rosenberg	Cetus	4	720,000 IU/kg, IV, every 8 h, days 1–5, 12–16	72	8	17	35	CR: 30[+], 27[+], 23[+], 15, 13, 11, 9, 6 PR: 36[+], 21[+], 19, 13, 11, 11, 9, 7, 7, 6, 6, 6, 6, 3, 2, 1, 1
ILWG	Cetus	19	600,000 IU/kg, IV, every 8 h, days 1–5, 12–16	35	2	3	14	CR: 54[+], 47[+] PR: 55[+,b], 47[+,b], 3
ILWG	Cetus	20	600,000 IU/kg, IV bolus, every 8 h, days 1–3, 18 MIU/m², CI[c], days 9–15	47	2	2	9	CR: 30[+], 21 PR: 10, 10
ILWG	Cetus	21	18 MIU/m², CI, days 1–5, 18–27 MIU/m², CI, days 11–15	25	2	2	16	CR: 37[+], 31[+] PR: 16, 7
ILWG	Cetus	22	600,000 IU/kg, IV, every 8 h, days 1–5, 11–15	46	2	7	20	CR: 19[+], 10 PR: 28[+], 25[+], 25[+], 22, 21[+], 19[+], 1

			18 MIU/m², CI, days 1–5 22.5 MIU/m², CI, days 11–15	48	2	5	15	CR: 26[+], 23[+] PR: 12, 12, 10, 6, 3
NBSG	Cetus	23	18 MIU/m², CI, days 1–5, 11–15	33	0	1	3	PR: 2
Negrier	Cetus	12	18 MIU/m²/day, CI, days 1–5, 11–15	53 (51)	5	9	27	Median progression-free survival > 7.2
Modified Group C	Cetus	7	600,000 IU/kg, IV, every 8 h, days 1–5, 11–15	32 (30)	0	4	12	PR: 28[+], 8, 3, 1[+]
Thompson	Hoffmann-LaRoche	24	18 MIU/m², CI, days 1–5 6–18 MIU/m², CI, days 12–16 or 10–19	29	4	5	31	CR: 28[+], 22[+], 11[+], 2[+] PR: 28[+], 9, 8[+], 3[+], 2[+]
Bajorin	Hoffmann-LaRoche	13	9 MIU/m², CI, days 1–4 × 4 weeks	21	1	1	10	CR: 21[+]

[a] Cetus IL-2 1 mg = 3 million Cetus units = 18 million International Units (IU). Hoffmann-LaRoche IL-2 units were arbitrarily converted to IU as 1 Hoffmann-LaRoche unit = 3 IU.
[b] Surgical resection to NED status.
[c] Continuous infusion.

179

greater than 1 year are still ongoing, with a range of $19^+–55^+$ months from entry on study.

The response rate in trials using LAK cells administered together with continuous-infusion IL-2 was 17.9% (37 of 207) (12,13,21–24). In contrast to the IV bolus studies, patients on the different continuous infusion regimens were not uniformly treated to maximum tolerance in an ICU-level setting. Complete and durable responses were observed, and in a subset of 21 responses for whom complete information on duration is currently available, 54% are projected to have progression-free intervals greater than 2 years.

V. IL-2 IN COMBINATION WITH INTERFERON-α OR INTERFERON-β

The major trials of IL-2 in combination with interferon-α or interferon-β in patients with RCC are listed in Table 5. The rationale for testing this combination extensively in patients with RCC is discussed in detail in several of the original reports. In brief, animal models demonstrated synergistic antitumor activity, and both IL-2 and the interferons have shown clinical activity as single agents in RCC.

Several doses and schedules for this combination cytokine treatment are represented in Table 5. In the most intense regimens, both IL-2 and interferon-α were administered by IV bolus every 8 h (5,25,26). Toxicity approximated that found with high-dose IL-2 alone or IL-2/LAK. In a phase I study, Rosenberg et al. reported a 31% response rate, including 4 complete responses, in 35 RCC patients (25). Based on this study, the NCI-sponsored extramural IL-2/LAK Working Group (ILWG) conducted phase II studies of IL-2 and interferon-α with and without LAK but were unable to show an improvement in antitumor activity compared with their previous and concurrent trials of similar regimens without interferon-α (5,26).

The combined response rate in three trials using more moderate, but still inpatient, doses and schedules was only 9.3% (27–29). However, response rates ranging from 17 to 32% were reported from six separate phase I or II studies in which the dose and schedule of IL-2 and interferon-α or β allowed outpatient treatment (30–35). A total of 150 patients were accrued in the latter trials, with 5 complete and 33 partial responses, for an overall response rate of 25%. Since the reports are preliminary and in some cases still have been reported only in abstract form, durability and sites of response and the demographic characteristics of the patients cannot be assessed.

Table 5 IL-2 in Combination with Interferon-α and β in RCC

Study	IL-2 supplier	Reference	Dose and schedule[a]	Patients: total no. entered (no. evaluable)	CR	PR	Response rate: (CR + PR)/N (%)	Duration (months)
Rosenberg	Hoffmann-LaRoche	25	IL-2: 3.0–13.5 MIU/m², IV, every 8 h, days 1–5, 15–19 IFN: 3–6 MU/m², IV, every 8 h, days 1–5, 15–19	35	4	7	31	CR: 14$^+$, 13$^+$, 10$^+$, 6 PR: 12$^+$, 11, 10$^+$, 8$^+$, 8$^+$, 7, 5$^+$
ILWG	Hoffmann-LaRoche	26	IL-2: 13.5 MIU/m², IV, every 8 h, days 1–5, 11–15 LAK: days 11, 12, 14 IFN: 3 MU/m², IV, every 8 h, days 1–5, 11–15	28 (24)	0	3	12.5	PR: 1, 3$^+$, 5$^+$
ILWG	Cetus	5	IL-2: 14.4 MIU/m², IV, every 8 h, days 1–5, 15–19 IFN: 3 MU/m², IV, every 8 h, days 1–5, 15–19	28	0	3	11	PR: 8$^+$, 5$^+$, 1$^+$
Lindermann	Hoffmann-LaRoche	27	IL-2: 9 MIU/m², CI, days 1–4, 15–18 IFN: 6 MU/m², SC, days 1, 4, 15, 18	40 (24)	1	0	4	CR: 7$^+$

Table 5 (Continued)

Study	IL-2 supplier	Reference	Dose and schedule[a]	Patients: total no. entered (no. evaluable)	CR	PR	Response rate: (CR + PR)/N (%)	Duration (months)
Ilson	Hoffmann-LaRoche	28	IL-2: 9 MIU/m², CI, days 1–4, 8–11, 15–18 IFN: 6 MU/m², IV, days 1–4, 8–11, 15–18	35 (32)	0	3	9	PR: 7, 5⁺, 5
NBSG	Cetus	24	IL-2: 18 MIU/m², CI, days 1–5 IFN: 3 MU/m², SC, qod	41	0	5	12	NA
Priest	Hoffmann-LaRoche	30	IL-2: 1.5–7.5 MIU/m², SC, days 1–5, 8–12, 15–19, 22–26 IFN: 2.5–12.5 MU/m², SC, 3 times/week	20	0	5	25	NA
Sznol	Hoffmann-LaRoche	31	IL-2: 4.5–9.0 MIU/m², SC, days, 1–5, 8–12, 15–19, 22–26	23	0	5	22	NA

Author		Company	Regimen					
Atzpodien	32	Cetus	IFN: 1.5–3.0 MU/m², SC, daily; IL-2: 18–27 MIU/m², SC, days 1, 2, then 3.6–4.8 MIU/m², days 1–5; IFN: 3–6, MU/m², SC, 3 times/week	34	4	6	29	19[+] in CR patients
Demchak	33	Hoffmann-LaRoche	IL-2: 6 MIU/m², IV, days 1–5; IFN: 9 MU/m², SC or IV, 3 times/week	39 (29)	0	5	17	PR: 11[+], 7[+], 5[+], 3[+], 3[+]
Figlin	34	Hoffmann-LaRoche	IL-2: 6 MIU/m², CI, days 1–4; IFN: 6 MU/m², IM or SC, days 1–4	27 (22)	0	7	32	NA
Krigel	35	Cetus	IL-2: 30 MIU/m², IV, 3 times/week; IFN-β: 6 MU/m², IV, 3 times/week	24 (22)	1	5	27	CR: 24; PR: 23[+], 24[+], 9, 5, 4

[a] Cetus IL-2 1 mg = 3 million Cetus units = 18 million International Units (IU). Hoffmann-LaRoche IL-2 units were arbitrarily converted to IU as 1 Hoffmann-LaRoche unit = 3 IU. IFN, interferon.

VI. ISSUES RELATED TO IL-2 TREATMENT

A. Dose Response of IL-2 in Patients with RCC

The outpatient studies, although small and preliminary, have produced responses in patients with RCC and thus raise an important question: are high doses of IL-2 that are associated with severe acute toxicity necessary for optimum clinical efficacy? Bradley et al. of Cetus Corporation reviewed their response data in all RCC patients treated with IL-2 and initially concluded that the activity of IL-2 was related to intensity (toxicity) of the treatment regimen, as predicted by preclinical studies (36). However, the characteristics of the patients selected for treatment in the moderate-dose or outpatient studies may have been less favorable for response than those entered to the intense, ICU-level regimens. Evidence has been presented that selection of patients may strongly influence response rates in phase II studies of RCC patients treated with biologic agents. Fisher et al., when attempting to explain the discrepancy in response rates of RCC patients to IL-2/LAK between the ILWG (16%) and the NCI Surgery Branch (33%), noted that the ILWG series contained fewer patients with disease restricted to lung or chest (19). An analysis undertaken by Cetus of all RCC patients treated with bolus IL-2 alone (see earlier) also showed that response rates are higher in patients with ECOG performance status 0 versus 1 and perhaps are higher in those patients with metastatic disease limited to the lungs.

A possible example of selection bias and differences in population of patients between primarily outpatient IL-2 studies and the ICU-level regimens can be seen in the study of Bukowski et al. conducted in the SWOG, which contained a high percentage of patients with ECOG performance status greater than 0 and who had not undergone a previous nephrectomy (16). In contrast, over 80% of patients entered to most high-dose IL-2 studies had a previous nephrectomy, and at least 60% were ECOG PS 0. To address the question of dose response to IL-2 more definitively and avert the difficulties in comparing separate phase II studies, the NCI Surgery Branch has initiated a randomized phase III trial of high-dose bolus IL-2 (720,000 IU/kg every 8 h) versus the same schedule of IL-2 at 72,000 IU/kg every 8 h. In this type of comparison, assessment of both durability of response and response rate are important in determining whether the lower doses are in fact equal in efficacy to the more toxic regimens.

B. Continuous Infusion Versus Bolus IL-2 Administration

Continuous-infusion IL-2 alone has been approved for the treatment of RCC in several European countries and remains the predominant mode of IL-2 administration there. Since the original report from West et al. describing a limited series of patients treated with continuous-infusion IL-2 and LAK cells (37), a number of investigators have proposed that continuous-infusion IL-2 has greater biologic activity and less toxicity than IL-2 administered by IV bolus every 8 h. On a unit-per-unit basis, IL-2 by continuous infusion clearly produces greater biologic effects and toxicity than IL-2 administered intermittently, such as in the every 8 h IV bolus schedule. However, the data in Tables 1, 2, and 4 suggest that IL-2 by continuous infusion, alone or with LAK cells, is not more active with regard to antitumor activity than the every 8 h IV bolus regimen.

When directly compared in a small randomized study and given to the same level of toxicity, the bolus and continuous-infusion regimens administered with LAK appeared to produce equivalent results, although the study was too small to detect anything but very large differences in response rates (22). Continuous-infusion regimens administered with less intensity and toxicity also produced rates and durability of clinical responses consistent with (but generally not greater) than the high-dose every 8 h IV bolus schedule. Although these data can be interpreted to mean that continuous-infusion regimens have greater biological activity and thus produce responses with less toxicity, the dose-response relationship for the IV bolus regimen has not been determined, and it is possible that lower, less toxic doses of IL-2 administered by IV bolus every 8 h could be equally active to the high doses currently in use. Thus, there are no convincing data that continuous-infusion IL-2 is either more active or less toxic than other schedules of administration. There is additionally some concern that continuous infusion may not be the optimal schedule of IL-2 administration to achieve best antitumor activity; when polyethylene glycol-IL-2, which has a prolonged in vivo half-life and thus mimics a continuous IL-2 infusion, is administered to tumor-bearing animals, antitumor activity is correlated with initial peak serum levels (38).

C. Contribution of LAK to the Clinical Activity of IL-2

The major IL-2/LAK trials in patients with RCC were conducted by the NCI Surgery Branch, the ILWG, and the Modified Group C centers. These same groups conducted the key trials of high-dose bolus IL-2 alone using the same dose and schedule administered in the IL-2/LAK studies. A subset of the NCI Surgery Branch RCC patients (39) and all patients entered in the Modified Group C trials were directly randomized to receive IL-2 alone versus IL-2/ LAK (Table 6) (7). Therefore, it appears reasonable to make tentative comparisons of the large IL-2-alone and IL-2/LAK data bases in which IL-2 was given by IV bolus every 8 h. The response rate to IL-2 alone (17%) is not

Table 6 Randomized Studies of IL-2 versus IL-2/LAK in RCC

Study	IL-2 supplier	Reference	Dose and schedule[a]	Patients: total no. entered (no. evaluable)	CR	PR	Response rate: (CR + PR)/N (%)
NCI Surgery Branch	Cetus	39	720,000 IU/kg, IV, every 8 h	48 (42)	3	7	24
			+ LAK				
Modified Group C	Cetus	7	600,000 IU/kg, IV, every 8 h	48 (46)	7	8	31
			+ LAK	37	1	2	8
Bajorin	Hoffmann-LaRoche	13	9 MIU/m^2, CI, days 1–4, × 4 weeks	32 (30)	0	4	13
				24	1	2	13
			+ LAK	21	1	1	10

[a] Cetus IL-2 1 mg = 3 million Cetus units = 18 million International Units (IU). Hoffmann-La Roche IL-2 units were arbitrarily converted to IU as 1 Hoffmann-La Roche unit = 3 IU.

substantially different from that seen in IL-2/LAK-treated patients (23%). For both IL-2 and IL-2/LAK responses, remissions can be quite durable, and approximately 40% of responding patients are progression-free at 2 years with a low risk of relapse subsequently. The data do not support a major contribution of LAK cells to the efficacy of high-dose bolus IL-2 in patients with RCC. A separate randomized multicenter trial of Hoffmann-LaRoche IL-2 by continuous infusion versus the same dose and schedule of IL-2 given with LAK also did not appear to show a benefit for RCC patients receiving LAK (13). Since preclinical models suggested the effect of LAK could be demonstrated best when used with lower and less toxic doses of IL-2, the lack of benefit attributed to LAK in the latter study, which used a relatively well-tolerated IL-2 dose and schedule, is particularly disappointing.

D. Contribution of Interferon-α or β to the Activity of IL-2 in Patients with RCC

The results of phase II studies adding interferon to high- and moderate-dose IL-2 regimens do not appear to show any substantial increase in activity over that expected with IL-2 alone. Although these disappointing results could be attributed to patient selection or chance, the number of patients cumulatively accrued to the IL-2/interferon-α studies has been substantial, and many of the studies were done by investigators experienced in giving similar IL-2-alone regimens.

In contrast, consistent response rates greater than 15% have been seen in outpatient IL-2/interferon-α studies. Although follow-up is short and most studies are yet to be completely documented in full articles, there is good evidence that complete and durable responses can be achieved with these regimens without the acute toxicities of the high-dose regimens. Randomized studies are required to determine if outpatient combination IL-2/interferon-α therapy is more effective than either agent administered alone at outpatient doses or whether it is equivalent to the high-dose, more toxic IL-2 regimens. Such randomized studies require large numbers of patients and may therefore be neither feasible nor of high priority, since IL-2/interferon-α response rates are still low and are unlikely to change median survival.

E. Does IL-2 Benefit Patients with RCC?

The preceding data clearly show that the response rate of high-dose IL-2 with or without LAK cells is in the range 15–20%. Even though this response rate is well below the 50% figure usually associated with a measurable increase in median survival, some investigators have considered the possibility that biologic agents may increase survival without producing objective tumor regression. Although these questions can only be answered in phase III randomized studies (which have not been done), the median survival of patients in phase II IL-2 studies generally falls in the same range as that found in similar patients treated with ineffective chemotherapeutic agents.

Since median survival of the population of patients under therapy is probably not significantly improved, on what basis can one conclude that IL-2 is beneficial to patients with RCC? IL-2 has been clearly shown to produce durable complete and partial responses in a subset of patients. Although responses may be occurring in patients who would have done well and survived longer anyway, the argument can be made that prolonged disease-free or progression-free survival induced by IL-2 represents a significant change in the clinical history of the tumor of the individual patient and is an improvement over survival with disease progression.

To gain perspective on the activity of IL-2 in patients with RCC, one must consider the natural history of the disease and also examine current treatment alternatives for these patients. Although no agent is approved by the the U.S. Food and Drug Administration for treatment of RCC, the activity of IL-2 is frequently compared to that of interferon-α, which is reported to produce similar response rates (15–20%) and can be administered with substantially less toxicity in the outpatient setting (40). Although a phase III comparison is required to determine the relative merits of the two treatments, a review of the literature suggests that interferon does not produce the frequency of complete or durable responses seen in IL-2 studies, even though overall response rates are similar. In a large series of RCC patients treated with recombinant interferon-α preparations in multiple phase II trials conducted in the United States (41–46), there were 4 complete and 30 partial responders in a cohort of 239 evaluable patients (14.2%). Follow-up was sufficient to determine response duration in four of the studies (41–44). No more than 12 of the 30 responses (40%) in this series lasted greater than 12 months, and only 6 of those 12 were still ongoing (range 12^{+}–31^{+} months). In contrast, 35–40% of responders to high-dose IL-2 or IL-2/LAK given by the every 8 h IV bolus regimen are expected to remain in remission beyond 2 years. Although clearly not definitive, these data suggest IL-2 responses may be qualitatively better. Selection of patients in these series probably does not explain the difference in durability of response, since only responders are being compared, and these patients are likely to be similar with regard to performance status and sties of disease in both the interferon and IL-2 series. However, the difference between IL-2 and interferon-α, if it exists, appears to be small, thus requiring very large (and perhaps not feasible) phase III studies to detect meaningful clinical differences.

Given the relatively low response rates observed with both agents, future resources may be better directed at improving upon this single-agent activity rather than in extensive comparison of the two alternative treatment approaches. A discussion of potential future strategies to improve upon the therapeutic ratio of IL-2 in the treatment of RCC is beyond the scope of this review. However, it is likely that greater understanding of the mechanisms responsible for mediating tumor regression in vivo will be required before true therapeutic advances are made. Currently, there is a paucity of preclinical data suggesting simple strategies to enhance the clinical activity or decrease toxicity of IL-2. Recent findings with respect to the mechanisms of hypotension following administration of TNF suggest that inhibitors of the nitric oxide pathway may decrease IL-2 toxicity (47). With regard to efficacy, preliminary animal model data with IL-6 showed this agent to have impressive antitumor activity with little toxicity and suggest combinations with IL-2 may result in additional therapeutic benefit (48).

VII. SUMMARY

A total of 26 studies of interleukin-2 in patients with renal cell carcinoma were reviewed. The criteria for inclusion in this review were as follows: the number of evaluable RCC patients treated with an IL-2-based regimen was 15 or greater, an abstract or full publication was available and published in English, the studies used Cetus or Hoffmann-LaRoche IL-2, and IL-2 was administered alone, combined with LAK cells, or combined with interferon-α or interferon-β. A total of 1041 evaluable RCC patients were treated in the 26 studies: 152 received IL-2 alone by intravenous bolus every 8 h, 183 received a similar regimen with LAK cells, 56 were given continuous-infusion IL-2 alone, 207 received continuous-infusion IL-2 with LAK cells, 47 received a hybrid regimen of bolus IL-2 priming and continuous-infusion IL-2 with LAK cells, 62 were treated on primarily outpatient IL-2-alone trials, and 334 were given various dose and schedule combinations of IL-2 and interferon-α (one study was done with interferon-β).

High-dose IL-2 given by IV bolus every 8 h produced a response rate of 17%, including complete responses in 4%. Both partial and complete responses were durable, with approximately 40% of all responders expected to maintain the response beyond 2 years. Furthermore, longer follow-up available in the IL-2/LAK data base indicates that subsequent progression is uncommon in patients continuing in remission at 2 years. The addition of LAK and/or interferon-α to high-dose IL-2 alone does not appear to enhance the activity of the every 8 h IV bolus schedule. Continuous infusion of IL-2 also does not appear to enhance activity or decrease toxicity. Subset analysis of an IL-2-alone data base performed by Cetus Corporation indicates ECOG performance status 0 patients are more likely to respond to IL-2, and a trend is present for better response rates in patients with lung-only metastatic disease. Overall mortality for patients treated with high-dose bolus IL-2 approached 4%.

In summary, IL-2 appears to benefit a small subset of RCC patients by producing durable complete or partial remissions. The issues of dose response to IL-2 alone or the contribution of interferon-α to low-dose IL-2 in the treatment of RCC has not been settled. New therapeutic approaches are needed to enhance the activity and decrease the acute toxicity of IL-2.

REFERENCES

1. Rosenberg SA, Lotze MT, Muul LM, et al. Observations on the systemic administration of autologous lymphokine-activated killer cells and recombinant interleukin-2 to patients with metastatic cancer. N Engl J Med (1985); 313:1485.
2. Rosenberg SA, Lotze MT, Muul LM, et al. A progress report on the treatment of 157 patients with advanced cancer using lymphokine-activated killer cells and interleukin-2 or high-dose interleukin-2 alone. N Engl J Med (1987); 316:889.
3. Rosenberg SA. Adoptive immunotherapy of cancer using lymphokine activated killer cells and recombinant interleukin-2. In: DeVita VT, Hellman S, Rosenberg SA, eds. Important advances in oncology. Philadelphia: Lippincott, (1986); 55–92.
4. Rosenberg SA, Lotze MT, Yang JC, et al. Experience with the use of high-dose interleukin-2 in the treatment of 652 cancer patients. Ann Surg (1989); 210:474.
5. Atkins MB, Sparano J, Fisher RI, et al. Randomized phase II trial of high dose IL-2 either alone or in combination with interferon alpha 2B in advanced renal cell carcinoma. Proc Am Soc Clin Oncol (1991); 10:166.
6. Abrams JS, Rayner AA, Wiernik PH, et al. High-dose recombinant interleukin-2 alone: a regimen with limited activity in the treatment of advanced renal cell carcinoma. J Natl Cancer Inst (1990); 82:1202.
7. McCabe MS, Stablein D, Hawkins MJ. The modified group C experience—phase III randomized trials of IL-2 vs IL-2/LAK in advanced renal cell carcinoma and advanced melanoma. Proc Am Soc Clin Oncol (1991); 10:A714.
8. Poo WJ, Fynan T, Davis C, Flynn S, Durivage H, Todd M. High-dose recombinant interleukin-2 alone in patients with metastatic renal cell carcinoma. Proc Am Soc Clin Oncol (1991); 10:A557.
9. Siegel JP, Puri RK. Interleukin-2 toxicity. J Clin Oncol 1991; 9:694.
10. Margolin KA, Raynor AA, Hawkins MJ, et al. Interleukin-2 and lymphokine-activated killer cell therapy of solid tumors: analysis of toxicity and management guidelines. J Clin Oncol 1989; 7:486.
11. Lee RE, Lotze MT, Skibber JM, et al. Cardiorespiratory effects of immunotherapy with interleukin-2. J Clin Oncol 1989; 7:7.

12. Negrier S, Philip T, Stoter G, et al. Interleukin-2 with or without LAK cells in metastatic renal cell carcinoma: a report of a European multicentre study. Eur J. Cancer Clin Oncol (1989); 25:S21.

13. Bajorin DF, Sell KW, Richards JM, et al. A randomized trial of interleukin-2 plus lymphokine-activated killer cells versus interleukin-2 alone in renal cell carcinoma. Proc Am Assoc Cancer Res (1990); 31:A1106.

14. Creekmore SP, Harris JE, Ellis TM, et al. A phase I clinical trial of recombinant interleukin-2 by periodic 24-hour intravenous infusions. J Clin Oncol (1989); 7:276.

15. Perez EA, Schudder SA, Meyers FA, Tanaka MS, Paradise C, Gandara DR. Weekly 24-hour continuous infusion interleukin-2 for metastatic melanoma and renal cell carcinoma: a phase I study. J Immunother (1991); 10:57.

16. Bukowski RM, Goodman P, Crawford ED, Sergi JS, Redman BG, Whitehead RP. Phase II trial of high-dose intermittent interleukin-2 in metastatic renal cell carcinoma: a Southwest Oncology Group study. J Natl Cancer Inst (1990); 82:143.

17. Sleijfer D, Janssen R, Willemse P, et al. Subcutaneous interleukin 2 (Cetus) in patients with metastatic renal cell cancer. Proc Am Soc Clin Oncol (1991); 10:163.

18. Whitehead RP, Ward D, Hemingway L, Hemstreet GP, Bradley E, Konrad M. Subcutaneous recombinant interleukin 2 in a dose escalating regimen in patients with metastatic renal cell adenocarcinoma. Cancer Res (1990); 50:6708.

19. Fisher RI, Coltman CA Jr, Doroshow JH, et al. Metastatic renal cancer treated with interleukin-2 and lymphokine-activated killer cells. Ann Intern Med (1988); 108:518.

20. Parkinson DR, Fisher RI, Rayner AA, et al. Therapy of renal cell carcinoma with interleukin-2 and lymphokine-activated killer cells: phase II experience with a hybrid bolus and continuous infusion interleukin-2 regimen. J Clin Oncol (1990); 8:1630.

21. Gaynor ER, Weiss GR, Margolin KA, et al. Phase I study of high-dose continuous-infusion recombinant interleukin-2 and autologous lymphokine-activated killer cells in patients with metastatic or unresectable malignant melanoma and renal cell carcinoma. J Natl Cancer Inst (1990); 82:1397.

22. Weiss GR, Margolin K, Aronson FR, et al. A randomized phase II trial of continuous infusion interleukin-2 or bolus injection IL-2 plus lymphokine-activated killer cells for advanced renal cell carcinoma. J Clin Oncol (1992); in press

23. Dillman RO, Oldham RK, Tauer KW, et al. Continuous interleukin-2 and lymphokine-activated killer cells for advanced cancer: a National Biotherapy Study Group trial. J Clin Oncol (1991); 9:1233.

24. Thompson J, Benyunes M, Benz L, Lindgren C, Fefer A. Prolonged continuous intravenous infusion interleukin-2 and lymphokine-activated killer cell therapy for renal carcinoma. Proc Am Soc Clin Oncol (1991); 10:179.

25. Rosenberg SA, Lotze MT, Yang JC, et al, Combination therapy with inter-

leukin-2 and alpha-interferon for the treatment of patients with advanced cancer. J Clin Oncol (1989); 7:1863.

26. Aronson FR, Sznol M, Atkins MB, et al. A phase II trial of interleukin-2, interferon-alpha, and lymphokine-activated killer cells for advanced renal cell carcinoma. Proc Am Soc Clin Oncol (1990); 9:183.

27. Lindermann A, Monson JRT, Staher RA, et al. Low intensity combination treatment with r-interleukin-2 and r-interferon alfa-2A in renal cell carcinoma. A multicenter phase II trial. Proc Am Soc Clin Oncol (1990); 9:150.

28. Ilson D, Motzer R, Kradin R. A phase II study of recombinant interleukin-2 and alpha interferon (Roferon) for patients with advanced renal cell carcinoma. Proc Am Assoc Cancer Res (1991); 32:1116.

29. West W, Schwartzberg L, Blumenchein G, et al. Continuous infusion inter-leukin-2 plus subcutaneous interferon alpha 2B in advanced malignancy. Proc Am Soc Clin Oncol (1990); 9:191.

30. Priest ER, Ratain MJ, Janisch L, et al. Outpatient subcutaneous interleukin-2 and interferon alfa-2A: a phase I study. Proc Am Soc Clin Oncol (1991); 10:209.

31. Sznol M, Janik JE, Sharfman WH, et al. A phase 1a/1b study of subcutaneously administered interleukin-2 in combination with interferon-alfa 2a. Proc Am Soc Clin Oncol (1991); 10:209.

32. Atzpodien J, Korfer A, Menzel T, et al. Home therapy using recombinant human IL-2 and IFN-α2B in patients withh metastatic renal cell carcinoma. Proc Am Soc Clin Oncol (1991); 10:177.

33. Demchak P, Atkins M, Sell K, et al. Phase II study of interleukin-2 and interferon alpha-2a outpatient therapy for metastatic renal cancer. Proc Am Soc Clin Oncol (1991); 10:175.

34. Figlin R, Citron M, Whitehead R, et al. Low dose continuous infusion recombi-nant human interleukin-2 and Roferon-A; an active outpatient regimen for metastatic renal cell carcinoma. Proc Am Soc Clin Oncol (1990); 8:460.

35. Krigel RL, Padavic-Shaller KA, Rudolph AR, et al. Renal cell carcinoma: treatment with recombinant interleukin-2 plus beta-interferon. J Clin Oncol (1990); 8:460.

36. Bradley EC, Louie AC, Paradise CM, et al. Antitumor response in patients with metastatic renal cell carcinoma is dependent upon regimen intensity. Proc Am Soc Clin Oncol (1989); 8:A519.

37. West WH, Tauer KW, Yannelli JR, et al. Constant-infusion recombinant inter-leukin-2 in adoptive immunotherapy of advanced cancer. N Engl J Med 1987; 316:898.

38. Zimmerman RJ, Aukerman SL, Katre NV, Winkelhake JL, Young JD. Schedule dependency of the antitumor activity and toxicity of polyethylene glycol-modified interleukin 2 in murine tumor models. Cancer Res (1989); 49:6521.

39. Linehan WM, Shipley WU, Longo DL. Cancer of the kidney and ureter. In: DeVita VT, Hellman S, Rosenberg SA, eds. Cancer: principles and practice of oncology. Philadelphia: Lippincott, (1989); 979.

40. Muss HB. Renal cell carcinoma. In: DeVita VT, Hellman S, Rosenberg SA, eds. Biologic therapy of cancer. Philadelphia: Lippincott, (1991); 298.

41. Buzaid AC, Robertone A, Kisala C, Salmon SE. Phase II study of interferon alfa-2a, recombinant (Roferon-A) in metastatic renal cell carcinoma. J Clin Oncol (1987); 5:1083.

42. Muss HB, Costanzi JJ, Leavitt R, et al. Recombinant alfa interferon in renal cell carcinoma: a randomized trial of two routes of administration. J Clin. Oncol (1987); 5:286.

43. Figlin RA, deKernion JB, Mukamel E, Palleroni AV, Itri LM, Sarna GP. Recombinant interferon alfa-2a in metastatic renal cell carcinoma: assessment of antitumor activity and anti-interferon antibody formation. J Clin Oncol (1988); 6:1604.

44. Quesada JR, Rios A, Swanson D, Trown P, Gutterman JU. Antitumor activity of recombinant-derived interferon alpha in metastatic renal cell carcinoma. J Clin Oncol (1985); 3:1522.

45. Krown SE, Einzig AI, Abramson JD, Oettgen HF. Treatment of advanced renal cell cancer with recombinant leukocyte A interferon. Proc Am Soc Clin Oncol (1983); 2:C225.

46. Einzig AI, Krown SE, Oettgen HF. Recombinant leukocyte interferon in renal cell cancer. Proc Am Soc Clin Oncol (1984); 3:C209.

47. Kilbourn RG, Gross SS, Jubran A, et al. NG-methyl-L-arginine inhibits tumor necrosis factor-induced hypotension: implications for the involvement of nitric oxide. Proc Natl Acad Sci USA (1990); 87:3629.

48. Mule JJ, McIntosh K, Jablons DM, Rosenberg SA. Antitumor activity of recombinant interleukin 6 in mice. J Exp Med (1990); 171:629.

18

Interleukin-2 as a Single Agent in Advanced Renal Cell Cancer

Janice P. Dutcher

Albert Einstein College of Medicine, Bronx, New York

I. INTRODUCTION

As stated numerous times in this book, interleukin-2 (IL-2) or T cell growth factor is an extremely potent inducer of both proliferation and enhanced activity of T lymphocytes. In addition, it is capable of activating a nonspecific cytotoxic activity, LAK (lymphokine-activated killer) activity, which along with cytotoxic T cells and natural killer (NK) cells is capable of antitumor cytotoxicity (1,2). Clinical responses of significance have also resulted from this therapy, particularly striking in renal cell cancer (3–6).

Initial studies utilized both IL-2 infusion and ex vivo activation of primed lymphocytes, attempting to expand the specific population of activated killer cells. This approach requires substantial technical expertise and materials expense and is quite time consuming and possibly more toxic to patients.

It is therefore of substantial interest to demonstrate equivalent immunologic and clinical activity of therapy with IL-2 alone. That this may be the case has been suggested by a series of clinical trials sponsored by the National Cancer Institute and by private industry. These are summarized here, and a detailed description of the experience of the IL-2 Working Group is provided.

II. INTERLEUKIN-2

IL-2 has been shown to induce activation of natural killer and LAK cells (7). This in turn induces release of secondary cytokines, which may induce some of the therapeutic and toxic effects of these biologic agents (8–10).

There continues to be debate about whether the therapeutic effects are related to the cellular activation or to the effects of the release of secondary cytokines. It likely will be found to be both. Nevertheless, as we further elucidate the mechanism, we are attempting to capitalize on the clinical benefits.

III. ANIMAL STUDIES OF IL-2

Animal studies using models for metastatic tumors have shown benefit with both IL-2 and IL-2 plus LAK cells (1,2). However, these studies demonstrated both a dose response from IL-2 and added benefit in many nonimmunogenic tumors from the addition of LAK cells. The extent of both effects is less certain in humans. Clinical trials have been based initially on these models, but now variations are being investigated. A series of human clinical trials have attempted to study IL-2 versus IL-2 plus LAK cells to assess response rate and duration and to sort out the relative benefits of the addition of LAK cells.

IV. CLINICAL RESULTS OF IL-2-ALONE THERAPY

Two studies have directly compared high-dose bolus IL-2 versus IL-2 plus LAK cells (11,12). These have shown no difference in overall or the complete response rate in patients with renal cell cancer. From the data of Rosenberg, the response duration appears to be similar in the two arms (11,12).

The initial experience of the IL-2 Working Group with high-dose IL-2 alone in renal cell cancer was negative in a small group of patients (13). Statistically, however, this is still consistent with the relatively low response rate seen with either IL-2 or IL-2 plus LAK. Thus, further exploration of IL-2 alone was undertaken.

The IL-2/LAK Cell Working Group recently performed a study again evaluating high-dose bolus IL-2 or high-dose bolus IL-2 plus interferon-α (IFN-α) in patients with metastatic renal cell cancer. The goal was to reevaluate IL-2 alone, as well as to test the hypothesis that the addition of interferon-α may upregulate HLA-DR expression among other antigens and will enhance responsiveness to IL-2 therapy. The end point was to demonstrate a twofold greater response rate among patients treated with the combination than that seen with IL-2 alone. However, this study did not demonstrate clinical synergy between IL-2 and interferon-α when given at high dose (14). Nevertheless, a substantial response rate in metastatic renal cell cancer was observed with high-dose IL-2 given without LAK cells, either with or without interferon.

To summarize this study, patients were randomized to treatment with either IL-2 (30 patients) or IL-2/IFN (28 patients). The schedule of IL-2 is as described previously, at an intravenous (IV) dose of 1.33 $\mu g/m^2$ (24 × 10^6 IU/m^2 per dose) given every 8 h on days 1–5 and 15–19 (for a maximum of 28 possible doses). A 9-day break between IL-2 cycles allows almost total recovery from the initial treatment week and provides better tolerance during the second week of treatment.

The concurrent part of the study, when either IL-2 or IL-2 plus interferon was given, was not different in types of patients entered—performance status, age, or sites of disease—yet describes equivalent response rate and survival status. Fewer doses of IL-2 were given in the combination arm.

Toxicity was as expected with IL-2 therapy, with hypotension and capillary leak syndrome occurring to a similar extent in both arms of the study. Interferon toxicity appeared to limit the number of doses of IL-2 given in this study, and fewer mean numbers of doses were given than in the IL-2-alone arm. In the IL-2 alone arm, 2 complete responsers (CR), and 5 partial responses (PR) (3 nearly CR) were seen. This was a 27% response rate, compared to 11% with IL-2/IFN-α, with which there were no complete responders. This difference was not compared, and both results are within the range of response for IL-2 in renal cell cancer. There was no doubling of response rate with IL-2 plus interferon-α. This study again demonstrated the durability of responses to IL-2 in renal cell cancer, with patients continuing to respond at 16^+, 15^+, 14^+, 13^+, 12^+, 11^+, and 4 months.

Site of metastatic disease appeared to influence response, with a 36% response rate among patients having lung-only sites of disease and 28% among those with lung, lymph node, and soft tissue involvement. The majority of responders were of performance status 0.

V. OTHER STUDIES OF HIGH-DOSE IL-2

Other studies of high-dose IL-2 in renal cell cancer, as stated, have also demonstrated response, at a rate ranging from 0 to 27%. Rosenberg et al. (11), using the same dose and schedule, saw a 22% response rate, including durable responses lasting 27^+–34^+ months. The Modified Group C experience also demonstrated responses, primarily partial, but again durable (12).

Studies at lower doses of intravenous IL-2 or as a continuous infusion have also demonstrated responses, including complete responses (15–18). The data seems to suggest that with lower doses, the degree and duration of response are less durable.

The subcutaneous route of administration may provide comparable pharmacology to higher dose studies, however, and at least one report suggests complete responses with this approach (19). The response rate in the small study of 21 patients was 29%, with 2 complete responses. Duration of response was not available from the initial report.

VI. IL-2 VERSUS OTHER PHASE II AGENTS IN RENAL CELL CANCER

The question remains whether IL-2 or IL-2/LAK therapy enhances the natural history of the disease in patients with renal cell cancer. At Albert Einstein Cancer Center, we analyzed in a nonrandomized, retrospective fashion data from concurrent phase II studies carried out in patients with renal cell cancer: one IL-2 based and one with a new chemotherapeutic agent, taxol (20). The patients entered in either study were comparable in performance status and in sites of disease and time to metastatic disease. The taxol patients did not undergo cardiopulmonary screening (treadmill or pulmonary function tests) but were otherwise similar.

These were no responses in patients treated with taxol ($n = 22$), and among the concurrent IL-2 patients ($n = 14$), there were 6 responders. Median progression-free survival is different between the two groups, with a median of 6 months for those treated with taxol and 10 months for those treated concurrently with IL-2. Median overall survival was substantially different: 8 months for patients treated with taxol and 16 months for patients treated with IL-2-based therapy (20). There were no long-term survivors among those treated with taxol, whereas durable responses (4$^+$ years) were achieved with IL-2.

VII. SUMMARY

We and others have shown that high-dose IL-2 and the combination of high-dose IL-2 plus IL-2/IFN have activity against advanced renal cell cancer.

High-dose IL-2 alone produces a response ratio of 17–25%, with 10% complete responses. Durable (greater than 1 year) responses are seen among both complete and partial responders. This is similar to the results reported with high-dose IL-2 plus LAK cells and is substantially better than previous or concurrent data from chemotherapy trials.

Patients with Eastern Cooperative Oncology Group performance status 0 (no symptoms), disease confined to lung, lymph nodes, or nonhepatic abdominal masses appears to respond best. Within these subgroups, no difference was seen among those treated with or without the renal mass in place. Thus, pretreatment nephrectomy is not a requirement of the current IL-2 Working Group study. Toxicity is manageable, with substantial recovery from IL-2 side effects occurring between cycles of IL-2.

In conclusion, we find a response rate and duration of response in renal cell carcinoma with high-dose IL-2 similar to those reported with IL-2 plus LAK cells. Thus, at this point we consider high-dose IL-2 alone to be the standard therapy for metastatic renal cell cancer to which other therapies should be compared. Attempts at reducing doses and combining other cytokines at lower doses should be compared with results with high-dose IL-2 alone.

ACKNOWLEDGMENTS

Supported in part by Cancer Center Core Grant 5P30-CA13330-20 awarded by NIH and NIH Contract NCI-CM-73705-03.

The members of the Cytokine Working Group are Albert Einstein College of Medicine, Bronx; Tufts–New England Medical Center, Boston; Loyola University, Chicago; University of Texas, San Antonio; University of California, San Francisco; and City of Hope Medical Center, Duarte.

REFERENCES

1. Mule JJ, Shu S, Schwartz SL, et al. Adoptive immunotherapy of established pulmonary metastases with LAK cells and recombinant interleukin-2. Science 1984; 225:1487.
2. La Freniere R, Rosenberg SA. Successful immunotherapy of murine experimental hepatic metastases with lymphokine-activated killer cells and recombinant interleukin-2. Cancer Res. 1985; 45:3735.
3. Rosenberg SA, Lotze, MT, Muul LM, et al. Observations on the systemic administration of autologous lymphokine-activated killer cells and recombinant interleukin-2 to patients with metastatic cancer. N Engl J Med 1985; 313:1485.
4. Rosenberg SA, Lotze MT, Muul LM, et al. A progress report on the treatment of 157 patients with advanced cancer using lymphokine-activated killer cells and interleukin-2 or high-dose interleukin-2 alone. N Engl J Med 1987; 316:889.
5. Fisher RI, Coltman, Ca, Doroshow, JH, et al. A phase II clinical trial of interleukin-2 and lymphokine activated killer cells in metastatic renal cancer. Ann Intern Med 1988; 108:518.
6. West WH, Tauer, KW, Yannelli JR, et al. Constant-infusion recombinant

interleukin-2 in adoptive immunotherapy of advanced cancer. N Engl J Med 1987; 316:898.

7. Grimm EA, Robb RJ, Roth JA, et al. Lymphokine-activated killer cell phenomenon. III. Evidence that IL-2 is sufficient for direct activation of peripheral blood lymphocytes into lymphokine-activated killer cells. J Exp Med 1983; 158:1356.

8. Numerof RP, Aronson, FR, Mier JW. IL-2 stimulates the production of IL-1α and IL-1-β by human peripheral blood mononuclear cells. J Immunol 1988; 141:4250.

9. Gemlo, BT, Palladino MA, Jr, Jaffee HS, et al. Circulating cytokines in patients with metastatic cancer treated with recombinant interleukin 2 and lymphokine-activated killer cells. Cancer Res 1988; 48:5864.

10. Mier JW, Vachino G, Van der Meer J, et al. Induction of circulating tumor necrosis factor as the mechanism for the febrile response to interleukin-2 cancer patients. J Clin Immunol 1988; 8:426.

11. Rosenberg SA, Lotze, MT, Yang JC, et al. Experience with the use of high-dose interleukin-2 in the treatment of 652 cancer patients. Ann Surg 1989; 210:474.

12. McCabe MS, Stablein, D, Hawkins, MJ. The modified group C experience— phase III randomized trials of IL2 vs IL2/LAK in advanced renal cell carcinoma and advanced melanoma. Proc Am Soc Clin Oncol 1991; 10:714.

13. Abrams, J, Rayner, AA, Wiernik, PH, et al. High-dose recombinant interleukin-2 alone: a regimen with limited activity in the treatment of advanced renal cell carcinoma. J Natl Cancer Inst 1990; 82:1202.

14. Atkins M, Sparano J, Fisher RI, et al. Randomized phase II trial of high dose IL2 either alone or in combination with interferon alpha 2B (IFN) in advanced renal cell carcinoma (RCCA). Proc Am Soc Clin Oncol 1991; 10:166.

15. Bukowski RM, Goodman P, Crawford ED, et al. Phase II trial of high-dose intermittent interleukin-2 in metastatic renal cell carcinoma: a Southwest Oncology Group study. J Natl Cancer Inst 1990; 82:142.

16. Sleijfer D, Janssen R, Willemse P, et al. Subcutaneous interleukin 2 (Cetus) in patients with metastatic renal cell cancer. Proc Am Soc Clin Oncol 1991; 10:163.

17. Negrier S, Mercatello A, Tognet E, et al. Interleukin 2 (IL2) therapy in 64 patients with metastatic renal cell carcinoma. Proc Am Soc Clin Oncol 1990; 9:196.

18. Bajorin DF, Sell KW, Richards JM, et al. A randomized trial of interleukin-2 plus lymphokine-activated killer cells versus interleukin-2 alone in renal cell carcinoma. Proc Am Assoc Cancer Res 1990; 31:1106.

19. Aztpodien J, Korfer A, Menzel T, et al. Home therapy using recombinant human IL2 and IFN-2b in patients with metastatic renal cell carcinoma. Proc Am Soc Clin Oncol 1991; 10:177.

20. Walpole E, Dutcher JP, Sparano J, et al. Survival after phase II treatment of advanced renal cell cancer with taxol or high dose interleukin 2. Proc Am Assoc Cancer Res 1991; 32:186.

19

Interleukin-2 in Patients with Metastatic Renal Cell Carcinoma

Efficacy and Tolerance to a New Schedule

D. Prapotnich

Centre Médico-Chirurgical de la Porte de Choisy, Paris, France

B. Escudier

Institut Gustave-Roussy, Villejuif, France

M. Brandely

Roussel UCLAF, Romainville, France

I. INTRODUCTION

Each year, 65 patients are surgically treated in the Urology Department of CMC de la Porte de Choisy in Paris for renal cell carcinoma, and about 20% of these have metastatic disease. Immunotherapy utilizing recombinant interleukin-2 (rIL-2) in this latter group has been investigated in collaboration with the Institut Gustave-Roussy and the Roussel UCLAF Corporation.

Since the initial report by Rosenberg et al. (1) in 1985, no significant improvement has been noted in the efficacy of rIL-2 or tolerance to this type of therapy. The use of high-dose rIL-2 alone or in combination with LAK cells in patients with metastatic renal cell carcinoma has resulted in the production of reproducible tumor responses, with response rates between 20 and 25%. Toxicity remains high, however, and limits the use of this cytokine. Thus, the goal of new clinical trials should be to improve response rate and/or to decrease toxicity. The purpose of the present report is to outline our studies utilizing a different schedule for rIL-2 administration in patients with renal carcinoma.

Our approach is based on a schedule involving administration of IL-2 for 2 days a week, using a 24 h continuous infusion of this cytokine. During the initial year of this trial, rIL-2 was given with interferon-γ (IFN-γ). IFN-γ was given subcutaneously on the same 2 days rIL-2 was administered. The use of this combination was prompted by reports of the efficacy of interferon-α (IFN-α) as a single agent (2–4) and the production of objective tumor regressions during administration of IFN-γ (5). Finally, cytokine combinations, such as rIL-2 and IFN-α, have been used with encouraging clinical results.

II. MATERIALS AND METHODS

A total of 33 patients were treated from April 1989 to May 1990. All individuals had histologically proven metastatic renal cell adenocarcinoma with measurable disease. Eligibility criteria included age < 70 years, performance status < 2 Eastern Cooperative Oncology Group, white blood count > 3000 mm^{-3}, platelet count > 100,000 mm^{-3}, serum creatinine level < 140 μmol/ liter, liver enzymes < three times institutional normal values, and absence of brain metastases, cardiac dysfunction, respiratory failure, and active systemic infection. All patients were hospitalized in an intensive care unit. Central venous catheters were inserted before starting treatment and were maintained as long as necessary for intravenous therapy. rIL-2 (Roussel UCLAF) was administered as a continuous intravenous infusion at a dose of 24 × 10^6 IU/m^2/ day for 48 h. IFN-γ was given subcutaneously at a dose of 5 × 10^6 IU/m^2 on both days. Therapy was given weekly for a total of 5 weeks.

III. RESULTS

Toxicity was tolerable, with administration of 92.5% of the planned doses possible. Hypotension occurred in 58% of the cycles, requiring pressor agents in 13%. Patients were able to leave the hospital within 2 h after completion of the rIL-2 infusion in 95% of the cycles. A total of seven patients had partial responses (PR, 21%) and then received a combination of rIL-2 and lymphokine-activated killer (LAK) cells (7): three then improved their response to complete responses (CR). Of the remaining patients, two underwent pulmonary resection of residual disease; and two remained in stable PR but with some further reduction in tumor size.

In view of the lack of significant benefit associated with IFN-γ administration, a second trial was initiated in July 1990. rIL-2 was administered at the same dose level and schedule without IFN-γ. A total of 32 patients from our institution have been entered into this study, and a multicenter study is in progress. The patient characteristics: males-females 22:10 and a mean performance status (Karnofsky) 93. Of the 32 evaluable patients, six had a partial response (19%), 11 had stable disease (34%), and 15 (47%) had progression of disease.

IV. DISCUSSION

The results of these two trials suggest that rIL-2 given on a 2 day/week schedule, alone or in association with IFN-γ, can produce responses similar to those reported by other investigators (1) who utilized different schedules with substantially more toxicity. When rIL-2 is administered as a 48 h continuous infusion on a weekly basis, the tolerance and patient acceptability are quite good, and response rates of 21 and 19% appear similar to those in other reports (1). Continued investigation of this schedule is underway in a multi-institutional trial.

REFERENCES

1. Rosenberg SA, Lotze MT, Muul LM, et al. A progress report on the treatment of 157 patients with advanced cancer using lympokine activated killer cells and interleukin-2 or high dose interleukin-2 alone. N Engl J Med 1987; 316:889–97.
2. Fossa SD, DeGaris ST, Heier MS, et al. Recombinant interferon alpha-2a with or without vinblastine in metastatic renal cell carcinoma. Cancer 1986; 57:1700-4.
3. Buzaid AC, Robertone A, Kisala C, Salmon SE. Phase II study of interferon ala-2a, recombinant (Roferon-A) in metastatic renal cell carcinoma. J Clin Oncol 1987; 5:1083-9.
4. Bergerat JP, Herbrecht R, Dufour P, et al. Combination of recombinant interferon alpha-2a and vinblastine in advanced renal cell cancer. Cancer 1988; 62:2320-4.
5. Garnick MV, Reich SD, Maxwell B, et al. Phase I/II study of recombinant interferon gamma in advanced renal cell carcinoma. J Urol 1988; 139(2):251-5.
6. Atzpodien J, Korfer A, Franks CR, et al. Home therapy with recombinant IL-2 and recombinant interferon alpha 2b in advanced human malignancies. Lancet 1990; 335:1509-12.
7. Escudier B, Farace F, Charpentier F, et al. New approaches in interleukin-2 (IL-2) therapy for metastatic renal cell carcinoma. Proc Am Assoc Cancer Res 1990; (275): A1631.

20

Pharmacology of Recombinant Human Interleukin-6

Richard D. Huhn

Robert Wood Johnson Medical School, New Brunswick, New Jersey

Daniel Levitt

Sandoz Pharmaceutical Corporation, East Hanover, New Jersey

I. INTRODUCTION

Interleukin-6 (IL-6) is an endogenous 20–25 kD phosphoglycoprotein cytokine involved in many aspects of host defense mechanisms. IL-6 was identified independently by several investigators on the basis of its activities in widely different bioassays. Among other identities, IL-6 has previously been termed T cell replacement factor, B cell stimulatory factor 2, hybridoma growth factor, hepatocyte stimulatory factor, interferon-β_2 and monocyte-granulocyte inducer 2 (1–8). In addition, it was identified as a novel human growth factor for murine hematopoietic cells (9). The genetic sequences for these various protein factors were found to be identical, leading to the international nomenclature designation IL-6 (10). Biologic and clinical features of IL-6 have recently been reviewed (11,12). This review focuses on the preclinical pharmacology of IL-6 that forms the foundation for the potential therapeutic applications of recombinant human IL-6 (rhIL-6).

II. PHARMACOLOGY IN VITRO

A. Hematopoiesis

As shown by murine and human blast cell colony assays, IL-6 synergizes with IL-3 in the recruitment of quiescent hematopoietic stem cells (13,14). In addition, IL-6 and IL-3 together support the proliferation and differentiation of multilineage and early committed hematopoietic progenitor cells (15–17). In bone marrow culture systems, IL-6 interacts with other hematopoietic growth factors, such as granulocyte-macrophage colony-stimulating factor (GM-CSF), macrophage CSF (M-CSF), and IL-4, to support the formation of several lineages of blood cell colonies (18–20). Although combinations of IL-6 with other colony-stimulating factors synergize to support the formation of megakaryocyte colonies in vitro, IL-6 appears to have minimal activity on the proliferation of megakaryocyte progenitors by itself (21). On the other hand, IL-6 clearly influences megakaryocyte maturation in vitro and in vivo, as assessed by megakaryocyte size, nuclear ploidy, and several other parameters (22–26). IL-6 may directly affect platelet formation by megakaryocytes, but the cellular mechanisms of IL-6 action on megakaryocyte morphology and subcellular structures are not well understood.

B. Immune Regulation

IL-6 stimulates the proliferation of B lymphocytes and is essential for their terminal differentiation and immunoglobulin production (2,27). Furthermore, IL-6 enhances secondary antigen-specific antibody responses in vitro and in vivo (28,29). The responsiveness of peripheral blood T lymphocytes and mature thymocytes to IL-2 are enhanced by IL-6; this effect is synergistically increased by IL-1 (30,31). IL-6 is also involved in the activation of cytotoxic T lymphocytes and stimulates the cytotoxic potential of peripheral blood natural killer cells against heterologous cellular targets (32–34).

C. Expression of Acute-Phase Proteins

IL-6 regulates expression and secretion of several acute-phase serum proteins by hepatocytes in culture (35,36). Prominent increases are observed in C-reactive protein, α_2-macroglobulin (rodents), and serum amyloid A protein expression and secretion. Increases are also observed in the expression of fibrinogen, haptoglobin, ceruloplasmin, and α_1-antitrypsin, along with decreases in the production of albumin and transferrin.

D. Effects on Endocrine Tissues and Bone and Mineral Metabolism

IL-6 stimulates the secretion of glucocorticoids by adrenal cortical cells, both by itself and in synergy with adrenocorticotropic hormone (ACTH) (37). In addition, IL-6 induces ACTH secretion by pituitary cells, which may enhance its action on adrenal glucocorticoid secretion (38,39). IL-6 may also inhibit insulin secretion by pancreatic β cells; the potential biologic or clinical significance of this effect is unclear (40). Data on possible effects of IL-6 on osteoclast activity and bone and mineral metabolism conflict: some reports suggest that IL-6 may stimulate osteoclast activity and calcium mobilization; other reports refute effects on osteoclasts (41–43).

E. Growth and Differentiation of Primary Cells and Transformed Cell Lines in Culture

IL-6 is identical to MGI-2A, a factor identified by Sachs and coworkers that acts as a differentiation factor for normal and leukemic myeloid cells (8). IL-6 by itself may induce the differentiation of myeloid and monocytic cell lines in vitro (44,45). Although enhanced proliferation of CD34$^+$ cells from patients with myeloid leukemias has been observed in cultures containing combinations of IL-6 with IL-3 or IL-4, combinations of IL-6 with other cytokines, such as granulocyte CSF or IL-1, have induced the differentiation and suppressed the self-renewal of leukemic progenitors (46–50). Thus, the effects of IL-6 on myeloid leukemia cells are variable and may depend in part on culture conditions. IL-6 also supports the proliferation of myeloma and lymphoma cell lines in vitro; whether primary human myeloma cells are stimulated in controversial, however (51–53). The effects of IL-6 on growth and differentiation of cells derived from solid tumors are not well established. IL-6 may effect the differentiation of breast carcinoma cell lines in vitro (54). One report indicated that IL-6 may be an autocrine growth factor for renal cell carcinoma cells (55). For the most part, however, IL-6 has shown little effect on the growth of human solid tumor cell lines, including renal carcinoma (56).

III. PHARMACOLOGY IN VIVO

A. Hematopoiesis in Rodents and Nonhuman Primates

rhIL-6 prominently elevates circulating platelet counts in mice, rats, and monkeys (26, 57–59). In one study, rhIL-6 administered to normal cy-

nomolgus monkeys at dosages of 5–80 μg/kg/day by twice daily subcutaneous injection resulted in 2- to 3-fold dose-dependent elevations of
platelet counts (59). This effect peaked by treatment day 8 and persisted for
approximately 1 week beyond discontinuation of treatment. rhIL-6 administered to rhesus monkeys at dosages of 3, 10, and 30 μg/kg/day by twice daily
subcutaneous injection for 8 or 11 days resulted in platelet count increases of
2- to 2.5-fold above baseline (Fig. 1) (26,60). The thrombopoietic effects of
rhIL-6 have been associated with increases in parameters of megakaryocyte
maturation and platelet production in both rodent and primate studies
(22,26,61,62). Specifically, megakaryocyte size and nuclear ploidy (DNA
content), expression of maturation markers, glycoprotein II_b/III_a, and
acetylcholinesterase by megakaryocytes (MK), and incorporation of amino
acids into platelet proteins were increased.

In addition to its thrombopoietic effects, rhIL-6 induces elevations of total
leukocyte counts, comprised predominantly of neutrophils and monocytes.
Mild decreases in hemoglobin concentrations and peripheral lymphocyte
counts have also been observed during treatment with rhIL-6 (26,58–60). In
rhesus monkeys, rhIL-6 induced modest increases in circulating hematopoietic progenitor cells, reflected by assays of mixed-cell colony-forming units
(granulocytes, erythrocytes, and monocytes-macrophages—also known as
CFU-GEMM) and megakaryocyte burst-forming units (BFU-MK) (63). In

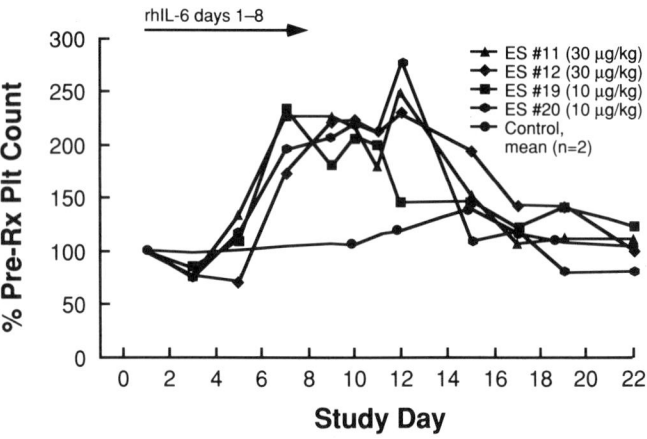

Figure 1 The effect of rhIL-6 on rhesus platelet counts. Adult rhesus monkeys
(two in each group) received either 10 or 30 μg/kg/day of rhIL-6 (SDZ ILS 969) or
control vehicle by twice daily subcutaneous injection on days 1–8. Platelet counts are
expressed as a percentage of pretreatment values. (Adapted from Ref. 63.)

murine models, the hematopoietic activity of rhIL-6 has promoted accelerated hematologic recovery following radiation-induced myelosuppression and bone marrow transplantation (64,65).

B. Acute-Phase Response

rhIL-6 induces prominent changes in serum proteins in rodents, rabbits, and monkeys that are consistent with its activities in vitro on hepatocytes (35,60,66). In rodents, dose-dependent increases in the hepatic expression of mRNA for fibrinogen, α_2-macroglobulin, cysteine proteinase inhibitor, haptoglobin, ceruloplasmin, thiostatin, and α_1-acid glycoprotein were observed following single intraperitoneal injections of IL-6. Concomitant increases in respective serum proteins were also observed. In monkeys in response to rhIL-6, there were dose-related increases in C-reactive protein, α_1-acid glycoprotein, and α_1-antitrypsin, as well as simultaneous decreases in serum albumin, prealbumin, and total cholesterol (Fig. 2).

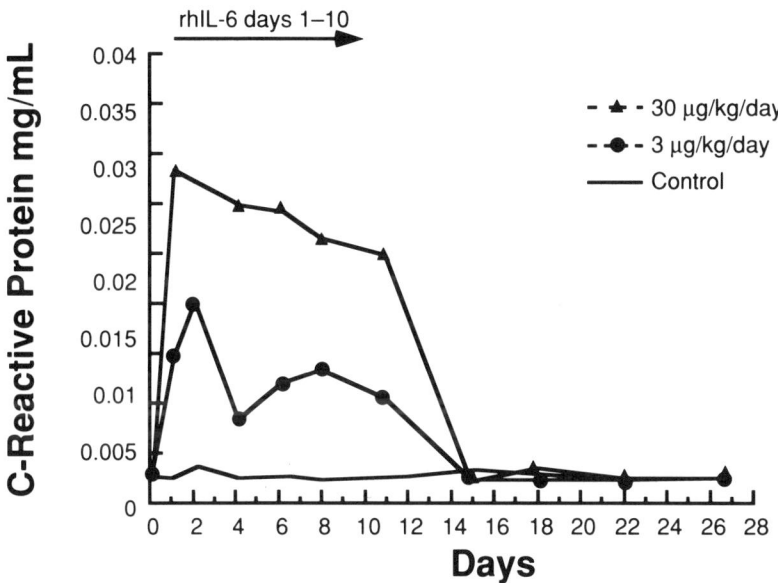

Figure 2 Elevation of C-reactive protein levels in rhesus monkey serum by rhIL-6 treatment. Rhesus monkeys (two in each group) were treated with 3 or 30 μg/kg/day of rhIL-6 or control vehicle by twice daily subcutaneous injection for 11 days. Serum C-reactive protein levels are shown (means of two subjects each). (Adapted from Ref. 60.)

C. Enhanced Resistance to Infection in Myelosuppressed Mice

SDZ ILS 969 (rhIL-6), either alone or in combination with recombinant murine GM-CSF, had a protective effect against bacterial infections in myelosuppressed mice (67). In these experiments, 100% of mice infected with *Escherichia coli* on day 4 following injection of 200 mg/kg of cyclophosphamide died by day 6. Daily administration of recombinant murine GM-CSF (rmGM-CSF), 5 µg/day beginning 24 h following cyclophosphamide, afforded protection to 20% of mice against a lethal intravenous inoculum of *E. coli*. Mice treated with rhIL-6 (5 µg/day) obtained 50% protection. The combination of rmGM-CSF with rhIL-6 resulted in 90% protection against the infection (Fig. 3). Similar protection was also observed against experimental infections with *Pseudononas aeruginosa* and *Staphylococcus aureus*.

D. Antitumor Activity

The effects of interleukin-6 on the development of experimental pulmonary or hepatic metastases were examined in mice receiving inocula of syngeneic

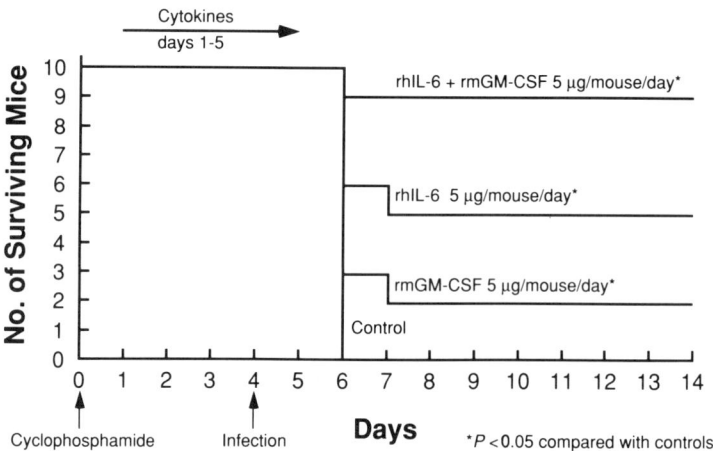

Figure 3 Effect of rhIL-6 and rmGM-CSF on the survival of neutropenic mice lethally infected with *E. coli*. On day 0, groups of 10 mice received SC cyclophosphamide at 200 mg/kg. Daily treatment with indicated doses of rhIL-6 and/or rhGM-CSF began on day 1 and was continued through day 4. On day 4, mice were infected with $1.2 \times LD_{95}$ (95% lethal dose) of *E. coli* by tail vein injection. Deaths were recorded daily. (Adapted from Ref. 67.)

methylcholanthrene-induced sarcoma cells (68). In each group six mice received tumor cells by injections into the tail vein or splenic vein on day 0. On days 3–7, the mice received rhIL-6 at various doses or control vehicle by three daily intraperitoneal injections. At rhIL-6 dosages of 10 μg per injection or greater, dramatic reductions in the number of metastases were observed at necropsy on day 14. Notably, the mice tolerated the interleukin-6 without signs of overt toxicity. In parallel experiments, rhIL-2 was administered by identical schedule to similarly prepared animals. rhIL-2 was less effective in reducing both pulmonary and hepatic metastases and caused a high frequency of toxic effects and therapy-related deaths. The effects of IL-6 and IL-2 against immunogenic tumors are thought to be mediated by the enhancement of host defenses, since total-body irradiation abrogated the antitumor activity.

Although IL-6 had a significant effect on reducing the number of metastases in mice in the 3 day experimental model, it did not significantly alter the survival of mice when administered 10 days after injection of tumor cells. However, a single 200 mg/kg dose of cyclophosphamide on day 10 after the inoculation of tumor cells, followed by rhIL-6, 100 μg three times per day for 15 doses, dramatically increased the long-term survival of mice bearing 10-day metastases of MCA-203 sarcoma (Fig. 4) (70).

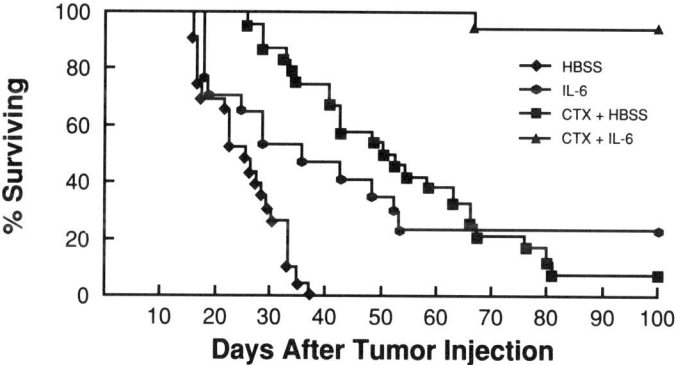

Figure 4 Effect of rhIL-6 and cyclophosphamide on the survival of mice bearing 10-day MCA-203 pulmonary metastases. On day 10 after inoculation of MCA-203 sarcoma cells, mice received 200 mg/kg of cyclophosphamide or control vehicle (Hanks' balanced salt solution) followed by 100 μg SC rhIL-6 or vehicle three times per day (15 doses). The pooled survival results of four experiments are shown. (From Ref. 70.)

In other experiments the effects of rhIL-6 on the growth of human mammary tumors in athymic mice were examined (69). On day 0, tumor cells of the human mammary carcinoma cell line MDA468 were injected subcutaneously into the flanks of athymic mice. From day 30 to day 40 following tumor cell inoculation, rhIL-6 or lipopolysaccharide (positive control) was administered by twice daily subcutaneous injection. Tumors on day 72 were 21–33% smaller in diameter in mice treated with 1 or 5 μg/day of rhIL-6 than in control mice.

IV. POTENTIAL THERAPEUTIC USES OF rhIL-6

A. Multilineage Hematopoiesis and Thrombopoiesis

The hematopoietic activities observed in vitro and in vivo (in both rodents and primates) may contribute to hematologic recovery following myelosuppressive antineoplastic chemotherapy and bone marrow transplantation (BMT) and enhanced hematopoiesis in congenital and acquired bone marrow failure. The thrombopoietic effect of rhIL-6 may help circumvent the persistent thrombocytopenia resulting from certain chemotherapeutic regimens and autologous BMT and potentially complement the myelopoietic effect of other hematopoietic growth factors in these clinical situations.

B. Host Defense Enhancement and Immunologic Regulation

rhIL-6 has effects related to host defense enhancement and immunologic regulation in vivo. These activities may be associated with protection against Gram-negative and Gram-positive infections in the setting of myelosuppression and thereby contribute to reducing morbidity and mortality following myelosuppressive antineoplastic chemotherapy and bone marrow transplantation.

C. Antitumor Activites

rhIL-6 has antineoplastic activities that are probably related to its effects on immune regulation and host defense mechanisms. On the basis of the antitumor activities observed in vitro and in vivo, rhIL-6 may have potential clinical antitumor activity in several neoplastic diseases.

REFERENCES

1. Kishimoto T, Ishizaka K. Regulation of antibody response in vitro. VII. Enhancing soluble factors for IgG and IgE antibody response. J Immunol 1973; 111:1194.

2. Hirano T, Yasukawa K, Harada H, et al. Complementary DNA for a novel human interleukin (BSDF-2) that induces B lymphocytes to produce immunoglobulin. Nature 1986; 324:73.

3. Van Damme J, Cayphas S, Van Snick J, et al. Purification and characterization of human fibroblast-derived hybridoma growth factor identical to T-cell-derived B-cell stimulatory factor-2 (interleukin-6). Euro J Biochem 1987; 168:543.

4. Simpson RJ, Moritz RL, Rubira MR, Van Snick J. Murine hybridoma/plasmacytoma growth factor. Complete amino-acid sequence and relation to human interleukin-6. Eur J Biochem 1988; 176:187.

5. Gauldie J, Richards C, Harnish D, Lansdorp P, and Baumann H. Interferon β_2/B-cell stimulatory factor type 2 shares identity with monocyte-derived hepatocyte-stimulating factor and regulates the major acute phase protein response in liver cells. Proc Natl Acad Sci U S A 1987; 84:7251.

6. Zilberstein A, Ruggieri R, Korn JH, Revel M. Structure and expression of cDNA and genes for human interferon-beta-2, a distinct species inducible by growth-stimulatory cytokines. EMBO J 1986; 5:2529.

7. Sehgal PB, May LT. Human interferon-β_2. J Interferon Res 1987; 7:521.

8. Shabo Y, Lotem J, Rubinstein M, et al. The myeloid blood cell differentiation-inducing protein MGI-2A is interleukin-6. Blood 1988; 72:2070.

9. Wong GG, Witek-Giannotti JS, Temple PA, et al. Stimulation of murine hemopoietic colony formation by human IL-6. J Immunol 1988; 140:3040.

10. Paul WE, Laughlin CA, Johnston MI. Report of nomenclature discussion. Ann N Y Acad Sci 1989; 557:579.

11. Hirano T, Akira S, Taga T, Kishimoto T. Biological and clinical aspects of interleukin 6. Immunol Today 1990; 11:443.

12. Van Snick J. Interleukin-6: an overview. Annu Rev Immunol 1990; 8:253.

13. Ikebuchi K, Wong GG, Clark SC, Ihle JN, Hirai Y, Ogawa M. Interleukin 6 enhancement of interleukin 3-dependent proliferation of multipotential hemopoietic progenitors. Proc Natl Acad Sci U S A 1987; 84:9035.

14. Leary AG, Ikebuchi K, Hirai Y, et al. Synergism between interleukin-6 and interleukin-3 in supporting proliferation of human hematopoietic stem cells: comparison with interleukin 1a. Blood 1988; 71:1759.

15. Suda T, Yamaguchi Y, Suda J, Miura Y, Okano A, Akiyama Y. Effect of interleukin-6 (IL-6) on the differentiation and proliferation of murine and human hemopoietic progenitors. Expo Hematol 1988; 16:891.

16. Koike K, Nakahata T, Takagi M, et al. Synergism of BSF-2/interleukin-6 and interleukin-3 on development of multipotential hemopoietic progenitors in serum-free culture. J Exp Med 1988; 168:879.

17. Okano A, Suzuki C, Takatsuki F, et al. In vitro expansion of the murine pluripotent hemopoietic stem cell population in response to interleukin-3 and interleukin-6. Transplantation 1989; 48:495.

18. Caracciolo D, Clark SC, Rovera G. Human interleukin-6 supports granulocytic differentiation of hematopoietic cells and acts synergistically with GM-CSF. Blood 1989; 73:666.

19. Rennick D, Jackson J, Yang G, Wideman J, Lee F, Hudak S. Interleukin-6 interacts with interleukin-4 and other hematopoietic growth factors to selectively enhance the growth of megakaryocytic, erythroid, myeloid, and multipotential progenitor cells. Blood 1989; 73:1828.

20. Bot FJ, van Eijk L, Broeders L, Aarden LA, Löwenberg B. Interleukin-6 synergizes with M-CSF in the formation of macrophage coloniues from purified human marrow progenitor cells. Blood 1989; 73:435.

21. Bruno E, Hoffman R. Effect of interleukin-6 on in vitro human megakaryocytopoiesis: its interaction with other cytokines. Exp Hematol 1989; 17:1038.

22. Ishibashi T, Kimura H, Uchida T, Kariyone S, Friese P, Burstein SA. Human interleukin-6 is a direct promoter of maturation of megakaryocytes in vitro. Proc Natl Acad Sci U S A 1989; 86:5953.

23. Navarro S, Debili N, Le Couedic J-P, et al. Interleukin-6 and its receptor are expressed by human megakaryocytes: in vitro effects on proliferation and endoreduplication. Blood 1991; 77:461.

24. Lotem J, Shabo Y, Sachs L. Regulation of megakaryocyte development by interleukin-6. Blood 1989; 74:1545.

25. Mei R-L, Burstein SA. Megakaryocytic maturation in murine long-term bone marrow culture: role of interleukin-6. Blood 1991; 78:1438.

26. Stahl CP, Zucker-Franklin D, Evatt BL, Winton EF. Effect of human interleukin-6 on megakaryocyte development and throbocytopoiesis in primates. Blood 1991; 78:1467.

27. Kishimoto T, Hirano T. Molecular regulation of B lymphocyte response. Annu Rev Immunol 1988; 6:485.

28. Takatsuki F, Okano A, Suzuki C, et al. Human recombinant IL-6/B cell stimulatory factor 2 augments murine antigen-specific antibody responses in vitro and in vivo. J Immunol 1988; 141:3072.

29. Takatsuki F, Okano A, Suzuki C, et al. Interleukin-6 perfusion stimulates reconstitution of the immune and hematopoietic systems after 5-fluorouracil treatment. Cancer Res 1990; 50:2885.

30. Lotz M, Jirik F, Kabouridis P, et al. B cell stimulating factor 2/interleukin 6 is a costimulant for human thymocytes and T lymphocytes. J Exp Med 1988; 167:1253.

31. Le J, Fredrickson G, Pollack M, Vilcek J. Activation of thymocytes and T cells by interleukin-6. Ann N Y Acad Sci 1989; 557:445.

32. Takai Y, Wong GG, Clark SC, Burakoff SJ, Herrmann SH. B cell stimulatory

factor-2 is involved in the differentiation of cytotoxic T lymphocytes. J Immunol 1988; 140:508.

33. Luger TA, Krutmann J, Kirnbauer R, et al. IFN-β_2/IL-6 augments the activity of human natural killer cells. J Immunol 1989; 143:1206.

34. Smyth MJ, Ortaldo JR. Comparison of the effect of IL-2 and IL-6 on the lytic activity of purified human peripheral blood large granular lymphocytes. J Immunol 1991; 146:1380.

35. Heinrich PC, Castell JV, Andus T. Interleukin-6 and the acute phase response. Biochem J 1990; 265:621.

36. Sehgal PB, Grieninger G, Tosato G, eds. Regulation of the acute phase and immune responses: interleukin-6. New York: Academy of Sciences, 1989.

37. Salas MA, Evans SW, Levell MJ, Whicher JT. Interleukin-6 and ACTH act synergistically to stimulate the release of corticosterone from adrenal gland cells. Clin Exp Immunol 1990; 79:470.

38. Naitoh Y, Fukata J, Tominaga T, et al. Interleukin-6 stimulates the secretion of adrenocorticotropic hormone in conscious, freely-moving rats. Biochem Biophys Res Commun 1988; 155:1459.

39. Perlstein RS, Mougey EH, Jackson WE, Neta R. Interleukin-1 and interleukin-6 act synergistically to stimulate the release of adrenocorticotropic hormone in vivo. Lymphokine Res 1991; 10:141.

40. Sandler S, Bendtzen K, Eizirik DL, Welsh M. Interleukin-6 affects insulin secretion and glucose metabolism of rat pancreatic islets in vitro. Endocrinology 1990; 126:1288.

41. Ishimi Y, Miyaura C, Jin CH, et al. IL-6 is produced by osteoblasts and induces bone resorption. J Immunol 1990; 145:3297.

42. Black K, Garrett IR, Mundy GR. Chinese hamster ovarian cells transfected with the murine interleukin-6 gene cause hypercalcemia as well as cachexia, leukocytosis and thrombocytosis in tumor-bearing nude mice. Endocrinology 1991; 128:2657.

43. Barton BE, Mayer R. IL 3 and IL 6 do not induce bone resorption in vitro. Cytokine 1990; 2:217.

44. Chen L, Novick D, Rubinstein M, Revel M. Recombinant interferon-$\beta2$ (interleukin-6) induces myeloid differentiation. FEBS Lett 1988; 239:299.

45. Miyaura C, Onozaki K, Akiyama Y, et al. Recombinant human interleukin 6 (B-cell stimulatory factor 2) is a potent inducer of differentiation of mouse myeloid leukemia cells (M1). FEBS Lett 1988; 234:17.

46. Akashi K, Harada M, Shibuya T, et al. Effects of interleukin-4 and interleukin-6 on the proliferation of CD34$^+$ and CD34$^-$ blasts from acute myelogenous leukemia. Blood 1991; 78:197.

47. Hoang T, Haman A, Goncalves O, Wong GG, Clark SC. Interleukin-6 enhances growth factor-dependent proliferation of the blast cells of acute myeloblastic leukemia. Blood 1988; 72:823.

48. Carlo-Stella C, Mangoni L, Almici C, Frassoni F, Fiers W, Rizzoli V. Growth

of CD34$^+$ acute myeloblastic leukemia colony-forming cells in response to recombinant hematopoietic growth factors. Leukemia 1990; 4:561.

49. Onozaki K, Akiyama Y, Okano A, et al. Synergistic regulatory effects of interleukin-6 and interleukin-1 on the growth and differentiation of human and house myeloid leukemia cell lines. Cancer Res 1989; 49:3602.

50. Metcalf D. Actions and interactions of G-CSF, LIF, and IL-6 on normal and leukemic murine cells. Leukemia 1989; 3:349.

51. Nilsson K, Jernberg H, Pettersson M. IL-6 as a growth factor for human multiple myeloma cells—a short overview. Curr Top Microbiol Immunol 1990; 166:3.

52. Anderson KC, Jones RM, Moromoto C, Leavitt P, Barut BA. Response patterns of purified myeloma cells to hematopoietic growth factors. Blood 1989; 73:1915.

53. Borinaga AM, Millar BC, Bell JB, et al. Interleukin-6 is a cofactor for the growth of myeloid cells from human bone marrow aspirates but does not affect the clonogenicity of myeloma cells in vitro. Br J Haematol 1990; 76:476.

54. Chen L, Mory Y, Zilberstein A, Revel M. Growth inhibition of human breast carcinoma and leukemia/lymphoma cell lines by recombinant interferon-β_2. Proc Natl Acad Sci U S A 1988; 85:8037.

55. Miki S, Iwano M, Miki Y, et al. Interleukin-6 (IL-6) functions as an in vitro autocrine factor in renal cell carcinomas. FEBS Lett 1989; 250:607.

56. Serve H, Steinhauser G, Oberberg D, Flegel WA, Northoff H, Berdel W. Studies on the interaction between interleukin-6 and human malignant non-hematopoietic cell lines. Cancer Res 1991; 51:3862.

57. Ishibashi T, Kimura H, Shikama Y, et al. Interleukin-6 is a potent thrombopoietic factor in vivo in mice. Blood 1989; 74:1241.

58. Ulich TR, del Castillo J, Guo K. In vivo hematologic effects of recombinant interleukin-6 on hematopoiesis and circulating numbers of RBCs and WBCs. Blood 1989; 73:108.

59. Asano S, Okano A, Ozawa K, et al. In vivo effects of recombinant human interleukin-6 in primates: stimulated production of platelets. Blood 1990; 75:1602.

60. Mayer P, Geissler K, Valent P, Ceska M, Bettelheim P, Liehl E. Recombinant human interleukin 6 is a potent inducer of the acute phase response and elevates the blood platelets in nonhuman primates. Exp Hematol 1991; 19:688.

61. Carrington PA, Hill RJ, Stenberg PE, et al. Multiple in vivo effects of interleukin-3 and interleukin-6 on murine megakaryocytopoiesis. Blood 1991; 77:34.

62. Hill RJ, Warren MK, Levin J. Stimulation of thrombopoiesis in mice by human recombinant interleukin 6. J Clin Invest 1990; 85:1242.

63. Winton EF. Preclinical studies with recombinant human interleukin-6. 1991. (Unpublished.)

64. Patchen ML, MacVittie TJ, Williams JL, Schwartz GN, Souza LM. Administration of interleukin-6 stimulates multilineage hematopoiesis and accelerates recovery from radiation-induced hematopoietic depression. Blood 1991; 77:472.

65. Okano A, Suzuki C, Takatsuki F, et al. Effects of interleukin-6 on hematopoiesis in bone marrow-transplanted mice. Transplantation 1991; 47:738.
66. Sakata Y, Morimoto A, Long NC, Murakami N. Fever and acute-phase response induced in rabbits by intravenous and intracerebroventricular injection of interleukin-6. Cytokine 1991; 3:199.
67. Mayer P. Enhanced resistance of combined treatment with rmGM-CSF and rhIL-6 in comparison to treatment with each cytokine alone on experimentally induced infections in myelosuppressed mice. Sandoz Forschungsinstitut study report, 1990.
68. Mulé JJ, McIntosh JK, Jablons DM, Rosenberg SA. Antitumor activity of recombinant interleukin 6 in mice. J Expo Med 1990; 171:629.
69. Jeney NV, Helm A. Therapeutic effect of rhIL-6 on the subcutaneous growth of the human mammary carcinoma cell line MDA-MB-468 in athymic nude mice. Sandoz Forschungsinstitut study report, 1989.
70. Mulé, JJ, Custer MC, Travis, WD, Rosenberg, SA. Cellular mechanisms of the antitumor activity of recombinant IL-6 in mice. J Immunol 1992; 148: 2622–2629.

21

Immunologic Effects and Antimetastatic Activity of Recombinant Human Interleukin-7 in Mice

Robert H. Wiltrout and Kristin L. Komschlies

National Cancer Institute–Frederick Cancer Research and Development Center, National Institutes of Health, Frederick, Maryland

Connie R. Faltynek

Sterling Winthrop Pharmaceuticals Division, Malvern, Pennsylvania

Giovanna Damia

Mario Negri Institute, Milan, Italy

I. INTRODUCTION

A. Background

Approximately 25,000 new cases of renal cell cancer are diagnosed each year in the United States, and many of these patients eventually develop disseminated disease (1). Renal cell cancer is relatively resistant to most chemotherapeutic drugs, which makes it a candidate for alternative treatment ap-

---

proaches, such as immunotherapy. In particular, the use of cytokines in conjunction with chemotherapeutic drugs that have shown some efficacy may be beneficial. One rationale for believing that such an approach may prove useful is based on the fact that primary renal cancers are often highly vascularized, and responses to biologic response modifiers (BRM), such as interferon-α (IFN-α) and interleukin-2 (IL-2), have been documented (2–4). These observations suggest that preclinical animal models for renal cancer could be useful for testing the ability of individual BRM, or BRM in combination with chemotherapeutic drugs or other BRM, to mediate antitumor responses.

B. RENCA Preclinical Model

The model chosen for preclinical study in our laboratory was the RENCA adenocarcinoma of BALB/c mice. The RENCA tumor arose spontaneously and was originally isolated by Stewart at the National Cancer Institute. Subsequently, Murphy and Hrushesky (5) extensively characterized the growth and progression of this tumor in syngeneic mice. The tumor spontaneously metastasizes from an intrarenal implant to the regional lymph nodes, lungs, liver, and spleen, as well as other organs. The immunogenicity of RENCA has been determined to be low to moderate (6,7), although some protection to rechallenge with viable RENCA cells following immunization with a membrane vaccine preparation has been reported (8). In our hands the RENCA tumor behaves as reported previously, with progressive metastases developing in the lymph nodes, lungs, and liver following the injection of 1×10^5 viable tumor cells under the capsule of the left kidney (9). Tumor-bearing mice routinely die between 35 and 45 days.

Previous studies from our laboratory demonstrated that various combinations of flavonoid compounds and IL-2 (10–14) or the combination of IL-2 and IFN-α (15) have potent antitumor effects against RENCA and that these effects are at least partially T cell mediated. Because of recent evidence that IL-7 has effects on T lymphocytes in vitro (16–19), studies were initiated to determine whether IL-7 had immunologic and antitumor effects in vivo.

II. BIOLOGIC EFFECTS OF IL-7

Interleukin-7 is 25 kD glycoprotein that was originally characterized as a product of a cloned murine bone marrow stromal cell line (20,21), and its mRNA has since been detected in the thymus and spleen (22). Recombinant human IL-7 (rhIL-7) exhibits a strong degree of homology with murine IL-7 (about 60%), with all six cysteine residues conserved (23). In vitro, IL-7 induces the proliferation of pro-B and pre-B lymphocytes (20,21) and affects the growth of both immature and mature cells of the T lymphocyte lineage (16–19). IL-7 has also been reported to induce lymphokine-activated killer (LAK) activity from peripheral blood leukocytes (24,25) and mouse splenocytes (26) in vitro. Much less is known about the in vivo effects of IL-7 on hematopoiesis, although a preliminary report suggested that splenic colony-forming units-granulocyte-macrophage (CFU-GM) are somewhat increased in mice treated with IL-7 (27). Thus, the aims of these studies are to (1) determine whether the administration of IL-7 to mice could alter the incidence or total number of single and multilineage myeloid progenitor cells, (2) determine whether IL-7 alters the number or subset composition of the T lymphocyte population, and (3) assess the antimetastatic effects of IL-7 against several mouse tumors.

III. HEMATOLOGIC EFFECTS OF rhIL-7 IN MICE

A. Induction of Leukocytosis

The twice daily intraperitoneal injection of C57Bl/6 mice with increasing doses of rhIL-7 (obtained from Sterling Drug, Malvern, PA; specific biologic activity of 2–5 $\times$ 10^7 U/mg) for various periods of time induced a profound leukocytosis in several lymphoid organs (Table 1). Optimal effects were achieved when rhIL-7 doses $\geq$ 5 μg per injection were administered twice daily for 4–7 days. Under these conditions there was about a threefold increase in the peripheral blood white cell (WBC) count and an even greater (fivefold) increase in the number of WBC in the spleen. Little change has been observed in the cellularity of the thymus or bone marrow.

Table 1 Hematologic Effects of rhIL-7 in Mice

Tissue site	Biologic effect
Peripheral blood	WBC increase by ~ 3-fold in a dose- and time-dependent manner
Bone marrow	Absolute white cell number not substantially altered; CFU-c and CFU-GEMM decreased by up to 90%
Spleen	WBC increased 5-fold in a dose- and time-dependent manner; CFU-c and CFU-GEMM increased up to 15-fold
Thymus	No significant change in cellularity
Lymph nodes	WBC increased up to 3-fold

B. Effects on Myeloid Progenitor Cells

When rhIL-7 is administered according to the preceding optimal regimen, there are striking changes (28) in the absolute number of both multipotential colonies containing granulocyte, erythroid, megakaryocyte, and macrophage lineages (CFU-GEMM), as well as single-lineage monocyte, myeloid, and myelomonocytic colonies (CFU-c). The number of both CFU-c and CFU-GEMM that can be cultured from the bone marrow decreases by > 90% after 7 days of rhIL-7 administration (Table 1). In contrast, the absolute number of both CFU types that can be cultured from the spleen increases up to 15-fold under the same conditions. One explanation for these results is an IL-7 induced exportation of CFU progenitors from the bone marrow to the spleen.

IV. EFFECTS OF rhIL-7 ON THE COMPOSITION OF LEUKOCYTE SUBSETS

Because of the general leukocytosis induced by rhIL-7 in mice (Table 1), studies were performed to determine which leukocyte subsets were altered. The results, summarized in Table 2, demonstrate that although the number of bone marrow CFU decreases there is also a corresponding decrease of several-alfold in the number of bone marrow cells that express the macrophage-granulocyte markers Mac-1 and 8C5. In contrast, there is about a threefold increase in the number of bone marrow cells that express the B220 antigen. These B220$^+$ cells are surface Ig negative (sIg$^-$), suggesting that they are B lymphocyte precursors.

In parallel with the increase in B220$^+$sIg$^-$ cells in the bone marrow, there is a similar increase in the number of these cells in the spleen. In addition, there also is a 2- to 3-fold increase in the number of CD8$^+$ cells. In the

Table 2 Alterations in Leukocyte Subset Composition Induced by Administration of rhIL-7 in Mice

Tissue site	Biologic effect
Bone marrow	3-fold increase in B220$^+$sIg$^-$ pre-B cells; 30–40% decrease in number of cells expressing Mac-1 and/or 8C5
Spleen	>30-fold increase in number of B220$^+$sIg$^-$ spleen cells; ~3-fold increase in number of CD8$^+$ T lymphocytes; Change in CD4/CD8 ratio from ~1.5:1 to 1:2

absence of a similar, parallel increase in CD4$^+$ lymphocytes, this results in a decrease in the CD4/CD8 ratio from about 1.5:1 to about 1:2.

V. ANTIMETASTATIC EFFECTS OF rhIL-7 IN MICE

Because administration of rhIL-7 causes an increase in CD8$^+$ T lymphocytes and CD8$^+$ T cells are known to contribute to various therapeutic combinations for treatment of RENCA, we speculated that rhIL-7 may have antimetastatic activity against RENCA. To date, the antimetastatic effects of rhIL-7 have actually been evaluated in five preclinical tumor models. Significant antimetastatic activity has been observed against pulmonary metastases established by either RENCA or the MCA-38 colon adenocarcinoma. Minimal or no antimetastatic activity has been detected against the B16 melanoma, the Lewis lung carcinoma, or the C-26 colon carcinoma.

The antimetastatic effects of rhIL-7 against RENCA are dose dependent, with a maximal inhibition of 75% in the number of metastases achieved when a dose of 100 μg is administered twice daily for 10 days (Fig. 1 and Table 3). An inhibition of 40–50% in the number of RENCA pulmonary metastases is achieved by the repeated administration of 25 μg rhIL-7. Similarly, the number of MCA-38 pulmonary metastases is reduced by up to 90% when 25 μg rhIL-7 is administered twice daily.

The mechanism for the observed antimetastatic effects of rhIL-7 is currently under investigation. Preliminary studies have shown that the number of splenic CD8$^+$ T cells increases by 5- to 10-fold and by about 15-fold in mice bearing RENCA and MCA-38, respectively. Interestingly, there is also a 9-fold increase in the number of CD8$^+$ lymphocytes that infiltrate into the lungs during the rhIL-7-induced regression of day 3 MCA-38 pulmonary metastases.

These results demonstrate that rhIL-7 can have antimetastatic activity against early metastases and suggest that T lymphocytes may play a role in these effects.

VI. CONCLUSIONS AND IMPLICATIONS

The studies presented here demonstrate that the twice daily administration of IL-7 preferentially stimulated bone marrow lymphopoiesis, induced a general leukocytosis, and increased the number of splenic CFU-GEMM and CFU-c. The number of bone marrow CFU-GEMM and CFU-c colonies were reduced in a manner that was dependent on IL-7 dose and duration of treatment. One hypothesis for the apparently opposing effects of rhIL-7 in the spleen and

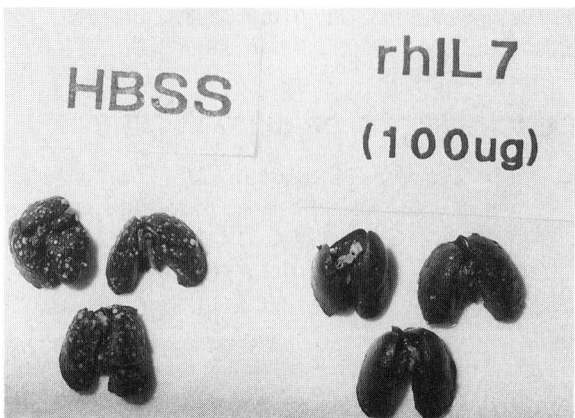

Figure 1 Antimetastatic effects of rhIL-7 in Mice. BALB/c mice were injected intravenously with one $\times$ 10^5 viable RENCA cells on day 0. On days 3–10, some of the mice were injected intraperitoneally twice daily with 100 μg rhIL-7. Control mice received the same number of injections of Hanks' balanced salt solution (HBSS).

bone marrow is that IL-7 has differential effects in those sites, such that hematopoietic precursor cells in the bone marrow are inhibited and those in the spleen are stimulated. A second hypothesis with regard to the effects of rhIL-7 on myelopoiesis is that rhIL-7 induces progenitors for CFU-c, CFU-GEMM, and/or even earlier progenitors to exit the bone marrow and localize in the spleen.

Recent evidence has shown that part of the leukocytosis induced in the spleens of normal (Ref. 29 and Komschlies et al., manuscript submitted for publication) or leukopenic (30) mice is due to an increase in cells with a pre-B cell phenotype. Our data support this conclusion in the bone marrow, where we observed an IL-7-induced increase in cells that were phenotypically identified as early B cells. In addition, the administration of rhIL-7 also preferentially increases the total number of splenic CD8$^+$ T cells. Thus, IL-7 may be of therapeutic value in promoting hematopoietic recovery in immunodeficient states, either iatrogenic in origin (e.g., bone marrow transplantation or chemotherapy and/or radiation therapy treatment of cancer) or disease-related (e.g., the acquired immunodeficiency syndrome). Preliminary studies from our laboratory suggest that rhIL-7 may accelerate the regeneration of the lymphoid compartment in both chemotherapy-treated (28) and irradiated mice (Boerman et al., manuscript in preparation).

Table 3 Antimetastatic and Immunomodulating Effects of rhIL-7 in Tumor-Bearing Mice

Tumor model	Biologic effect
RENCA	Reduction of 40–75% in number of early (day 3) pulmonary metastases; disproportionate increase in number of CD8$^+$ T cells in spleen; CD4/CD8 ratio in spleen changes from 2:1 to 1:1
MCA-38	Reduction of up to 90% in number of early (day 3) pulmonary metastases; Increase of approximately 15-fold in number of splenic CD8$^+$ T cells; CD4/CD8 ratio changes from 1.5:1 to 1:3 Increase of 9-fold in number of CD8$^+$ T cells present in lungs

Further studies have shown that rhIL-7 also induces significant increases in the CD8$^+$ T cell subset in both the spleens and lungs of mice bearing either RENCA or MCA-38 pulmonary micrometastases. This increase in CD8$^+$ T cells coincides with an rhIL-7-induced decrease of 40–90% in the number of preexistent metastatic tumor foci in the lungs. Studies are in progress to determine whether these CD8$^+$ T cells actually contribute to the therapeutic efficacy of rhIL-7. Because IL-7 has also been reported to activate monocytes and to induce the expression of monokine genes (31), studies are in progress to assess the possible role of pulmonary macrophages in the antimetastatic effects of rhIL-7 in mice.

ACKNOWLEDGMENTS

Research sponsored by the National Cancer Institute, DHHS, under Contract No. N01-C0-74102 with PRI/DynCorp. The contents of this publication do not necessarily reflect the views or policies of the Department of Health and Human Services, nor does mention of trade names, commercial products, or organizations imply endorsement by the U.S. Government.

REFERENCES

1. Silverberg BS, Lubera JA. Cancer statistics, CA 1989; 39:3.
2. Clark JW, Longo DL. Interferons in cancer therapy. In: DeVita VT Jr, Hellman S, Rosenberg, RA, eds. Cancer: principles and practice of oncology. Philadelphia: Lippincott 1987; 1–16.

3. Buzaid AC, Robertone A, Kisala C, Salmon SE. Phase II study of interferon alpha-2a, recombinant (Roferon-A) in metastatic renal cell carcinoma. J Clin Oncol 1987; 5:1083.

4. Rosenberg SA. Clinical immunotherapy studies in the surgery branch of the U.S. National Cancer Institute: brief review. Can Treat Rev 1989; 16(Suppl A):115.

5. Murphy GP, Hrushesky WJ. A murine renal cell carcinoma. J Natl Cancer Inst 1980; 50:1013.

6. Williams PD, Pontes EJ, Murphy GP. Studies on the growth of a murine renal cell carcinoma and its metastatic patterns. Res Commun Chem Pathol Pharmacol 1981; 34:345.

7. Hrushesky WJ, Murphy GP. Investigation of a new renal tumor model. J Surg Res 1973; 15:327.

8. Huben RP, Connelly R, Goldrosen MH, Murphy GP, Pontes JE. Immunotherapy of murine renal cancer. J Urol 1983; 129:1075.

9. Salup R, Herberman RB, Wiltrout RH. Role of natural killer activity in development of spontaneous metastases in murine renal cancer. J Urol 1985; 134:1236.

10. Salup RR, Back TA, Wiltrout RH. Successful treatment of advanced murine renal cell cancer by bicompartmental adoptive chemoimmunotherapy. J Immunol 1987; 138:641.

11. Wiltrout RH, Boyd MR, Back TC, Salup RR, Arthur JA, Hornung RL. Flavone-8-acetic acid augments systemic natural killer cell activity and synergizes with interleukin 2 for treatment of murine renal cancer. J Immunol 1988; 140:3261.

12. Hornung RL, Back TC, Zaharko DS, Urba WJ, Longo DL, Wiltrout RH. Augmentation of natural killer (NK) activity, induction of interferon and development of tumor immunity during the successful treatment of established murine renal cancer using flavone acetic acid (FAA) and interleukin 1. J Immunol 1988; 141:3671.

13. Mace KF, Hornung RC, Wiltrout RH, Young HA. Induction of cytokine gene expression in vivo by flavone acetic acid: strict dose dependency and correlation with therapeutic efficacy against murine renal cancer. Cancer Res 1990; 50:1742.

14. Futami H, Hornung RL, Back TT, Gruys ME, Wiltrout RH. Effect of systemic alkalinization on biologic response modification and therapeutic antitumor efficacy of flavone acetic acid plus recombinant interleukin 2. Cancer Res 1990; 50:7926.

15. Sayers TJ, Wiltrout TA, McCormick K, Husted C, Wiltrout RH. Antitumor effects of IFnα and IFN on a murine renal cancer (RENCA) in vitro and in vivo. Cancer Res 1990; 50:5414.

16. Watson JD, Morrissey PJ, Namen AE, Conlon PJ, Widmer MB. Effect of IL-7 on the growth of fetal thymocytes in culture. J Immunol 1989; 143:1215.

17. Conlon PJ, Morrissey PJ, Nordan RR, et al. Murine thymocytes proliferate in direct response to interleukin 7. Blood 1989; 74:1368.

18. Morrissey PJ, Goodwin RG, Nordan RP, et al. Recombinant interleukin 7, pre-B

cell growth factor, has costimulatory activity on purified mature T cells. J Exp Med 1989; 169:707.

19. Welch PA, Namen AE, Goodwin RG, Armitage R, Cooper MD. Human IL-7: a novel T cell growth factor. J Immunol 1989; 143:3562.
20. Namen AE, Lupton S, Hjerrild K, et al. Stimulation of B-cell progenitors by cloned murine interleukin-7. Nature 1988; 333:571.
21. Namen AE, Schmierer AE, March CJ, et al. B cell precursor growth-promoting activity—purification and characterization of a growth factor active on lymphocyte precursors. J Exp Med 1988; 167:988.
22. Goodwin RG, Namen AE. The cloning and characterization of interleukin-7. In: Cruse JM, and Lewis RE Jr, eds. Basel: Karger, *The year in immunology*, Vol. 6. 1990; 127.
23. Goodwin RG, Lupton S, Schmierer A, et al. Human interleukin 7: molecular cloning and growth factor activity on human and murine B-lineage cells. Proc Natl Acad Sci U S A 1989; 86:302.
24. Alderson MR, Sassenfeld HM, Widmer MB. Interleukin 7 enhances cytolytic T lymphocyte generation and induces lymphokine-activated killer cells from human peripheral blood. J Exp Med 1990; 172:577.
25. Stötter H, Custer MC, Bolton ES, Guedez L, Lotze MT. IL-7 induces human lymphokine-activated killer cell activity and is regulated by IL-4. J Immunol 1991; 146:150.
26. Lynch DH, Miller RE. Induction of murine lymphokine-activated killer cells by recombinant IL-7. J Immunol 1990; 145:1983.
27. Namen AE, Williams DE, Goodwin RG. A new hematopoietic growth factor. In: Spivak J, Drohan W, Dooley D, eds. *Hematopoietic growth factors in transfusion medicine*. New York: Wiley-Liss, 1990; 65.
28. Damia G, Komschlies KL, Faltynek CR, Ruscetti FW, Wiltrout RH. Administration of recombinant human interleukin 7 alters the frequency and number of myeloid progenitor cells in the bone marrow and spleen of mice. Blood 1992; 79:1121.
29. Morrissey PJ, Conlon P, Charrier P, et al. Administration of IL-7 to normal mouse stimulates B-lymphopoiesis and peripheral lymphadenopathy. J Immunol 1991; 147:567.
30. Morrissey PJ, Conlon P, Brackly S, Williams DE, Namen AE, Mochizuki DY. Administration of IL-7 to mice with cyclophosphamide-induced lymphopenia accelerates lymphocyte repopulation. J Immunol 1991; 146:1547.
31. Alderson MR, Tough TW, Ziegler SF, Grabstein KH. Interleukin 7 induces cytokine secretion and tumoricidal activity by human peripheral blood monocytes. J Exp Med 1991; 173:923.

VI

Combination Therapy with Cytokines

22

Tumor Necrosis Factor and Interferon-α_2

A Successful Approach to Metastatic Renal Cell Carcinoma

Ullrich Otto, Stefan Conrad, Andreas W. Schneider, and Herbert Klosterhalfen

University of Hamburg, Hamburg, Germany

I. INTRODUCTION

During the last few years, an increasing number of authors have reported about positive experiences in the therapy of metastatic renal cell carcinoma (RCC) with recombinant interferon-α_2 and γ (1–22). Using optimal doses, objective response rates of 30% and even more were achieved. Thus, the use of interferons in metastatic RCC is safe, effective, and well established. Nevertheless, response rates of 30% can only indicate a step in the right direction in the treatment of this malignancy. Interferon treatment is so far the only reasonable therapy for metastatic RCC, but this treatment still achieves fairly low response rates. Perhaps the combination of interferon with other immunomodulatory agents will improve tumor response.

In a preclinical study we evaluated the efficacy of treating RCC with tumor necrosis factor (TNF) in combination with various other cytokines or cytostatic agents. We found the combination of TNF and interferon-α_2 (IFN-α_2) to be more effective than any other combined or monotherapy leading to objective responses (23). Studies of proliferation kinetics revealed a synergistic antiproliferative and cytotoxic effect of TNF and IFN-α_2 (24). We therefore evaluated whether these encouraging preclinical results could be transferred to clinical therapy of metastatic RCC.

Because few data are published concerning the use of TNF in monotherapy in human malignancies and there is a lack of information about the toxicity and side effects of combined treatment with TNF and IFN-α_2, we initiated a randomized phase I clinical trial in patients with histologically confirmed renal cell carcinoma on therapy with multiple intravenous infusions of recombinant tumor necrosis factor (rhTNF) alone or in combination with intramuscular IFN-α_2. In an escalating dose schedule, we primarily studied the toxicity and potential side effects of recombinant TNF and evaluated the maximum tolerated dose (MTD). Moreover, the study aimed to detect the toxicity of combined application of rhTNF and IFN-α_2 in comparison to monotherapy with either cytokine alone. The study was therefore designed as a three-arm randomized trial. Furthermore, the antitumoral activity of all three treatment regimens was assessed.

Based on this experience in the use of tumor necrosis factor in the initial phase I study, we then designed an open, nonrandomized clinical phase II trial to further evaluate the efficacy of combined therapy with rhTNF and IFN-α_2 in the treatment of metastatic RCC. We intended to answer the question of whether it is possible to achieve an increased response rate by combining those cytokines than either one would produce in monotherapy.

II. MATERIALS AND METHODS

A. Clinical Phase I/II Study

Between 1987 and 1988, we conducted a prospective randomized three-arm clinical phase I/II trial on the therapy of metastatic RCC. Patients with a histologically proven metastatic RCC were included in the study. Inclusion criteria were history of radical nephrectomy, age more than 18 years, and estimated time of survival of at least 3 months with an Eastern Cooperative Oncology Group (ECOG)-Zubrod status of 2 or more. Patients who received IFN-α_2 before inclusion were not randomized, but they could receive combined treatment with rhTNF and IFN-α_2 outside the study. Further criteria of inclusion and exclusion are listed in Tables 1 and 2.

The study was designed to include a total of 16 patients, who were randomized into three different treatment arms: six patients in regimen A, six patients in regimen B, and four patients in regimen C.

Table 1 Inclusion Criteria for the Phase I/II Study

Histologically proven metastatic renal cell carcinoma
History of radical nephrectomy
Age $\geq$ 18 years
Estimated survival $>$ 3 months
ECOG-Zubrod performance status $\leq$ 2
Written informed consent

Regimen A consisted of a continuous intravenous infusion of rhTNF for 2 h, five times per week every 3 weeks. The initial dose was 0.02 mg/m^2. After each treatment cycle, the dose of rhTNF was escalated as shown in Figure 1 up to the individual maximum tolerated dose.

In regimen B patients received intramuscular (IM) recombinant IFN-α$_2$ at 12 $\times$ 10^6 units three times per week every week for the entire treatment period. After 3 weeks of IFN-α$_2$ monotherapy, rhTNF was given as a 2 h intravenous (IV) infusion, 5 days/week every 3 weeks. Doses and dose escalations were similar to those in regimen A.

In regimen C patients received recombinant human IFN-α$_2$ at 12 $\times$ 10^6 units—three times per week every week as a monotherapy.

Synthetic rhTNF was provided by Knoll AG (Ludwigshafen, Germany). For the intravenous infusion, 1 mg lyophilized rhTNF were suspended in 3 ml

Table 2 Exclusion Criteria for the Phase I/II Study

Pregnancy
Pretreatment with TNF or IFN-α$_2$
History of radiotherapy, chemotherapy, or major operations within 4 weeks of therapy
Central nervous system metastases
Diabetes requiring insulin treatment
Coagulation disorders
Severe infections within 4 weeks of therapy
Severe cardiovascular diseases within 6 months of therapy (e.g., myocardial infarction, uncontrolled hypo- or hypertension)
Weight loss more than 10% within 4 weeks of therapy
Laboratory values outside defined limits

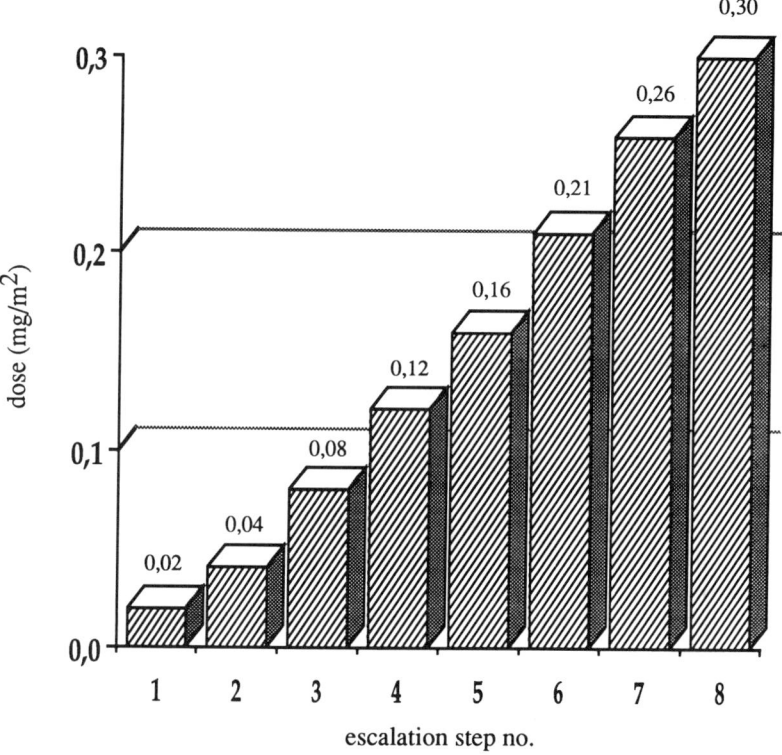

Figure 1 Dose escalation for rhTNF, phase I/II study.

sterile water. An aliquot of this solution was diluted with 5% human serum albumin to a total volume of 50 ml. The infusion was done by electronically controlled infusion pump over 2 h. Recombinant IFN-α_2 (Roferon) was purchased from Hoffmann-LaRoche (Grenzach/Wyhlen, Germany).

Before, during, and after therapy, potential side effects were documented by physical and laboratory examinations. Before and after each TNF infusion, patients were asked about their subjective complaints and were clinically examined.

Grading of toxicity was performed according to World Health Organization (WHO) guidelines. The maximum tolerated dose was defined as either reversible grade III or IV toxicities or irreversible grade II toxicities. Therapy was then continued on a dose level one step below the MTD.

Response to therapy was evaluated at the beginning of each cycle by clinical and radiologic examinations. Response criteria were complete remission (CR), partial remission (PR), stable disease (SD), and progressive disease (PD) according to WHO criteria.

Therapy was discontinued for disease progression, unexpected or life-threatening complications, or withdrawal of informed consent. In grade II toxicity, treatment was withheld until complete normalization of the side effects.

B. Clinical Phase II Study

Since 1988 we have conducted an open nonrandomized clinical phase II trial with the combination of rhTNF and IFN-α_2 in the therapy of metastatic renal cell carcinoma. Inclusion and exclusion criteria in the study resembled those of the preceding phase I study (see Figs. 1 and 2). Before initiation of therapy, an objective tumor progression was confirmed by repeated radiologic studies. In addition to the inclusion and exclusion criteria of the phase I/II study, patients with bone metastases only and patients with an ECOG-Zubrod performance status less than one were excluded.

A minimum of 14 patients was required for inclusion in the study. For each patient with objective response, an additional number of patients were included to a maximum of 25 patients.

All patients received initially 18×10^6 units IFN-α_2 three times a week IM. After a week of pretreatment with interferon-α_2 they received additionally a continuous infusion of 160 μg rhTNF per m^2 body surface area for 2 h on 5 consecutive days every 3 weeks. The preparation and application of TNF were performed as described earlier for the phase I/II study. Before, during, and after therapy, possible side effects were evaluated by physical and laboratory examinations. As in the phase I/II study, the patients received a complete physical examination after each single TNF infusion. Temperature, respiratory rate, heart rate, and blood pressure were noted before and 2, 6, and 24 h after administration of TNF. Toxicity was again classified according to WHO grading.

Response to therapy was evaluated after every third cycle. Response criteria were again CR, PR, SD, and PD according to WHO criteria.

Therapy was discontinued for progressive disease after a minimum of three cycles of combined therapy with TNF and IFN-α_2, as well as in patients who experienced unexpected or life-threatening complications and those who withdrew their consent.

III. RESULTS

A. Clinical Phase I/II Study

A total of 16 patients was included in the three-arm randomized phase I/II trial: seven patients received therapy in regimen A (rhTNF monotherapy), five patients were randomized in regimen B (combined therapy with rhTNF and IFN-α_2), and four patients received therapy according to regimen C (IFN-α_2 monotherapy).

Another two patients were treated with IFN-α_2 before inclusion without objective response. Both patients received combined therapy according to regimen B, outside the study.

1. Patient Characteristics

The mean age of 14 male and four female patients was 57.8 years (range 40–72). Of 18 patients 15 had lung metastases, one patient had exclusively bone metastases, and two lymph node metastases only (see Table 3). In six cases, RCC was primary metastatic; in all other patients, metastases had developed 1–45 months after radical nephrectomy.

2. Toxicity

During therapy with rhTNF and IFN-α_2, almost all patients developed fever and chills, frequently accompanied by nausea and vomiting during TNF infusions (see Table 4). Long-term toxicity, especially after numerous steps of dose escalation, included fatigue, malaise, and weight loss. These acute and chronic toxicities could be managed by additional medication and did not

Table 3 Patient Characteristics, Phase I/II Study

	Regimen			
	A	B	C	Overall
Mean age, years	62	51	51	56
Site of metastases				
Lung	6/7	1/5	2/4	9/16
Bone	0/7	1/5	0/4	1/16
Combined	1/7	1/5	2/4	6/16
Tumor grade				
1	0/7	0/5	0/4	0/16
2	6/7	5/5	3/4	14/16
3	1/7	0/5	1/4	2/16

Table 4 Toxicity of rhTNF and IFN-α_2 Therapy, Phase I/II Study[a]

	Grade 1	Grade 2	Grade 3	Grade 4
Hematotoxity				
Anemia	29 / 60 / –	– / – / –	– / – / –	– / – / –
Leukopenia	42 / 60 / 75	– / 40 / 25	– / – / –	– / – / –
Granulopenia	– / – / 25	– / – / –	– / – / –	– / – / –
Thrombopenia	42 / 20 / 25	14 / – / –	– / – / –	– / – / –
Bleeding	– / – / –	– / – / –	– / – / –	– / – / –
Gastrointestinal toxicity				
Bilirubin	– / – / 25	– / – / –	– / – / –	– / – / –
GOT/GPT	57 / 60 / 75	14 / 40 / –	– / – / –	– / – / –
(γ-GT)[b]	14 / – / 50	29 / 40 / 25	42 / 40 / –	14 / – / –
Alkaline phosphatase (AP)	42 / 80 / 50	14 / 40 / 25	– / – / –	– / – / –
Oral	– / – / 25	– / – / –	– / – / –	– / – / –
Nausea, vomiting	14 / 20 / 50	57 / 60 / 25	– / – / –	– / – / –
Diarrhea	29 / – / –	– / – / –	– / – / –	– / – / –
Cardiotoxicity				
Rhythm	42 / 40 / –	– / 20 / –	– / – / –	– / – / –
Function	– / – / –	– / – / –	– / – / –	– / – / –
Pericarditis	– / – / –	– / – / –	– / – / –	– / – / –
Neurotoxicity				
Conciousness	– / – / –	– / – / –	14 / 20 /–	– / – / –
Peripheral	– / – / –	– / – / –	– / – / –	– / – / –
Constipation	– / – / –	– / – / –	– / – / –	– / – / –
Nephrotoxicity				
BUN	42 / – / –	– / – / –	– / – / –	– / – / –
Creatinine	42 / 20 / 25	14 / – / –	– / – / –	– / – / –
Proteinuria	86 / 100 / 50	– / – / –	– / – / –	– / – / –
Hematuria	29 / – / –	14 / 40 / –	– / – / –	– / – / –
Pulmonary toxicity	14 / – / 25	– / 20 / –	– / – / –	– / – / –
Fever	14 / 20 / 25	71 / 60 / 50	14 / – / –	– / – / –
Chills	– / – / 50	71 / 100 / –	– / – / –	– / – / –
Allergic reactions	– / – / –	– / – / –	– / – / –	– / – / –
Cutaneous reactions	– / 20 / 25	14 / – / 50	– / – / –	– / – / –
Hair loss	– / – / 25	– / – / –	– / – / –	– / – / –
Infections	– / – / –	– / – / –	– / – / –	– / – / –
Pain				
Headaches	14 / 20 / –	– / – / –	– / – / –	– / – / –
Other	29 / 20 / –	14 / – / –	– / – / –	– / – / –
Fatigue	57 / 40 / 100	29 / 40 / –	14 / – / –	– / – / –
Anorexia	57 / 40 /25	– / 20 / –	– / – / –	– / – / –

[a] Numbers indicate incidence of maximum toxicities (%) regimen A / regimen B / regimen C. Grading according to WHO classification.
[b] GT, Glutamyltransferase.

Table 5 Response to rhTNF and IFN-α_2 Therapy, Phase I/II Study[a]

Regimen	CR + PR	SD	PD	Duration of SD (months)
A: TNF	0	4	2	5.4
B: TNF/IFN-α_2	0	3	4	6.8
C: IFN-α_2	0	3	1	9.6

[a] $n = 17$, including 1 nonrandomized patient in regimen B.

urge us to discontinue therapy in any patient. The limiting factors for dose escalation, defining the maximal tolerated dose, were changes in the following laboratory values: 14 of 18 patients developed grade I–II leukopenia, and there were also episodes of therapy-induced thrombopenia. A rise in the hepatic enzymes GOT, GPT, γ-GT, and AP occurred in 17 of 18 patients, including several grade III toxicities. All changes in laboratory values normalized quickly after cessation of the TNF infusion. Less often, anemia, nephrotoxicity characterized by a rise in creatinine or blood urea nitrogen (BUN), proteinuria, and hematuria, as well as tachycardia, reduced consciousness, hair loss, and cutaneous reactions, were noted. Nevertheless, none of these other side effects were dose limiting. All toxic reactions are listed in Table 4.

3. Response
Of 16 randomized and two nonrandomized patients, 17 were evaluable concerning response to therapy. A total of 10 patients showed a stable disease lasting for 3–13 months. There were 4 SD in regimen A, 3 SD in regimen B, and 3 SD in regimen C. The remaining seven patients showed tumor progression despite therapy (see Table 5).

B. Clinical Phase II Study

So far, 16 patients with metastatic RCC have been included in this open nonrandomized clinical phase II trial on the therapy of metastatic RCC with the combination of rhTNF and IFN-α_2.

1. Patient Characteristics
The mean age of 11 male and five female patients was 58.4 years (range 32–71). Of 16 patients 11 showed lung metastases, either alone (6) or in combination with metastases of the bone, vagina, trachea, thyroid gland, or retroperitoneal lymph nodes (see Table 6). In five patients, metastases were noted

Table 6 Patient Characteristics, Phase II Study

Mean age, years	58.4 (32–71)
Number of patients	16
Male	11
Female	5
Metastatic sites	
Lung	
Overall	11
Only	6
Bone	
Overall	2
Only	0
Lymph nodes and local recurrences	
Overall	7
Only	3

before nephrectomy; in the remaining 11 patients, the interval between nephrectomy and initial diagnosis of metastatic disease ranged between 1 and 96 months.

2. Toxicity

Under combined therapy with rhTNF and IFN-α₂, all patients developed fever and chills, frequently accompanied by nausea or, less often, by vomiting. These side effects were therefore similar to those previously noted in the phase I/II study. Because there was no dose escalation, these side effects mainly occurred during the first treatment cycles. When therapy was continued, patients adapted to these toxicities aided by nonsteroidal anti-inflammatory drugs and antiemetics. Nevertheless, fatigue, malaise, and weight loss became more frequent after repeated numbers of TNF infusions.

In two cases, therefore, we prolonged the outpatient interval from 2 to 3 or 4 weeks (see Table 7). The changes in laboratory values were similar to those in the phase I/II study. Almost regularly, a leukocytopenia was obvious at the end of TNF infusions, and mild thrombocytopenias and mild to moderate elevations of hepatic enzymes were also noted. Therapy was withheld only once, for 2 days, after a grade IV leukopenia. The white blood count normalized completely within these 2 days. Therapy could then be continued with a reduction in the TNF dose to 120 μg/m² and only reversible episodes of grade III leukopenia occurred. All toxic effects are listed in Table 7.

Table 7 Toxicity of Combined rhTNF and IFN-α_2 Therapy, Phase II Study[a]

	Grade 1	Grade 2	Grade 3	Grade 4
Hematotoxicity				
Anemia	43	7	–	–
Leukopenia	36	29	14	7
Granulopenia	14	7	–	–
Thrombopenia	21	7	7	–
Bleeding	–	–	–	–
Gastrointestinal toxicity				
Bilirubin	7	–	–	–
GOT/GPT	50	7	7	–
γ-GT	7	7	14	–
AP	50	42	7	–
Oral	7	–	–	–
Nausea, vomiting	50	50	–	–
Diarrhea	–	–	–	–
Cardiotoxicity				
Rhythm	85	–	–	–
Function	–	–	–	–
Pericarditis	–	–	–	–
Neurotoxicity				
Conciousness	–	7	–	–
Peripheral	–	–	–	–
Constipation	–	–	–	–
Nephrotoxicity				
BUN	14	–	–	–
Creatinine	29	–	–	–
Proteinuria	71	29	–	–
Hematuria	–	–	–	–
Pulmonary toxicity	–	7	–	–
Fever	7	93	–	–
Chills	–	100	–	–
Allergic reactions	–	–	–	–
Cutaneous reactions	7	21	–	–
Hair loss	7	–	–	–
Infections	14	–	–	–
Pain				
Headaches	71	–	–	–
Other	–	–	–	–
Fatigue	7	85	–	–
Anorexia	21	71	–	–

[a] Numbers indicate incidence of maximum toxicities (%). Grading according to WHO classification.

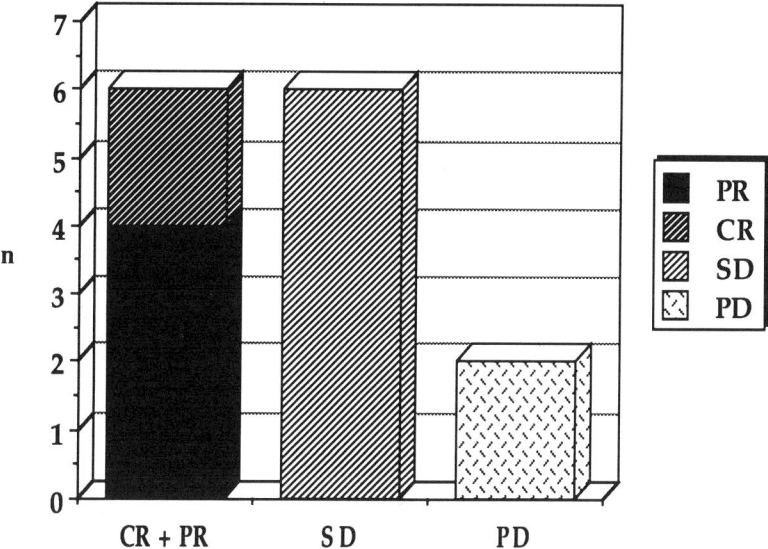

Figure 2   Response to combined rhTNF and IFN-α_2 therapy, phase II study.

3. Response

At the moment, 14 of 16 patients included in the study so far are evaluable for response. In six patients (43%), an objective response was achieved (2 CR and 4 PR). In six patients, a stable disease was achieved and in only two patients, the tumor progressed. Only patients with lung or soft tissue metastases and a small tumor burden responded to therapy. Objective responses were not seen in bone metastases or local recurrences. The medium duration of the responses cannot yet be defined, because no tumor relapse has occurred under maintenance therapy (see Figure 2).

IV. DISCUSSION

Our highly promising preclinical results in the therapy of human RCC xenografts in nude mice with the combination of TNF-α and IFN-α_2 (23) encouraged us to conduct two clinical phase I or phase II trials in patients with metastatic RCC. In our initial phase I study we were able to show that therapy with TNF alone or combined with IFN-α_2 is a tolerable treatment modality with mostly dose dependent side effects. The phase II study proved that with such a therapy response rates can be achieved that other therapeutic strategies can hardly produce.

The phase I study was primarily intended to find the maximum tolerated dose of TNF alone or in combination with IFN-α_2. The results of this phase I study were then used to design a phase II study to evaluate the antitumoral efficacy of the combination of TNF-α and IFN-α_2.

In the phase I study 18 patients received either continuous intravenous infusion of TNF with intraindividual dose escalation up to the MTD, IFN-α_2 alone, or both cytokines in combination. We showed that all three treatment regimens produced side effects that can in general be anticipated when using biologic response modifiers, including fever, flulike symptoms, nausea, vomiting, and chills. All these symptoms were more pronounced with TNF-α alone or in combination therapy compared to IFN-α_2 monotherapy. In most patients, hepatotoxicity was the dose-limiting factor, but the mechanisms responsible for the elevation of hepatic enzymes remain unclear.

No objective responses were seen in the phase I study, in contrast to a fairly high response rate in the phase II trial. We believe that four reasons are responsible for this difference:

First, only patients with advanced and progressive metastatic RCC who were not considered candidates for more established forms of therapy, including IFN-α_2 monotherapy were included into the phase I study. All these patients had either wide spread metastatic disease with a large tumor burden or a reduced performance status, or both. Our own experiences in IFN-α_2 or IFN-γ monotherapy demonstrate clearly that only patients with a good performance status respond to therapy with biologic response modifiers (15). When treated with IFN-α_2 in combination with vinblastine, objective responses were noted only in patients with a Karnofsky index of 80% or higher (15). Furthermore we believe that a cytokine therapy is effective only in patients with a smaller tumor burden. Clinical data supporting this belief have repeatedly been published for IFN-α_2 monotherapy (25). As shown by the results of our phase II study, this seems also to be true for combined TNF-α and IFN-α_2.

The second reason for the obvious differences in the response rates between the phase I and the phase II studies is possibly the dose escalation performed in the phase I study to determine the individual MTD. Our preclinical studies in the nude mouse model showed a clear dose dependence of the antitumoral effect of TNF. It should therefore be anticipated that extremely low doses of TNF-α, which were used in the first dose escalation cycles, are ineffective (26). In most patients with progressive disease, the tumor progressed during the first treatment cycles, when low doses of TNF-α were used.

The third reason may be the relatively low doses of IFN-α_2 in the phase I study. It is well known from the literature that only intermediate doses produce acceptable remission rates and are significantly more effective than low or high doses (25). Nevertheless, a dose of 12×10^6 units IFN-α_2 three times a week was chosen because of the unpredictability of severe side effects during combined treatment with TNF-α and IFN-α_2. As stated earlier, no prior experiences with a combination of these two cytokines in humans have been reported.

The final reason to explain the differences between the preclinical results in the nude mouse model and the clinical experiences in the phase I study is that the maximum tolerated dose for nude mice was much higher than for humans, given a conversion factor of 14 between laboratory animals and humans.

These explanations were therefore reflected in the design of the phase II study. Only patients with an ECOG-Zubrod performance status of 0–1 were included. No intraindividual dose escalation was performed. Therapy was conducted with 0.16 mg/m^2 of TNF-α, which was the average MTD in the phase I study. The IFN doses was elevated to 18 MU units three times a week. These changes resulted in the achievement of a 33% response rate. Comparable results have not yet been achieved by any other treatment mortality in patients with metastatic RCC.

Three observations during the phase II study should influence the treatment strategy of metastatic RCC in general. First, we clearly showed that the objective response rate was higher in patients with low tumor burden and only in these patients did complete remissions occur. These results are clearly correlated with our preclinical data (23). Up to 80% of all patients who underwent radical nephrectomy for initially nonmetastatic RCC develop metastases and finally die of their disease (24). The correlation between tumor burden and response rate with a potential of complete response in patients with low tumor burden and a good performance status might also qualify such combined cytokine treatment for adjuvant therapy after radical nephrectomy. Micrometastases may even respond better than small, visible secondaries.

The second observation is that only pulmonary and, to a smaller degree, soft tissue metastases responded to combined TNF-α/IFN-α_2 treatment, but local recurrences or bone metastases were treated without any effect. A similar tendency has been described for interferon monotherapy earlier (15). Nevertheless, the probability of an objective response was lower in IFN-α_2 monotherapy than in TNF-α/IFN-α_2 therapy. This observation therefore stresses the necessity for a clearly radical approach to nephrectomy in RCC, including a regional lymphadenectomy. A local recurrence or retroperitoneal lymph node metastases must be prevented by any means, because they are almost inaccessible to any kind of cytokine treatment.

The third observation is consistent with our preclinical findings: responses occurred promptly, leaving only murine fibrous tissue a few days after initiation of combined therapy in responding mice. Similarly, in the phase II study, several patients responded quickly after a few treatment cycles but a small amount of residual disease persisted in radiologic examinations without further decrease, but also without tumor relapse. Some of these patients may in fact be histologically complete responders, with only small areas of fibrous tissue left at the site of former metastases. These cases therefore lead to a diagnostic dilemma—whether to continue or discontinue therapy after a long-lasting partial response with small residual disease—that at present cannot be resolved. In the future, only proper histologic evaluation of these cases by biopsy or surgical removal of residual disease will provide proper information on this topic.

In conclusion, our results seem to qualify the combined systemic therapy with TNF-α and IFN-α_2 as a reasonable concept in the treatment of metastatic renal cell carcinoma. Further preclinical evaluation and growing experience in clinical therapy will help us to improve this therapeutic strategy further, possibly with the inclusion of a third cytokine into combined therapy.

REFERENCES

1. Buzaid AC, Robertone A, Kisala C, Salmon SE. Phase II study of interferon alpha-2a, recombinant (Roferon-A) in metastatic renal cell carcinoma. J Clin Oncol 1987; 5:1083–9.
2. Creagan ET, Buckner JC, Hahn RG, Richardson RR, Schaid DJ, Kovach JS. An evaluation of recombinant leukocyte A interferon with aspirin in patients with metastatic renal cell carcinoma. Cancer 1988; 61:1787–91.
3. DeKernion JB, Sarna G, Figlin R, Lindner A, Smith RB. The treatment of renal cell carcinoma with human leukocyte alpha-interferon. J Urol 1983; 130: 1063–6.
4. de Mulder PRM, Debruyne FMJ, Geboers ADH, Strijk S, Damsma O. Recombinant (r) alpha- and gamma-interferon (IFN) in the treatment of advanced renal cell carcinoma (RCC) abstract 528. J Urol 1989; 141 (part 2):294A.
5. Fossa SD, De Garis ST, Heier MS, et al. Recombinant interferon alpha-2a with or without vinblastin in metastatic renal cell carcinoma. Cancer 1986; 57(Suppl):1700–4.
6. Fujita T, Asano H, Naide Y, et al. Antitumor effects of human lymphoblastoid interferon on advanced renal cell carcinoma. J Urol 1988; 139:256–8.
7. Garnick MB, Reich SD, Maxwell B, Coval-Goldsmith S, Richie JP, Rudnick SA. Phase I/II study of recombinant interferon gamma in advanced renal cell carcinoma. J Urol 1988; 139:251–5.

8. Huber C, Aulitzky WA, Aulitzky WO, Frick J, Gastl G, Tilg H. Interferone gegen Krebs: Weg von der Holzhammer-Methode. Med Trib 1989; 33:33.
9. Kirkwood JM, Harris JE, Vera R, et al. A randomized study of low and high doses of leukocyte alpha-interferon in metastatic renal cell carcinoma: the American Cancer Society Collaborative Trial. Cancer Res 1985; 45:863–71.
10. Krown SE, Einzig AI, Abramson JD, et al. Treatment of advanced renal cell cancer (RCC) with recombinant leukocyte A interferon (rIFN-alpha-A). Proc Am Soc Clin Oncol 1983; 2:58.
11. Marumo K, Murai M, Hayakawa M, Tazaki H. Human lymphoblastoid interferon therapy for advanced renal cell carcinoma. Urology 1984; 24:567–71.
12. Muss HB, Costanzi JJ, Leavitt R, et al. Recombinant alpha interferon in renal cell carcinoma: a randomized trial of two routes of administration. J Clin Oncol 1987; 5:286–91.
13. Neidhart JA, Gagen MM, Young D, et al. Interferon-alpha therapy of renal cancer. Cancer Res 1984; 44:4140–3.
14. Otto U, Huland H, Zschaber R. Recombinant interferon gamma: first results of a clinical phase II study in patient with metastatic renal cell carcinoma and experimental studies of human renal cell carcinoma transplanted into nude mice (abstract 168). J Urol 1985; 133 (part 2):155A.
15. Otto U, Schneider A, Denkhaus H, Conrad S. Die Behandlung des metastasierenden Nierenkarzinoms mit rekombinantem alpha 2- oder gamma-Interferon. Ergebnisse zweier klinischer Phase-II-bzw. III. Studien. Onkologie 1988; 11:185–91.
16. Quesada JR, Swanson DA, Trindade A, Guttermann JU. Renal cell carcinoma: antitumor effects of leukocyte interferon. Cancer Res 1983; 43:940–7.
17. Rizzo M, Bartoletti R, Selli C, Sicignano A, Criscoulo D. Interferon alpha-2a and vinblastine in the treatment of metastatic renal cell carcinoma. Eur Urol 1989; 16:271–7.
18. Schornagel JH, Verweij J, ten Bokkel Huinink WW, et al. Phase II study of recombinant interferon alpha-2a and vinblastine in advanced renal cell carcinoma. J Urol 1989; 142:253–6.
19. Strayer DR, Weisband J, Carter WA, et al. Renal cell carcinoma and leukocyte interferon: correlation between sensitivity in a clonogenic assay and clinical response (abstract C-619). Proc Am Soc Clin Oncol 1984; 3:158.
20. Takaku F, Kumamoto Y, Koiso K., et al. Phase II study of recombinant human interferon gamma (S-6810) on renal cell carcinoma. Cancer 1987; 60:929–33.
21. Trump D, Harris H, Tuttle R, et al. Phase II trial of high dose human lymphoblastoid interferon (Wellferon) in advanced renal cell carcinoma (aRCC) (abstract). Proc Am Soc Clin Oncol 1985; 3:153.
22. Vugrin D, Hood L, Taylor W, Laszlo J. Phase II study of human lymphoblastoid interferon in patients with advanced renal carcinoma. Cancer Treat Rep 1985; 69:817–20.
23. Otto U, Baisch H, Hammerer P, Schneider A. Influence of tumor necrosis factor, interleukin II, alpha-2-interferon and gamma-interferon alone and in

combination on human renal cell and bladder carcinoma transplanted into NMRI nu/nu mouse. J Urol 1987; 137:253A.

24. Baisch H, Otto U. Cell kinetic effects of alpha-interferon and tumor necrosis factor (TNF) on human renal cell carcinomas transplanted into nude mice. Cytometry 1988; Suppl 2:18.

25. Krown SE. Interferon treatment of renal cell carcinoma. Current status and future prospects. Cancer 1987; 59:647–51.

26. Otto U, Baisch H, Klöppel G, Klosterhalfen H. Influence of TNF alone and in combination with alpha-2-IFN, gamma-IFN or IL II on human renal cell and bladder carcinoma after transplantation into NMRI nu/nu mice. J Interferon Res 1986; 6:136.

23

Trials with Tumor Necrosis Factor and Interferon-γ in Renal Carcinoma

Michael H. H. Sohn and Susanne Markos-Pusztai

University Clinic RWTH, Aachen, Germany

I. INTRODUCTION

Of all patients with renal cell carcinoma, 25–50% present with clinically apparent distant metastases (1). The overall survival of these patients is 53% at 6 months, 43% at 12 months, and 10–26% at 24 months. The 5-year cumulative survival rate is approximately 5–10% in most studies (2–5).

Fowler stated the following in 1987: "The pressures to do something, that might conceivably prolong or improve the quality of survival, whether self-imposed or exerted by the patient and family, may be overwhelming" (6). This need for adjuvant medical therapy exists in the vast majority of patients, since less than 10% present with solitary, surgically resectable metastases (4). In contrast to promising results in these few radically resected patients (25–50% 5-year survival rates), medical treatment of advanced metastatic spread remains an unsolved challenge (4,7–10).

The number of metastatic lesions, grade of tumor, general performance status, and weight loss determine survival rates and response to therapy (11). Since the first report on successful interferon-α treatment of advanced renal cell carcinoma by Quesada in 1983 (12), a broad variety of immunotherapeutic regimens has been designed and applied in this disease. Biologic response modifiers (BRM) were given alone, in combination, or combined with chemotherapeutic agents. Response rates vary between 6 and 28% for interferon-α monotherapies and between 22 and 50% for interleukin-2 (IL-2)-containing combination therapies (13,14). Until now, no standard therapy has emerged from all these studies, mainly because of high toxicities and variable prognostic selection criteria. Timing, dosage, and route of administration seem to have an important impact on toxicity and response.

II. TUMOR NECROSIS FACTOR-α

With the introduction of recombinant DNA technology, the cytotoxic monokine tumor necrosis factor-α (TNF-α) is now available in large quantities. Its antitumor effects were described by Carswell et al. in 1975 (15).

Decades before its isolation and description, Coley published a large series of 1200 advanced cancer patients treated with filtered medium from bacterial cultures. A response rate of 22% was reported (16). Experimental animal studies continued with bacterial extracts and finally led to Carswell's discovery that not bacterial endotoxin per se, but a reactive host factor, called TNF, was responsible for the antitumor efficiency. In the intervening 10 years before the TNF gene could be cloned, experimental studies showed that TNF was mainly produced by macrophages and that it killed some tumor, but not normal cells.

Isolation and purification revealed a trimeric structure with a molecular weight of 45,000. Each TNF-α monomer consists of 157 amino acids. Its β-barrel, or jelly roll, configuration is shown by many viral coat proteins. Bacterial endotoxin (lipopolysaccharide, LPS) is one of the most potent inducers of TNF-α production in mononuclear phagocytes (monocytes-macrophages). Other cytokines such as IL-1 and IL-2, also act as inducers, as well as interact with natural killer (NK) cells, T lymphocytes, mast cells, and fibroblasts (17).

The effects of TNF on other cells are mediated by specific TNF receptors on the cell surface, which are present on many normal and tumor cell lines varying from a few hundred up to about 20,000 per cell. Early events following TNF receptor occupation include increased plasma membrane permeability with subsequent Ca^{2+} influx and activation of phospholipase A_2, resulting in production of arachidonic acid and prostaglandin E_2 (PGE_2), as well as activation of respiratory burst oxidase. For lymphocytes TNF-α acts as costimulant for cell proliferation and functional activities, such as IL-2 receptor expression. In high doses TNF-α has demonstrated enhancement of IL-2-dependent T cell proliferation and T cell-derived interferon-γ (IFN-γ) production.

TNF-α also enhances cell surface major histocompatibility complex (MHC) expression in synergy with IFN-γ. Like IFN-γ, TNF-α probably acts as a maturation factor for cytolytic functions of cytotoxic T lymphocytes (CTL) and natural cytotoxic cells, such as non–MHC-restricted lymphokine-activated killer (LAK) cells. Beside these numerous effects, TNF-α acts in an autocrine manner on monoctyes-macrophages to enhance tumor cell cytotoxicity and production of other cytokines, such as IL-1, IL-6 and macrophage colony-stimulating factor (M-CSF). As a result of phospholipase A_2 activation, PAF is synthesized and released. Neutrophil granulocytes show enhanced phagocytosis, degranulation, and respiratory burst activity (17).

Endothelial cells respond to TNF-α with enhanced adhesion to lymphocytes and monocytes and enhanced procoagulant activity (17). IFN-γ and TNF-α are both potent antiproliferative agents in certain tumor cells. TNF-α acts cytostatic rather than cytotoxic. Furthermore, a synergistic effect of both cytokines has been observed in various tumor cell lines, probably initiated by the observed IFN-γ-mediated TNF receptor expression of tumor cells (18,19). The action of IL-2 in boosting NK and LAK cell cytotoxicity is probably dependent on autocrine and paracrine IFN-γ and TNF-α stimulation. IFN-γ and TNF-α further act synergistically in MHC class I antigen expression, thus augmenting CTL cytolytic functions in vitro (17).

Summing all known mechanisms of TNF-α antitumor activity, the following three pathways of action may be defined:

1. Direct cytostatic and cytotoxic activity of TNF-α in synergy with IFN-γ
2. Immunostimulatory effects of TNF-α, especially in combination with IFN-γ, on most cell populations involved in tumor defense
3. Endothelially transmitted procoagulation and vascular "leakiness," resulting in vascular malnutrition of tumors and metastasis

III. IFN-γ AND TNF-α IN RENAL CELL CARCINOMA MODEL SYSTEMS

In contrast to other interferons (α and β), IFN-γ is the product of a single gene and is produced by activated T lymphocytes. Its immunomodulatory effects are closely linked to TNF-α. Several authors tested the synergistic effects of these two cytokines on a variety of renal carcinoma cell lines in models in vivo and in vitro (20–22). In vitro, combinations of TNF-α and IFN-γ or INF-α showed synergistic cytotoxic effects compared to monotherapies and INF-α/γ combinations (19,20,23).

In vivo, several human renal carcinoma cell lines were implanted subcutaneously in rats and nude mice (24). Combinations of both α and γ IFN with TNF-α resulted in significant growth inhibition of most tumors (24). Subcutaneous drug administration was more effective than intravenous or intramuscular application, in analogy to experience with IFN-α in patients with renal cell carcinoma (25). In another study with xenotransplanted human renal cell carcinoma into nude mice, a combination of IFN-α and TNF-α given intraperitoneally resulted in a response rate of 86%, with one complete tumor eradication (26). Interferons or TNF alone was far less effective (27).

In a rat model the synergistic effect of TNF-α and IFN-γ could be confirmed (24). Monotherapies could not inhibit tumor growth of an established tumor. It should be mentioned that during most in vivo and in vitro studies, different tumor cells showed varying effects of immunotherapy, confirming the heterogeneity of renal cell carcinoma.

IV. CLINICAL TRIALS WITH TNF-α AND IFN-γ

IFN-α has been extensively used as a monotherapeutic agent in advanced renal cell carcinoma. A median response rate of 15% has been seen (28). Reports of IFN-γ as monotherapy are less frequent (28–31), and overall response rates were less than 10%. In an interesting report by Aulitzky et al. (32), however, low-dose subcutaneous application (100 μg once per week) produced a 30% response rate. When combined with IFN-α, similar results have been seen with response rates from 0 to 26% (33).

Published clinical trials using TNF-α in renal cell carcinoma are scarce. In other malignancies, TNF-α has been given by intravenous, subcutaneous, intraperitoneal, intratumoral, and intracavity routes (34–41). Although initial phase I and phase II studies showed the expected toxicity, only minimal antitumor effects could be observed. Two phase I trials with a combination of TNF-α and IFN-γ were reported in 1989 and 1990 (42,43). To our knowledge, only four study groups have published results with TNF-α-containing therapies in advanced renal cell carcinoma (44–47).

Figlin et al. treated 27 patients by daily intramuscular (IM) injections of human recombinant TNF-α (45). Of 25 evaluable patients, none responded; three patients had stable disease. De Mulder et al. (44) treated 21 patients and combined 50 μg/m^2 IM with 100 μg/m^2 of subcutaneous (SC) IFN-γ. A total of seven patients dropped out of the study because of toxicity. Of 14 evaluable patients, four showed a minor response and two patients stable disease. No complete or partial response was reported.

Otto et al. (46) combined 0.16 mg/m^2 of intravenous (IV) TNF-α, five times per week every 3 weeks with IFN-α$_{2A}$ at 18×10^6 U, three times per week IM. Of 19 evaluable patients, two achieved a complete and seven a partial response, resulting in a 47% response rate.

In parallel with these studies, we started a multicenter phase I/II trial of IFN-γ, 0.05 or 0.1 mg/m^2 sc, combined with TNF-α, 0.05 or 0.1 mg/m^2 IV (47).

At all four dose levels, TNF was administered as a 24 h infusion once weekly after 3 weeks of subcutaneous IFN-γ monotherapy. Combined application was maintained for 8 weeks. All patients had documented progressive metastatic disease *after* nephrectomy without previous chemo-, radio-, or immunotherapy. Toxicity monitoring included tolerable grade I and II side effects according to World Health Organization (WHO) grading (see Table 1). In the highest dose group (cohort D), transient grade III toxicities, mainly due to fever, were observed in up to 38% of the courses. The maximum tolerated dose (MTD) was not reached in this study.

Restaging was performed after 12 weeks. When progressive disease (PD) developed, patients were withdrawn from further treatment. During the first course, three patients refused further therapy, and two patients showed rapid progression during combined treatment and also were excluded.

After the first combined treatment cycle, 22 patients were evaluable for response. We defined only complete response (CR), partial response (PR), stable disease (SD), and progressive disease. Minor regressions were considered stable disease: three patients showed CR, one patient PR, 10 patients SD, and eight patients PD. Only eight patients accepted a second treatment cycle: two patients remained in CR, one patient in PR, and two in SD, and the remaining three patients developed PD. The two CR patients developed symptoms of intracerebral metastases during treatment. Because pretreatment

Table 1 Toxicity (WHO) Grading[a]

Grade	Group (%)			
	A	B	C	D
I	0–86	0–57 ECOG index	0–27 nausea	0–38
II	0–86 fever	0–57 consciousness	0–45 fever	0–50 nausea
III	0–14 fever	0–14 nausea	0–18 nausea, fever	0–38 fever
IV	0	0	0	0

[a] Percentage rates represent number of courses during which toxicities occurred. Dose groups: A, 0.05 mg/m^2 BS (body surface area) IFN-γ, 0.05 mg/m^2 BS TNF-α; B, 0.05 mg/m^2 BS IFN-γ, 0.1 mg/m^2 BS TNF-α; C, 0.1 mg/m^2 BS IFN-γ, 0.05 mg/m^2 BS TNF-α; D, 0.1 mg/m^2 BS IFN-γ, 0.1 mg/m^2 BS TNF-α.

Table 2   Correlation Response of Metastasis Location

Site of metastasis	CR	PR	SD	PD	
Lung	2	0	8	3	13
Lung and others	1	0	1	1	3
Lymph nodes	0	0	1	3	4
Local recurrence	0	1	0	1	2
	3	1	10	8	22

computed tomography (CT) of the head was not performed, it remains uncertain whether intracerebral metastases were present before starting treatment. A total of 26 patients are evaluable for survival, and overall 15 of 26 patients are still alive, some of them more than 30 months after starting treatment. The median survival has not been reached but will exceed 17 months. There is a significant correlation between response and prolongation of survival time when SD is included in the response group ($p < 0.05$ by log rank test). It must be mentioned that six patients who withdrew from further treatment because of PD later received other immuno- or chemotherapy. As expected from previous studies, lung metastases responded best to TNF/IFN-γ treatment (see Table 2), without reaching significance levels.

V. IMMUNOLOGY

In six patients, extensive immunologic monitoring of peripheral blood was performed in our institution. Peripheral blood (60 ml) was taken before IFN-γ monotherapy, 3 weeks after starting IFN-γ, directly before the first TNF-α application, and 24 h after finishing TNF-α infusion. The results are summarized in Table 3.

According to previous reports (48,49), an activation of monocytes-macrophages was noted after IFN-γ and combined TNF/IFN-γ treatment (see Fig. 1). The postulated effect of both cytokines on NK cell activation was less than expected (50).

In detail, an augmented expression of the NK marker CD56 was noted after IFN-γ monotherapy, which remained stable after TNF-α application. Other NK markers (CD16 and CD56) did not change with IFN-γ or TNF-α therapy. IL-2 receptor expression on lymphocytes was stimulated significantly by IFN-γ but not further increased after TNF-α. In vitro induction of lymphocyte-IL-2 receptor expression was also enhanced by IFN-γ but not by TNF-α.

Table 3 Immunologic Monitoring During TNF-α/IFN-γ[a]

Lymphocyte subpopulations	IFN-γ	IFN-γ/TNF-α
IL-2R$^+$	+	Stable
NK marker CD16	Stable	Stable
NK marker CD57	+	Stable
NK marker CD56	Stable	Stable
CD3, 4, 8, 19, 45	Stable	Stable
In vitro induction IL-2R expression	+	Stable
Chemiluminescence assay, monocytes	+	+
Serum toxicity on U-937 cells	Stable	Stable
LPS- and IFN-induced IL-2 expression of monocytes	0	+

[a] Only significant changes are depicted.

On the other hand, LPS- and IFN-induced IL-2 receptor expression on monocytes was stimulated by TNF-α but not by IFN-γ. Monocytes-macrophages showed a significant increase in activity in chemiluminescence assays after IFN-γ and even more under combined TNF-α/IFN-γ treatment.

In general, a decrease in lymphocytes and monocytes occurred with IFN/TNF-α treatment but returned slowly to normal values after several weeks of treatment. Because of the small number of patients, no correlation between immunologic parameters and response was attempted. During IFN-γ and TNF/IFN-γ application, antibodies against TNF-α were not detected in repeated examinations.

Serum inhibitors of TNF-α were excluded by studying the proliferative and cytotoxic effect of patient sera on the growth of U-937 cell lines after adding TNF-α to the culture. It seems notable that under prolonged TNF-α therapy a growth stimulation on U-937 cells occurred after adding patient sera *without* in vitro addition of TNF-α (30–60% rise in counts per minute).

VI. DISCUSSION

In contrast to previous published studies using TNF-α-containing immunotherapies in renal cell carcinoma (RCC), a favorable response rate could be established in our multicenter study (44,45). Of the patients, 18% showed CR or PR and 45.5% had at least SD after 12 weeks. Before entering the study all patients had proven progressive disease after nephrectomy, as determined by two computed tomographic scans at 6-week intervals. Thus, spontaneous regressions after nephrectomy could be excluded. Most of our patients had

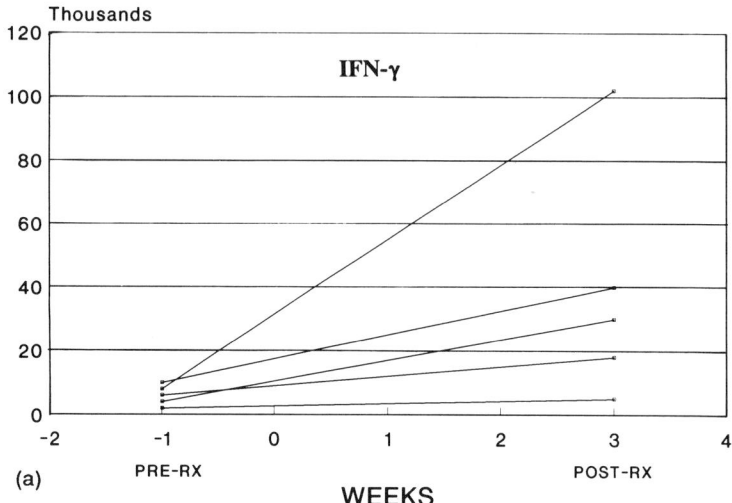

(a)

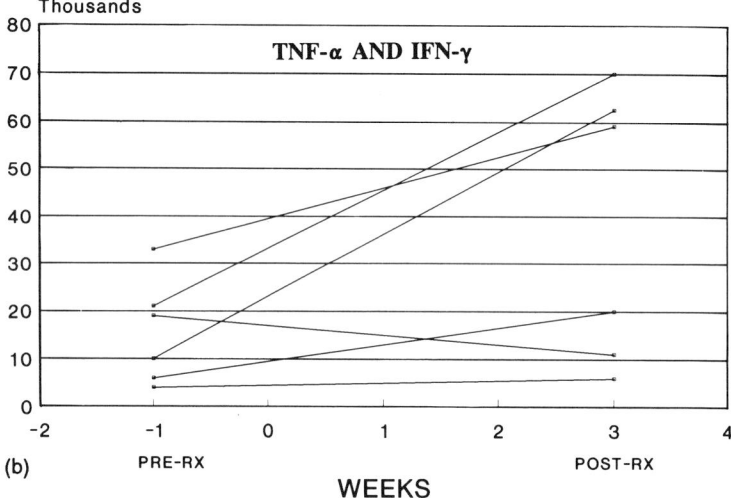

(b)

Figure 1 Phorbolmyristate (PMA)-stimulated monocyte chemiluminescence (CL, counts/minute): (a) Five patients IFN-γ monotherapy and (b) six patients TNF-α/ IFN-γ combined therapy. Values are given as integral CL activity. CL counts in 25 minutes (luminometer).

multiple progressive metastases. Generally, an 18% response rate is not an exciting success in metastatic RCC; a recently published response rate of IL-2-containing immunotherapies reached 30% and more (14,51).

From the accessible protocol information of other studies, it remains unclear whether comparably strict exclusion criteria have always been used. When placebo-controlled randomized studies are ethically impossible, the effect of a "positive superselection" may be misleading. One should keep in mind that patients can reach 5 year survival rates between 25 and 50%, if isolated lung metastases are surgically excised. Perhaps these patients should remain candidates for surgery. A short-term CR or PR is less important than prolongation of survival time, irrespective of response.

Prolongation of survival time has only rarely been used as a response parameter in previous studies, probably it means more to the incurable patient than short-term success under high treatment toxicity. Especially in the field of immunotherapy, dosage, mode of application, and dosage intervals have a strong impact on cytotoxic and immunoactivating effects (32).

This may explain the striking differences in response and toxicity between various TNF-α-containing studies (44–47). After our own preliminary experience with a TNF-α/IFN-α combination, presented by Otto et al. in Chapter 22, we must recognize that 2 h infusions with even higher doses of TNF-α (0.16 mg/m^2) for 5 days are better tolerated than 24 h infusions once a week.

Immunologic monitoring of patients receiving TNF-α-containing therapies remains another point of debate. Several studies have shown a significant decrease in macrophage activation in patients with metastatic disease (52,53). TNF-α is a potent activator of macrophage-monocyte function, which was confirmed by our immunologic monitoring. Macrophages and monocytes showed statistically significant activation in chemiluminescence assays and in LPS- and IFN-induced IL-2 receptor expression. T cell IL-2 receptor expression was augmented by IFN-γ, but not by TNF-α, but enhanced NK cell activity could not be identified 24 h after TNF-α treatment. In is interesting to note that sera of TNF-treated patients enhanced the spontaneous proliferation rates of U-937 cell lines. These findings confirm previous observations on macrophage activation during TNF-α therapy (48,49). TNF-α-mediated NK cell activation remains a point of discussion: contradictory findings may be explained by different dosages, application forms, and intervals for immunologic monitoring (50,54).

TNF-α certainly has procoagulant activity, which results in vascular leak and leukocyte adhesion to the endothelial layer. This generalized effect after systemic TNF-α application may explain the disappearance of leukocytes from peripheral blood samples directly after TNF-α application, as described by other authors (42,49). In this case the discrepancy between locally active lymphocyte populations and their representation in the peripheral circulation becomes obvious and hampers conclusions concerning the immunologic effect of applied immunostimulations. These phenomena may explain the difficulties in various immunotherapeutic studies in comparing clinical and immunologic response.

VII. CONCLUSIONS

TNF-α and IFN-γ have shown synergistic effects in models of renal cell carcinoma in vivo and in vitro. Clinically, however, few studies have been performed in metastatic renal carcinoma (44–47). Treatment protocols, inclusion criteria, administration routes, intervals, and dosages of TNF-α differ, and conclusions are not possible.

The only multicenter study combining TNF-α and IFN-γ was performed under guidance of our institution and demonstrated an 18% response rate (CR and PR) in 22 evaluable patients. Toxicity was tolerable, and possible significant prolongation of survival time even in stable disease was noted. Immunologically, a significant rise in monocyte/macrophage activation was found, whereas NK cell activity remained stable after TNF-α application. Immunologic monitoring of TNF-α-containing therapies remains problematic because of PAF- and PGE_2-mediated enhanced leukocyte adherence to vascular endothelium and consequent peripheral leukocyte deprivation. A promising multicenter study on the combination of TNF-α and IFN-α, based on monocenter data from Otto et al. (46), is underway at our institution.

REFERENCES

1. Linehan WM, Shipley WU, Longo DL. Cancer of the kidney and ureter. In: De Vita VT, Hellmann S, Rosenberg SA, eds. Cancer, principles and practice of oncology. Philadelphia: Lippincott, 1989; 979–998.
2. DeKernion JB, Ramming KP, Smith RB. The natural history of metastatic renal cell carcinoma: a computer analysis. J Urol 1978; 120:148–52.
3. Silverberg E. Statistical and epidemiologic data on urologic cancer. Cancer 1987; 60:692–717.
4. Golimbu M, Al-Askari S, Tessler P, Morales P. Aggressive treatment of metastatic renal cancer. J Urol 1986; 136:807.
5. Linehan WM. Introduction. In: Debruyne FMJ, Bukowski RM, Pontes JE, de Mulder PHM, eds. Immunotherapy of renal cell carcinoma. Berlin: Springer-Verlag, 1991; 1–3.

6. Fowler JE. Nephrectomy in metastatic renal cell carcinoma. Urol Clin North Am 1987; 14:749–52.

7. Trasher JB, Clark JR, Cleland BP. Surgery for pulmonary metastases from renal cell carcinoma. Urol 1990; 35:487–91.

8. Flanigan RF. Operative Behandlung des metastasierten. Nierenzellkarzinoms Extracta Urol 1991; 14:8–14.

9. DeKernion JB. Treatment of advanced renal cell carcinoma. Traditional methods and innovative approaches. J Urol 1983; 130:2–7.

10. Tolia BM, Whitmore WF Jr. Solitary metastases from renal cell carcinoma. J Urol 1975; 114:836–8.

11. Neves RJ, Zincke H, Taylor WF. Metastatic renal cell cancer and radical nephrectomy: identification of prognostic factors and patient survival. J Urol 1988; 139:1173–6.

12. Quesada JR, Swanson DA, Trinidade A, Gutterman JV. Renal cell carcinoma: antitumor effects of leucocyte interferon. Cancer Res 1983; 43:940–5.

13. Wirth M. Stellenwert der Interferone, des Interleukin 2 und des Tumornekrosefaktors in der Therapie des Nierenzellkarzinoms. Urologe A 1991; 30:77–80.

14. Bergmann L, Weidmann E, Mitron PS. Immuntherapie des fortgeschrittenen. Nierenzellkarzinoms Dtsch Med Wochenschr 1991; 116:384–90.

15. Carswell EA, Old LJ, Kassel RL, et al. An endotoxin-induced serum factor that causes necrosis of tumors. Proc Natl Acad Sci U S A 1975; 72:3666–70.

16. Balkwill FR. Does tumor necrosis factor have a future in cancer therapy? In: Broden EJ, ed. Progress in oncology. Updates in cytokines. Basel: Hoffmann-LaRoche, 1990; 11–8.

17. Meager A. Cytokines. Buckingham: open university press, 1990; 144–242.

18. Fransen L, van der Heyden J, Ruysschaert R, Fiers W. Recombinant tumor necrosis factor: its effect and its synergism with interferon-gamma on a variety of normal and transformed human cell lines. Eur J Cancer Clin Oncol 1986; 22:419–22.

19. Van Moorselaar RJA, Beniers AJMC, Schalken JA, Debruyne FMJ. In: Debruyne FMJ, Bukowski RM, Pones JE, deMulder PHM, eds. Interferon and tumor necrosis factor in renal cell carcinoma model system. Berlin: Springer-Verlag, 1991: 47–54.

20. Kavaussi LR, Ruesing RA, Hudson MA, et al. Effect of tumor necrosis factor and interferon gamma on human renal carcinoma cell line growth. J Urol 1989; 142:875–8.

21. Sugarman BJ, Aggarual BB, Hass PE, et al. Recombinant human tumor necrosis factor: effects on proliferation of normal and transformed cells in vitro. Science 1985; 230:943–8.

22. Fox B, Mule J, Kasid A, et al. Treatment of murine tumor targets with TNF and interferon gamma but not with interferon alpha unmasks specific cytotoxicity by a long-term cultured tumor infiltrating lymphocyte (TIL) line. Proc Am Assoc Cancer Res 1989; 30 (1497):377.

23. Dubois MF, Ferrieux C, Lebon P. Synergistic cytotoxic effects of recombinant human tumor necrosis factor, interferons and heat-stress. Cancer Res 1989; 49:5618–22.

24. Van Moorselaar RJA, Beniers AJMC, Hendriks BTH, et al. In vivo Antiproliferative Effects of Gamma Interferon and tumor necrosis factor alpha in a rat renal cell carcinoma model system. J Urol 1990; 143:1247–51.

25. Aulitzky W, Gastl G, Aulitzky WE, et al. Successful treatment of metastatic renal cell carcinoma with a biologically active dose of recombinant interferon gamma. J Clin Oncol 1989; 7:1875–8.

26. Baisch H, Otto U, Kloppel G. Antiproliferative and cytotoxic effects of single and combined treatment with tumor necrosis factor or interferon on a human renal cell carcinoma, xenotransplanted into nu/nu mice: cell kenetic studies. Cancer Res 1990; 50:6389–95.

27. Bregman MD, Meyskens FL. Human recombinant alpha- and gamma-interferons enhance the cytotoxic properties of tumor necrosis factor on human melanoma. J Biol Response Mod 1988; 7:384–9.

28. Horaszewicz JS, Murphy GP. An assessment of the current use of human interferons in therapy of urological cancers. J Urol 1989; 142:1173–80.

29. Research group on renal cell carcinoma. Recombinant Human Interferon Gamma (S-6810). Phase II study of recombinant human interferon gamma on renal cell carcinoma. Cancer 1987; 60:929–33.

30. Laszlo J, Goldstein D, Gockerman J, et al. Phase I studies of recombinant interferon. J Biol Response Mod 1990; 9:185–93.

31. Garnick MB, Reich SD, Maxwell B, et al. Phase I/II study of recombinant interferon gamma in advanced renal cell carcinoma. J Urol 1988; 139:251–5.

32. Aulitzky W, Gastl G, Aulitzky WE, et al. Successful treatment of metastatic renal cell carcinoma with a biologically active dose of recombinant interferon/gamma. Eur Urol 1990; 18/51:260A.

33. De Mulder PHM, Franssen MPH, Punt CJA, et al. Monotherapy and combination therapy with interferon-α, interferon-γ, and tumor necrosis factor-α in metastatic renal cell carcinoma. In Dubruyne FMJ, Bukowski RM, Pontes JE, de Mulder PHM, eds. Immunotherapy of renal cell carcinoma. Berlin: Springer-Verlag, 1991; 82–90.

34. Retsas S, Leslie M, Bottomley D. Interlesional tumor necrosis factor combined with interferon gamma in metastatic melanoma. Br Med J 1989; 298:1290–1.

35. Moritz T, Niederle N, Baumann J, et al. Phase I study of recombinant human tumor necrosis factor alpha in advanced malignant disease. Cancer Immunol Immunother 1989; 29:144–50.

36. Freund M, Kleine HD, Steinmeier O, et al. Treatment of patients with AML and advanced CML with recombinant tumor necrosis factor (TNF-α). Ann Hematol 1991; Suppl 1:123A.

37. Breth U, Schmidt H, Karck V, et al. Phase II-trial of recombinant human tumor necrosis factor alpha in patients with malignant ascites from ovarian carcinomas and non-ovarian tumors with intra-peritoneal spread. Proc ASCO 1991; 10:187.

38. Wanebo HJ. Tumor necrosis factors. Semin Surg Oncol 1989; 5:402–13.
39. Fudimoto S, Itano S, Kimura T, et al. Phase I and early phase II clinical study of a new anti-tumor lymphokine (OH1) produced by stimulated B-cell leukemia Line, BALL-1. Proc ASCO 1986; 5:232.
40. Chapman PB, Lester TJ, Casper ES, et al. Clinical pharmacology of recombinant human tumor necrosis factor in patients with advanced disease. J Clin Oncol 1987; 5:1942–51.
41. Pfreundschuh MG, Steinmetz HT, Tuschen R. Phase I study of intratumoral application of recombinant human tumor necrosis factor. Eur J Cancer Clin Oncol 1989; 25:379–88.
42. Demetri GD, Spriggs DR, Sherman ML. A phase I trial of recombinant human tumor necrosis factor and interferon-gamma: effects of combination cytokine administration in vivo. J Clin Oncol 1989; 7:1545–53.
43. Schiller JH, Alberti DB, Arzoomaion RZ. Phase I trial of combination of recombinant gamma interferon and recombinant tumor necrosis factor alpha. Proc Am Assoc Cancer Res 1990; 31:183.
44. DeMulder P, Debruyne F, Rikken G, et al. Recombinant tumor necrosis factor alpha and interferon-gamma in the treatment of advanced renal cell carcinoma (RCC). Proc ASCO 1989; 8:144.
45. Figlin R, deKernion J, Sarna G, et al. Phase II study of recombinant tumor necrosis factor in patients with metastatic renal cell (RCC). Proc ASCO 1988; 7:169.
46. Otto U, Conrad S, Schneider AW. Combined therapy with TNF-alpha and IFN-alpha 2A in metastatic renal cell carcinoma. Promising preclinical and clinical results. In: Deicher H et al., eds. How to optimize IFN-therapy. VI European Interferon Workshop, February 27–March 1, 1991, Hannover.
47. Sohn M, Levens W, Rubben H, et al. Phase I/II trial with TNF/GAMMA-interferon in metastatic renal cell carcinoma. J Cancer Res Clin Oncol 1990; 116:1058.
48. Conkling PR, Chua CC, Nadler P, et al. Clinical trials with human tumor necrosis factor: in vivo and in vitro effects of human mononuclear phagocyte function. Cancer Res 1988; 48:5604–9.
49. Schiller JH, Storer BE, Witt PL. Biological and clinical effects of intravenous tumor necrosis factor-α administered three times weekly. Cancer Res 1991; 51:1651–8.
50. Mannel PN, Kist A, Ho AD. Tumor necrosis factor production and natural killer and activity in periperal blood during treatment with recombinant tumor necrosis factor. Br J Cancer 1989; 60:585–8.
51. Atzpodien JA, Korfer CR, Franks H, et al. Home therapy with recombinant interleukin 2 and interferon alpha 2b in advanced human malignancies. Lancet 1990; 335:1509–12.
52. Boetcher DA, Leonard EJ. Abnormal monocyte chemotactic response in cancer patients. J Natl Cancer Inst 1974; 52:1091–9.

53. Kleinermann ES, Honeser D, Yaung RC, et al. Defective monocyte killing in patients with malignancies and restoration of function during chemotherapy. Lancet 1980; 2:1102–5.

54. Kist A, Ho AD, Roth V, et al. Decrease of natural killer cell activate and monokine production in periperal blood of patients treated with recombinant tumor necrosis factor. Blood 1988; 72:344–8.

24

Immunotherapy of Patients with Metastatic Renal Cell Carcinoma Using an Outpatient Regimen of Interleukin-2 and Interferon-α

UCLA School of Medicine

Robert A. Figlin, William C. Pierce, Nancy Moldawer, Jean B. deKernion, and Arie Belldegrun

UCLA School of Medicine, Los Angeles, California

I. INTRODUCTION

Renal cell carcinoma (RCC) is the most common malignancy of the kidney. Approximately 24,000 cases of RCC occurred in 1991, which accounts for nearly 3% of all adult neoplasms. Nearly 50% of patients with localized renal cell carcinoma are cured by surgery, but the treatment of metastatic renal cell carcinoma has been in the most part ineffective, with a median survival of approximately 10 months. The Eastern Cooperative Oncology Group identified performance status, time from initial diagnosis, number of metastatic sites, prior cytotoxic chemotherapy, and recent weight loss as important indicators for survival (1). Many cytotoxic agents have been utilized as single agents in an attempt to impact metastatic RCC, but response rates with all agents is low, usually less than 10% (2,3). Chemotherapy has not been demonstrated to improve survival for these patients. Early reports with progesterone therapy generated some enthusiasm (4), but subsequent studies failed to produce a significant number of objective responses (5). The ineffectiveness of standard modalities of therapy led to the early application of immunotherapy for metastatic RCC and has helped to usher in a new era in cancer therapy.

II. IMMUNOTHERAPY

A. General Principles

Although clinically apparent RCC leads to patient death in the absence of effective therapy, the natural history of RCC is not fully understood. A carefully performed study revealed 235 unrecognized cases of RCC in 16,294 autopsies performed in Malmo, Sweden (6). This behavior can be explained by immunologic surveillance of RCC. Advances in immunology and molecular biology have generated a vast array of active substances commonly known as biologic response modifiers. These agents are capable of enhancing the immune destruction of tumors by altering the immunogenicity of tumor cells or by increasing the effectiveness of the immune response.

The immunologic approach to therapy can be classified as active or passive. An example of passive or adoptive immunotherapy is the transfer to the tumor-bearing host of active immunologic agents, such as cells with antitumor activity, that can directly destroy tumor. Active immunotherapy refers to methods used to directly stimulate the immune system of the host to improve tumor destruction. Examples of immune stimulators include bacillus Calmette-Guérin vaccine, autologous tumor cells or antigens, and cytokines. Cytokines are a class of proteins that are crucial to the activation, regulation, communication, and effector functions of the immune system. An attractive means by which the immunologic destruction of tumor might be enhanced is by providing the tumor-bearing host with both active and passive immunotherapy.

B. Interferons

The interferons constitute a complex family of inducible cellular glycoproteins. The three major classes of interferons are designated α, β, and γ. In 1983, two groups simultaneously reported the regression of metastatic RCC in response to partially purified human leukocyte interferon (7,8). Subsequent studies revealed a response rate of 15–20%, establishing the interferons as one of the most effective single agents for metastatic renal cell carcinoma (9,10). The mechanism(s) by which the interferons display antitumor effects in vivo are not known. They may enhance the immunogenicity of tumor cells by enhancing the expression of major histocompatibility complex (MHC) class I and class II antigens. Malignant proliferation may be slowed by the inhibition of oncogene expression (11). Cytotoxicity by effector cells may be enhanced.

Recent in vitro and xenograft models of RCC suggest that interferon-α (IFN-α) may inhibit RCC by preventing the expression of a 160 kD kidney-restricted glycoprotein (gp160). RCC cell lines that express gp160 are interferon-α-resistant, and those that are gp160 negative are sensitive (12).

C. Interleukins

The discovery of the T cell growth factor interleukin-2 (IL-2) has ushered in a new era in the field of cancer immunotherapy and has opened new avenues of approach for the treatment of metastatic RCC. IL-2 is a lymphokine produced and secreted by T lymphocytes. This important glycoprotein molecule is intimately involved in most if not all of the immune responses in which T lymphocytes play a role. High-dose IL-2 was used to treat 54 patients with RCC at the National Cancer Institute (NCI), and 4 complete responses (CR) plus 8 partial responses (PR) occurred, for a response rate of 22% (13). Some of the responses were durable, a phenomenon not observed with interferon treatment. The treatment resulted in frequent and severe toxicity, however, which greatly diminishes its potential clinical utility. It has been demonstrated that low-dose continuous-infusion IL-2 has clinical efficacy and can be administered with acceptable toxicity (14).

III. COMBINATION BIOLOGIC THERAPY

Many of the most effective cytotoxic chemotherapeutic regimens involve combinations of chemotherapeutic agents. This basic concept, together with the probability that the immunologic destruction of tumor cells is most likely a multistep process, has led to combination cytokine therapy. Interferons α and γ have demonstrated synergistic antiproliferative effects against RCC in vitro (15). This observation when applied clinically demonstrated that sequentially administered interferons α and γ resulted in 2 CR and 6 PR of 30 assessable patients (15).

IL-2 and lymphokine-activated killer (LAK) cells have been combined in immunotherapy. LAK cells are generated when resting lymphocytes are incubated in IL-2 for 3–4 days. These cells become capable of lysing a variety of fresh natural killer (NK) cell-resistant tumor cells in vitro. There are several reports of the efficacy of IL-2 and lymphocyte-activated killer cells in metastatic RCC (16–18). A total of 72 patients with metastatic RCC received LAK plus high-dose IL-2 at the NCI. There was a 35% response rate, with 8 CR plus 17 PR (13). There was, in addition, significant toxicity. In some reports, however, the addition of LAK cell infusions to IL-2 regimens did not produce a noticeable change in antitumor response rate compared to IL-2 alone but resulted in more severe toxicity (16). Thus, the contribution of LAK to the clinical responses associated with high-dose IL-2 is yet to be defined.

The improved response of metastatic RCC to biologic therapy led to the development at the University of California–Los Angeles (UCLA) of an outpatient-based combination biologic therapy protocol. The documented modest activity of both interferon-α and IL-2 in the treatment of metastatic RCC in combination with their differing biologic activities led us to combine these agents in our phase II protocol. Patients received either continuously infused or subcutaneously administered IL-2 together with subcutaneously administered interferon-α. For the continuous-infusion patients, the first course of IL-2 was administered in the hospital; all other therapies were given on an outpatient basis. The remainder of this chapter describes the UCLA experience with outpatient-based combination biologic therapy for metastatic RCC.

IV. PHASE II STUDY

A. Materials and Methods

A group of 52 eligible patients with histologically confirmed metastatic RCC were consecutively entered in the trial (19,20). All patients had bidimensionally measurable disease, adequate blood counts (hemoglobin $\geq$ 10 g/dl, granulocytes greater than 1500 mm^{-3}, and platelets greater than 100,000 mm^3), adequate renal and hepatic function (serum creatinine less than 2 mg/dl, serum bilirubin less than 1.6 g/dl, and SGOT less than 150 IU or less than four times the upper limits of normal), prothrombin and partial thromboplastin time within 50% of normal, and a performance status greater than 70% (Karnofsky scale). Exclusion criteria for this trial included prior therapy with IL-2 or IFN-α; anticancer therapy within 4 weeks of initiation of therapy; clinically significant pulmonary dysfunction; pleural effusion; ascites; cardiac disease (e.g., congestive heart failure, symptomatic coronary artery disease, cardiac arrhythmias, prior myocardial infarction, or hypertension requiring β-adrenergic or calcium channel blockers); active infection; serum calcium greater than 12 mg/dl; major surgery within the preceding 3 weeks; prior malignancy; active peptic ucler disease; corticosteroid use; and central nervous system disease (e.g., brain metastasis, psychiatric illness, or seizure disorder). Patients were provided with and signed an informed consent approved by the University of California at Los Angeles Human Subject Protection Committee.

Recombinant human interleukin-2 (rhIL-2; Teceleukin, Ro 23-6019) was provided by Hoffmann-La Roche (Nutley, NJ) as a lyophilized powder in sterile 5 ml vials. The vials contained approximately 1 or 5 million units of rhIL-2 and were reconstituted with 1 ml sterile preservative-free isotonic saline. The specific activity of rhIL-2 was $1.5-2.0 \times 10^7$ U/mg protein based on an rhIL-2 bioassay using a calorimetric determination of cell growth.

In all the patients who received continuous-infusion IL-2, an indwelling double-lumen central venous catheter (Davol, Inc., Cranston, RI) was inserted before initiating treatment. Prophylactic antibiotic support was not used. rhIL-2 was administered for 4 consecutive days on days 1–4 of each treatment week as a continuous intravenous (IV) infusion (96 h) in 100 ml normal saline via the Strato micropump (Strato Medical Corporation, Beverly, MA): eight patients received fixed-dose IL-2, 4 MU/day; 30 patients received infusional IL-2 at 2 MU/m^2/day. Patients on infusional IL-2 received rhIFN-α_{2A} at 6 MU/m^2/day, with each dose of interferon-α administered subcutaneously or intramuscularly on days 1 and 4 of each treatment week before bedtime. A total of 14 patients were placed on a subcutaneous regimen of IL-2 and interferon-α. Pharmacokinetic studies have demonstrated that IL-2 can be safely administered via a subcutaneous route and measurable levels can be obtained in the serum (21). Subcutaneous administration of IL-2 abrogates the necessity of central line placement as well as the cost of the pump apparatus necessary for continuous-infusion IL-2 administration. Patients enrolled on the subcutaneous protocol received 4 MU IL-2 subcutaneously each day, given as a single daily dose on 4 consecutive days; no treatment was rendered on days 5, 6, and 7 of each treatment week. Interferon-α 9 MU was administered subcutaneously as a single evening dose on days 1 and 4. Dose escalation was not permitted at any time. Patients were closely monitored for changes in clinical status, including vital signs, body weight, and physical examination on a weekly basis while receiving therapy. Treatment was withheld from patients with grade III toxicity until symptoms improved, and treatment was resumed at a lower dose of IL-2 with no modification to the rhIFN-α_{2A} dose. Treatment was withheld from patients with a second grade III toxicity until symptoms improved, and treatment was resumed at a lower dosage of rhIL-2 and rhIFN-α_{2A}. Development of any grade IV nonhematologic toxicity required discontinuation of therapy. Toxicities were evaluated according to a modified World Health Organization toxicity grading scale. Courses of rhIL-2 and rhIFN-α_{2A} were continued until disease progression, unacceptable toxicity, or a maximum of six courses (36 weeks).

Patients received acetaminophen, 650 mg orally every 4 h as needed for fever, indomethacin, 25–50 mg orally 30 minutes before and 4 h following the rhIFN-α_{2A} injection, 50 mg oral meperidine 30 minutes following the rhIFN-α_{2A} injection and as needed to control rigors throughout the course of treatment, diphenhydramine at 25–50 mg orally as needed for rash and pruritus, and diphenozylate hydrochloride with atropine sulfate, 10 mg orally as needed for nausea and vomiting. Postural hypotension and volume depletion were managed with fluid administration.

A complete response was defined as the complete disappearance of all clinically detectable disease for a minimum of 4 weeks. A partial response was defined as a 50% or greater decrease in the sum of the products of the two longest perpendicular diameters of all measurable lesions for at least 4 weeks with no simultaneous progression of evaluable disease, or the appearance of new lesions. Stable disease (SD) was defined as a less than 25% increase or a less than 50% decrease in tumor size with no simultaneous progression of evaluable disease, or the appearance of new lesions. Progressive disease was defined as an increase of greater than 25% in measurable lesions, or the appearance of new lesions. A pathologic complete remission was defined as clinically apparent disease that upon surgical resection revealed no pathologic evidence of renal cell carcinoma. A surgical complete remission was defined as clinically apparent disease that, upon surgical resection, rendered the patient clinically disease free but that renal cell carcinoma was found in the pathologic specimen. Patients were evaluated for response after each 6-week course of treatment. Response duration was calculated from the date of the initial response to the most recent evaluation of that response or to documentation of progression. Survival duration was calculated as the length of survival from the initiation of treatment.

Serum samples for the measurement of rhIFN-α_{2A} antibodies were collected before treatment, after every two courses of treatment, and at study termination or withdrawal. The samples were obtained approximately 48–72 h following the completion of therapy to minimize potential assay interference by cytokine presence in the serum. An enzyme immunoassay (EIA) was used to screen all serum samples for rhIFN-α_{2A} (21) and rhIL-2 (Gallati, personal communication). Those sera found to be positive for antibodies by the EIA were subsequently tested for the presence of neutralizing antibody by a neutralization bioassay.

B. Results

A total of 52 patients were evaluated, including 38 men and 14 women: 50 patients were evaluable for response and 51 for toxicity. The ages ranged from 29 to 79, with a median of 57. The median Karnofsky performance status was 90. Of all patients 75% had received nephrectomy before initiation of immunotherapy. An initial disease-free interval of greater than 12 months was experienced by 42% of patients. Sites of metastatic disease included lung and other sites in 44% of patients, lung only (parenchyma) in 35% of patients, local recurrence in 29% of patients, bone in 21% of patients, liver in 21% of patients, and peripheral lymph nodes in 12% of patients. Prior chemotherapy or hormonal or radiation therapy occurred in only 8% of patients. No patients received prior biologic therapy. There were 14 objective responders of 50 evaluable patients who received combination biologic therapy (28%); two patients (4%) achieved a pathologic complete remission, and 1 (2%) achieved a surgical complete remission. The two patients who achieved a pathologic complete remission appeared to have residual tumor on restaging but, upon surgical exploration, had no viable tumor in the resected specimen. The patient who had a surgical complete remission had viable tumor in the lesion persisting upon restaging. A total of 11 patients (22%) showed a partial response; seven (14%) patients had stable disease and 29 (58%) had progressive disease on combination biologic therapy. The median duration of response for patients who achieved a complete remission is 18^+ months ($15^+ - 28^+$) and for partial response patients is 5^+ months ($1^+ - 24^+$). No complete responders have yet relapsed.

C. Toxicity

Toxicities were frequent but for the most part manageable. All patients developed fever greater than 38°C and chills, and all patients also developed a pruritic, erythematous rash during the first week of the first cycle of biologic therapy, which slowly resolved but did not recur with subsequent courses of therapy. Most (98%) patients experienced fatigue and anorexia, 92% experienced diarrhea, and 96% experienced nausea and vomiting. Reversible thyroid dysfunction characterized by hypo- and hyperfunction occurred in 91% of evaluated patients (23). The incidence of thyroid dysfunction increased with increased numbers of treatment cycles. Thyroid function normalized following therapy in all patients and was not dose limiting. Hypotension requiring the administration of IV fluids between cycles occurred in 17% of patients. Myalgias and arthralgias occurred in 19% of patients. Neurologic dysfunction, including somnolence and disorientation, occurred in 13%, paresthesias in 17%, and carpal tunnel syndrome in 2% of patients. Pulmonary toxicity, including dyspnea at rest, occurred in only one (2%) patient. Cardiovascular events, including arrhythmias and pericarditis, occurred in 6%. A single patient with cardiac toxicity died (2%). Abnormal renal function characterized by a creatinine of 2.1–5 times normal occurred in 25% of patients. Liver dysfunction reflected by a SGOT greater than four times normal or a bilirubin greater than 1.7 times normal occurred in 22% of patients. Hematologic toxicities included anemia requiring transfusions in 19%, neutrophil counts less than 1000 μl^{-1} in 14%, and platelet counts less than 100,000 μl^{-1} in 8% of patients. Central line sepsis occurred in 6% of patients, and six (11%) patients experienced symptoms of fever, chills, nausea, and pruritus similar to symptoms experienced while on IL-2 therapy following IV contrast administration for the routine follow-up of measurable disease by computed tomographic imaging (24). Despite the frequency of toxicities, grade III or IV toxicities requiring dosage modifications were rare. Severe nausea and vomiting required dosage modification in 17% of patients. Severe fatigue occurred in 15%. Somnolence and disorientation requiring dosage modification occurred in 10%. Significant arrhythmias occurred in 4%. Intractable diarrhea occurred in 4%, and significant pulmonary dysfunction occurred in 2% of patients. Severe granulocytopenia requiring dosage modification occurred in one (2%) patient. All patients were evaluated for the development of antibodies to rhIFN-α_{2A} and rhIL-2 antibodies. No patient developed antibodies as measured by the EIA.

V. DISCUSSION

There is clearly a role for biologic therapy in the management of metastatic renal cell carcinoma (25). Single-agent interferon-α has a reproducible, modest effect on the disease. The combination of several biologic agents is a logical extension of this single-agent activity. In experimental murine models, the combination of IL-2 and interferon-α has resulted in enhanced efficacy compared to either agent alone (26–28). Multiple phase I trials have reported on this combination of agents and have demonstrated activity in renal cell carcinoma (29–36). Our phase II trials demonstrate that an outpatient-based regimen of IL-2 and interferon-α can be safely administered and in our hands resulted in a response rate of 28%. IL-2 can be administered via continuous infusion or by subcutaneous injection. Responses were noted in the lung, mediastinum, perirenal and peripheral lymph nodes, and renal fossa. Although by standard clinical criteria all responses were partial, complete pathologic remissions were noted and none of these remissions has relapsed to date.

We have demonstrated that combination biologic therapy can be safely and effectively utilized in the treatment of metastatic renal cell carcinoma and that the treatment can be effectively administered on an outpatient basis. We are currently attempting to expand on this modality of therapy by incorporating tumor-infiltrating lymphocytes and additional biologic agents in the therapeutic regimen.

REFERENCES

1. Elson JB, Witte RS, Trump DL. Prognostic factors for survival in recurrent or metastatic renal cell carcinoma. Cancer Res 1978; 48:7310.
2. Yagoda A. Chemotherapy of renal cell carcinoma. Sem Urol 1989; 7:199.
3. deKernion JB. Treatment of advanced renal cell carcinoma. Traditional and innovative approaches. J Urol 1983; 130:2.
4. Hrushesky WJ, Murphy GP. Current status of the therapy of advanced renal carcinoma. J Surg Oncol 1977; 9:277.
5. deKernion JB, Ramming KD, Smith RB. The natural history of metastatic renal cell carcinoma: a computer analysis. J Urol 1978; 120:148.
6. Hellsten S, Berge T, Wehlin L. Unrecognized renal cell carcinoma: clinical and diagnostic aspects. Scand J Urol Nephrol 1981; 8:269.
7. deKernion JB, Sarna G, Figlin RA, et al. The treatment of renal cell carcinoma with human leukocyte alpha-interferon. J Urol 1983; 130:1063.
8. Quesada JR, Swanson DA, Trinidade A, et al. Renal cell carcinoma: antitumor effects of leukocyte interferon. Cancer Res 1983; 43:940.
9. Figlin RA, deKernion JB, Mukamel E, et al. Recombinant interferon alpha-2a in metastatic renal cell carcinoma: assessment of antitumor activity and anti-interferon antibody formation. J Clin Oncol 1988; 6:1604.
10. Sarna G, Figlin RA, deKernion JB. Interferon in renal cell carcinoma: the UCLA experience. Cancer 1987; 59:610.
11. Kirkwood JM, Ernstoff MS. Interferons in the treatment of human cancer. J Clin Oncol 1984; 2:352.
12. Nanus, DM, Pfeffer LM, Bander NH, et al. Antiproliferative and antitumor effect of alpha-interferon in renal cell carcinoma: correlation to expression of a kidney associated differentiation glycoprotein. Cancer Res 1990; 50:4190.
13. Rosenberg SA, Lotze MT, Yang YC, et al. Experience with the use of high-dose interleukin-2 in the treatment of 652 cancer patients. Ann Surg 1989; 210:474.
14. Sosman JA, Kohler PC, Hank J, et al. Repetitive weekly cycles of recombinant human interleukin-2: responses of renal cell carcinoma with acceptable toxicity. J Natl Cancer Inst 1988; 80:60.
15. Ernstoff MS, Nair S, Bahnson RR, et al. A phase IA trial of sequential administration recombinant DNA-produced interferon: combination recombinant interferon gamma and recombinant interferon alpha in patients with metastatic renal carcinoma. J Clin Oncol 1990; 8:1637.
16. Albertini MR, Sosman JA, Hank JA, et al. The influence of autologous lymphokine-activated killer cell infusion on the toxicity and antitumor effect of repetitive cycles of interleukin-2. Cancer 1990; 66:2457.

17. Clark JW, Smith JW II, Steis RG, et al. Interleukin-2 and lymphokine-activated killer cell therapy: analysis of a bolus interleukin-2 and a continuous infusion interleukin-2 regimen. Cancer Res 1990; 50:7343.

18. Gaynor ER, Weiss GR, Margolin KR, et al. Phase I study of high-dose continuous-infusion interleukin-2 and autologous lymphokine-activated killer cells in patients with metastatic or unresectable malignant melanoma and renal cell carcinoma. J Natl Cancer Inst 1990; 82:1397.

19. Figlin RA, Belldegrun A, Moldawer N, et al. Concomitant administration of recombinant human interleukin-2 and recombinant interferon alpha-2A: an active outpatient regimen in metastatic renal cell carcinoma. J Clin Oncol 1992; 10:414.

20. Figlin RA, Belldegrun A, deKernion J. Immunotherapy of patients with metastatic renal cell carcinoma (RCCa) using an outpatient regimen of interleukin-2 (IL-2) and interferon-alpha (IFN) administered either alone or with in vivo primed tumor infiltrating lymphocytes (pTIL): the UCLA experience (abstract) ASCO. Proc Am Soc Clin Oncol 1992; 11:197.

21. Whitehead RP, Ward D, Hemmingway L, et al. Subcutaneous recombinant interleukin 2 in a dose escalating regimen in patients with metastatic renal cell adenocarcinoma. Cancer Res 1990; 50:6708.

22. Hennes U, Jucker W, Fisher EA, et al. The detection of antibodies to recombinant interferon alpha-2A in human serum. J Biol Stand 1987; 15:231.

23. Jacobs EL, Clare-Salzler MJ, Chopra IJ, et al. Thyroid function abnormalities associated with the chronic outpatient administration of recombinant interleukin-2 and recombinant interferon-alpha. J Immunother 1991; 10(6):448.

24. Abi-Aad S, Figlin RA, Belldegrun A, et al. Metastatic renal cell cancer: Interleukin-2 toxicity induced by contrast agent injection. J Immunother (in press) 10(4):292.

25. Quesada JR. Biologic response modifiers in the therapy of metastatic renal cell carcinoma. Semin Oncol 1988; 15:396.

26. Cameron RB, McIntosh JK, Rosenberg SA. Synergistic antitumor effects of combination immunotherapy with recombinant interleukin-2 and a recombinant hybrid alpha-interferon in the treatment of established murine hepatic metastases. Cancer Res 1988; 48:5810.

27. West WH, Tauer KW, Yannelli JR, et al. Constant-infusion recombinant interleukin-2 in adoptive immunotherapy in advanced cancer. N Engl J Med 1987; 316:898.

28. Sosman JA, Kohler PC, Hank J, et al. Repetitive weekly cycles of recombinant human interleukin-2: responses of renal carcinoma with acceptable toxicity. J Natl Cancer Inst 1988; 80:60.

29. Rosenberg SA, Lotze MT, Yang JC, et al. Combination therapy with interleukin-2 and alpha-interferon for the treatment of patients with advanced cancer. J Clin Oncol 1989; 7:1863.

30. Hirsh M, Lipton A, Harvey H, et al. Phase I study of interleukin-2 and recombinant interferon alpha 2A: an outpatient therapy for patients with advanced malignancy. J Clin Oncol 1990; 8:1657.

31. Mittelman A, Huberman MJ, Puccio C, et al. A phase I study of recombinant human interleukin-2 and alpha-interferon-2A in patients with renal cell cancer, colorectal cancer and malignant melanoma. Cancer 1990; 66:664.

32. Lee RH, Talpaz M, Rothberg HM, et al. Concomitant administration of recombinant human interleukin-2 and recombinant interferon alpha-2A in cancer patients: a phase I study. J Clin Oncol 1989; 7:1726.

33. Budd GT, Osgood B, Barna B, et al. Phase I clinical trial of interleukin-2 and alpha-interferon: toxicity and immunologic effects. Cancer Res 1989; 49:6432.

34. Sznol M, Mier JW, Sparano J, et al. A phase I study of high dose interleukin-2 in combination with interferon-alpha-2b. J Biol Response Mod 1990; 9:529.

35. Bukowski RM, Murphy S, Sergi J, et al. Phase I trial of continuous infusion recombinant interleukin-2 and intermittent interferon-alpha-2A: clinical effects. J Biol Response Mod 1990; 9:538.

36. Belldegrun A, Koo AS, Bochner B, et al. Immunotherapy for advanced renal cell cancer: the role of radical nephrectomy. Eur Urol 1990; 18:42.

25

Phenotypic and Functional Analysis of Lymphoid Cells in the Peripheral Blood and Tumor of Cancer Patients Treated with Recombinant Interleukin-2 plus Interferon-α

G. Thomas Budd, James H. Finke, Raymond R. Tubbs, Mark Edinger, Jill Stanley, Siva R. Murthy, James S. Sergi, Sharon V. Medendorp, Vicki Gibson, Laurie Bauer, and Ronald M. Bukowski

The Cleveland Clinic Foundation, Cleveland, Ohio

I. INTRODUCTION

Recent clinical trials have demonstrated that the combination of recombinant interleukin-2 (rIL-2) and recombinant human interferon-α_{2A} (rhIFN-α_{2A}) has therapeutic activity in patients with advanced cancer (1–3). Significant durable clinical responses were seen in patients with metastatic malignant melanoma and renal cell carcinoma treated with this combination of cytokines. These responses have been noted in clinical trials utilizing a variety of doses and schedules of rIL-2 and rhIFN-α_{2A} (1–4).

Studies in animal models suggest that tumor regression produced by rIL-2 and IFN-α therapy requires the participation of the host immune system because this combination was not effective in irradiated mice or in mice bearing nonimmunogeneic tumors (5). Natural killer (NK) involvement as a possible effector cell, was suggested because rIL-2 and IFN-α was not effective in NK-deficient beige mice bearing the reticulum cell sarcoma

273

M5076 (6). However, other studies suggest T cells are important in the antitumor activity of rIL-2 and IFN-α therapy (7,8) because the effectiveness of this combination was abrogated by in vivo depletion of Lyt-2$^+$ T cells in tumor-bearing mice and therapy was inactive in athymic mice (7,8).

The immunologic changes induced by treatment with rIL-2 plus rhIFN-α_{2A} in cancer patients have not been well characterized. Buss et al. (1) found that bolus rIL-2 given with rhIFN-α_{2A} augmented NK activity in the peripheral blood, and the degree of activity appeared to be inversely related to the dose of rhIFN-α_{2A} administered.

The data presented here extend our previous work (1). We detail the effect of this therapy on lymphoid cell phenotype and function in the tumor itself in patients who have received several different schedules of rIL-2 and rhIFN-α_{2A}. Our data demonstrate that T cells, and to a lesser degree macrophages, represent the predominant infiltrate before therapy in biopsied tumor and that T cells, not NK cells, increase in some tumors during treatment. Finally, T cells were cloned from small tumor biopsies during therapy, and some of these clones had lytic activity for the autologous tumor.

II. MATERIALS AND METHODS

A. Patient Population and Treatment Schedules

Patients who were treated with one of three different rIL-2 plus rhIFN-α_{2A} regimens were included in this study. The three treatment programs are outlined in Table 1 and involved either continuous infusion (CI) or bolus administration of rIL-2 and intramuscular (IM) administration of rhIFN-α_{2A}. Eligible patients included those with malignancies refractory or unresponsive to conventional therapy and who had adequate hematologic, cardiovascular, pulmonary, and renal function as described previously (1). Patients treated in the phase I trial with CI underwent detailed studies of lymphocyte phenotypes and cytolytic activity in peripheral blood. In patients from all three trials tumors were biopsied at various time intervals for immunohistochemical and cloning investigations. Informed consent was obtained in accordance with institutional and National Cancer Institute guidelines.

B. Quantitation of Lymphocyte Subpopulations

Immunocytometric analysis of peripheral blood leukocytes (PBL) was performed using a modification of a previously described method (9). Studies were performed on two to three pretreatment samples on days 5, 12, 19, and 26 of therapy. FITC, phycoerythrin (PE), and biotin-conjugated monoclonal

Table 1   Summary of Treatment Programs Utilizing rIL-2 and rhIFN-α_{2A}

| Protocol number[a] | Patients entered | Cytokine treatment | | | |
| | | rIL-2 | | rhIFN-α_{2A} | |
		Dose (U/m^2 $\times$ 10^6)	Schedule (days)	Dose (U/m^2 $\times$ 10^6)	Schedule (days)
2376[b]	23	3.0–4.5 CI	1–5 8–12 15–19 22–26	5.0–10.0 3 times/week IM	
2681[c] 2682[c]	21	3.0 CI	1–4 8–11 15–18 22–25	5.0 IM	1–4 8–11 15–18 22–25
1964[b]	112	0.1–26.0 IV bolus	3 times/week (4 weeks)	0.1–10.0 IM	3 times/week (4 weeks)

[a] The Cleveland Clinic Foundation.
[b] Phase I dose escalation trials.
[c] Phase II trials in metastatic renal carcinoma and malignant melanoma.

antibodies were employed to phenotypically identify and quantitate lymphocytic subsets. These included FITC–anti-CD4, PE–anti-CD8, biotin–anti-CD3, FITC–anti-CD3, PE–anti-CD25, biotin–anti-HLADR, PE–anti-CD56, biotin–anti-CD8, FITC–anti-CD11a, and PE–anti-CD16c (Becton Dickinson, BD; Gentrac and Coulter).

Labeling of biotin-bound antibody was done using duochrome (DC) plus phycoerythrin Texas red (BD). Antibody titers were adjusted according to the fluorescence sensitivity of the flow cytometer (FACScan, BD). Isotypically matched controls for each particular subclass of immunoglobulin and system employed were utilized to allow the most accurate delineation of positive and autofluorescent populations and to control for nonspecific binding by a particular subclass of immunoglobulin compared to autofluorescent background.

Analyses on the FACScan were performed utilizing an argon ion laser (Cyonics) with 15 MW of 488 nm excitation. Live gating of the forward and orthogonal scatter channels, as determined by fluorescence (CD45$^+$CD14$^-$) backgating, was employed to this same end and to selectively acquire events for lymphocytes. Polymorphonuclear leukocytes and monocytes were quantitated as nongated events derived from the gating tube (FITC-aCD45, PE-aCD14, and DC-aCD2). Individual fluorescence populations were determined through the use of acquisition and contouring and quadrant analysis software (FACScan Research Software LYSYS and II, Becton Dickinson), as well as simultaneous multiparameter analysis software (Paint-a-Gate, BD) run on a HP310 workstation (Hewlett-Packard). Results for selected subpopulations were reported as a percentage of total lymphocytes and as the absolute number $\times$ 10^3 ml^{-1} whole blood corrected for nonspecific binding by isotypic controls.

C. Biopsy Immunohistology

Pretreatment and posttreatment tumor biopsy tissue were rapidly frozen in isopentane to $-130°C$ in liquid nitrogen on a chuck and stored at $-70°C$ until sectioning. Sections (6 μm) were fixed in reagent-grade acetone (Fisher) for 10 minutes, air dried, and immunostained with the avidin-biotinylated peroxidase complex method (10). Mouse monoclonal antibodies to the following determinants were incubated with the sections at dilutions optimized for tonsillar sections (30 minutes, ambient temperature): CD3, CD4, CD8, CD14, CD16b, HLA-DR, HLA-A, B, C, CD22. Sequential incubation was done with biotinylated affinity-purified horse antimouse IgG (Vector), preformed avidin-biotinylated peroxidase complex (Elite ABC, Vector), and the chromogenic substrate 3-amino-9-ethylcarbazole and 0.003% H_2O_2. The sections were then counterstained with hematoxylin. Results were expressed using a semiquantitative scoring system (see Table 3).

D. Evaluation of NK and LAK Activity

The cytolytic activity of mononuclear lymphocytes derived from Ficoll-Hypaque separation of heparinized blood was evaluated in 4 h ^{51}Cr release assay. NK activity was determined against ^{51}Cr-labeled NK-sensitive K562 erythroleukemia cells (American Type Culture Collection), as previously described (11). Lymphokine-activated killer (LAK) cell activity was evaluated using ^{51}Cr-labeled NK-resistant Daudi lymphoma cells (American Type Culture Collection) (12). Assays were performed in microtiter trays using 5000 target cells per well and effector-target ratios of 1.5:1–50:1. The percentage specific lysis at each ratio was determined after harvesting with a Skatron device (Skatron, Sterling, VA). Results were expressed as lytic units per 1×10^7 MNL, with one lytic unit (LU) defined as the number of effector cells producing 30% specific lysis of target cells in 4 h.

E. Cloning of Lymphocytes from Biopsies

Single-cell suspensions from tumor biopsies were performed by subjecting tissue to enzyme digestion, as previously described (13). A limiting dilution microculture system described by Moretta et al. (14) was employed for cloning of tumor-infiltrating lymphocytes (TIL). Lymphocytes in the biopsy specimen were plated at one lymphocyte per well in 96-well round-bottomed Costar plates containing irradiated (2000 R) autologous PBL (1×10^5) as feeders in a final volume of 200 ml RPMI supplemented with 10% fetal calf serum, 5 μg/ml of phytohemaggluttinin-P, and 100 U/ml of rIL-2. After 7 and 14 days, half the medium was replaced with fresh medium containing 100 U/ml of rIL-2 and 1×10^5 irradiated PBL. After 3–4 weeks, clones were transferred to 24-well plates and fed with rIL-2, irradiated PBL, and autologous tumor. Clones of sufficient size were phenotyped and tested for lytic activity.

F. Statistical Analysis of Data

Multiple determinations for various immunologic parameters in the peripheral blood were performed in selected patients before and during treatment with CI infusions of rIL-2 and rhIFN-α_{2A}. Data analysis was performed in a manner similar to that in our previous publication (1). Two pretreatment readings were averaged to obtain a pretreatment mean value. The percentage change from baseline was examined individually for each treatment day. Mean percentage changes from baseline for NK activity and mean absolute changes from baseline for LAK activity were calculated for individual patients. These changes were compared for patients treated at three different dose levels and for responding and nonresponding patients. All comparisons were made using nonparametric statistical techniques, including the Kruskal-Wallis (15), and the Wilcoxon rank-sum and signed-rank tests (16).

Absolute lymphocyte subset values were plotted throughout the follow-up period to examine their longitudinal behavior. The drop-in value from baseline to day 5 was calculated. Differences were examined within dose and response levels and across dose and response groups. Values for study days 6–26 were then averaged to examine what was considered a rebound effect of rIL-2 therapy. Differences between baseline values and the treatment means were calculated and compared within dose and response groups, as well as across dose and response groups.

III. RESULTS

A. NK and LAK Activity in Peripheral Blood

Previously we reported that intravenous bolus administration of rIL-2 combined with rhIFN-α_{2A} enhances NK activity in the peripheral blood (1). Here we assessed NK and LAK activity in peripheral blood of patients receiving rIL-2 by CI and rhIFN-α_{2A} by IM injection. Lytic activity was studied in four to six patients at the three dose levels on the days outlined previously.

The NK and LAK activity at various time points for patients treated at two dose levels (rIL-2, 3.0 × 10^6 U/m^2, and rhIFN-α_{2A}, 5.0 or 10.0 × 10^6 U/m^2) are illustrated in Figure 1. When percentage changes from baseline on each study day (all patients studied) were examined, increased activity was noted on day 12 for these two dose levels ($p = 0.03$ and $p = 0.06$), respectively. After day 12 the data obtained were too sparse for valid comparisons. When these two dose levels were compared, patients receiving 10.0 × 10^6 U/m^2 of rhIFN-α_{2A} showed increased NK activity on day 12 ($p = 0.04$); however, this effect was not seen at other time points. Finally, the mean percentage change from baseline was calculated for each patient. No significant differences in the percentage change were detected between the various dose levels or in the responding and nonresponding patients.

Changes in the number of cells expressing the marker for MHC-nonrestricted cytotoxic effectors (CD56$^+$) as a result of therapy are also presented in Figure 1. After an initial decrease in lymphocyte numbers, the total CD56$^+$ and CD3$^-$CD56$^+$CD8$^-$ populations appeared to increase above baseline levels during weeks 2–4 of treatment (p values $= 0.03$). Less dramatic and consistent were the increases in cells expressing the NK marker CD16c. The increase in CD56$^+$ cells coincided with the increase in LAK and NK activity (Fig. 1). In subsequent experiments we determined that the CD56$^+$ cells within the peripheral blood were responsible for much of the observed LAK activity. PBL were isolated on day 9 of study from a patient receiving rIL-2 CI and rhIFN-α_{2A}. At this time the percentage of CD56$^+$ was increased over prestudy values and the cytolitic activity of NK cells (CD5$^-$CD56$^+$) was compared to that of the T cell population (CD5$^+$CD56$^-$). In a preliminary experiment we found that sorted CD5$^-$CD56$^+$ PBL displayed potent lytic activity for Daudi (599 LU/10^6 cells) and the renal cell carcinoma line CCF-RC-2 (89.0 LU per 10^6 cells), whereas the CD5$^+$CD56$^-$ T cells showed only low levels of lytic activity for the same targets (3.0 and 1.2 LU/10^6). These results are preliminary but suggest that in rIL-2 plus rhIFN-α_{2A}-treated patients the CD5$^-$CD56$^+$ cells in peripheral blood have significant LAK activity compared to the CD5$^+$CD56$^-$ population.

B. Changes in T Cell Subsets as a Consequence of Combined Therapy

As previously reported, with CI rIL-2 (17), the combination of rIL-2 and rhIFN-α_{2A} produced a decrease in lymphocytes during week 1 of treatment, and lymphocytosis developed as therapy was continued. Changes from base-

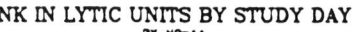

NK IN LYTIC UNITS BY STUDY DAY
RX_NO=1A

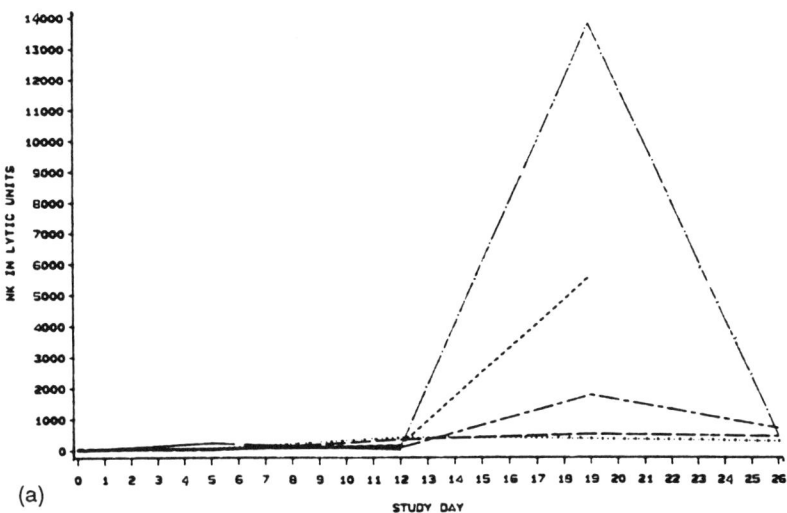

(a)

NK IN LYTIC UNITS BY STUDY DAY
RX_NO=1B

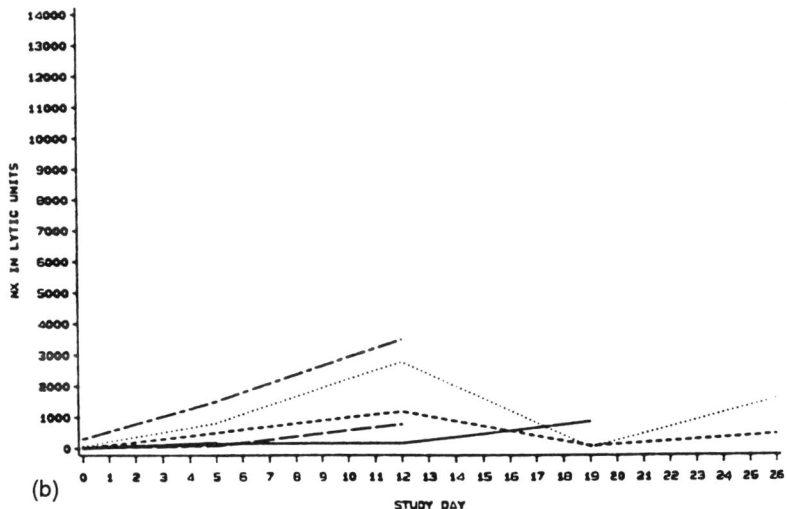

(b)

Figure 1 Evaluation of NK (a and b) and LAK (c and d) activity in the peripheral blood of patients treated with rIL-2 and rhIFN-α_{2A}. Lytic response to K562 (NK) and Daudi (LAK) was assessed prestudy and on days 1, 5, 15, and 26 of study. On the same days, PBL were analyzed for the presence of $CD56^+$ cells (e and f). (a, c, and e) Results from dose level a (rIL-2, 3×106 U/m^2 /24 h and rhIFN-α_{2A}, 5×10^6 U/m^2, IM). (b, d, and f) Results from dose level b (rIL-2, 3×10^6 U/m^2/24h and rhIFN-α_{2A}, 10×10^6 U/m^2, IM). The data are from protocol 2376, listed in Table 1. Each line represents data from a different patient.

LAK IN LYTIC UNITS BY STUDY DAY
RX_NO=1A

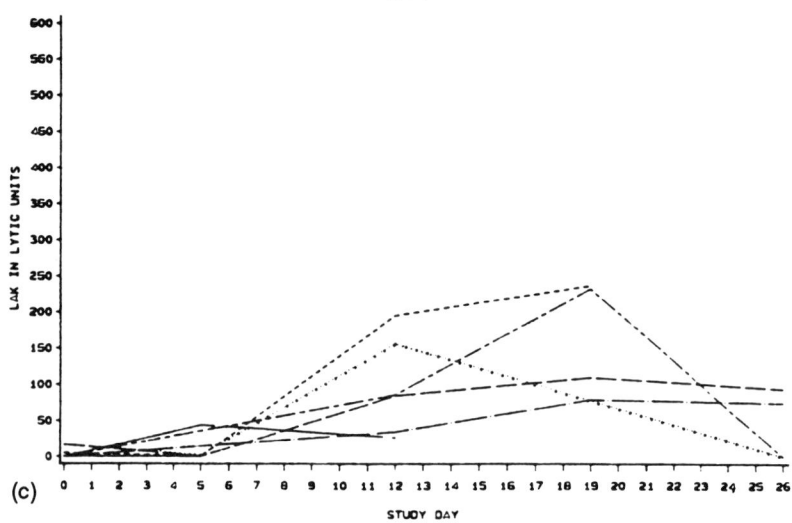

(c)

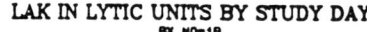

LAK IN LYTIC UNITS BY STUDY DAY
RX_NO=1B

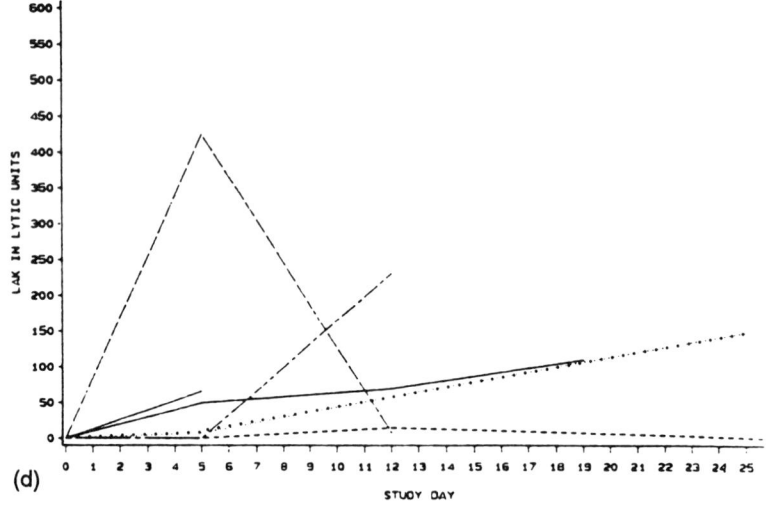

(d)

Figure 1   (Continued)

ABSOLUTE NUMBER OF CD56 BY STUDY DAY
RX_NO=1A

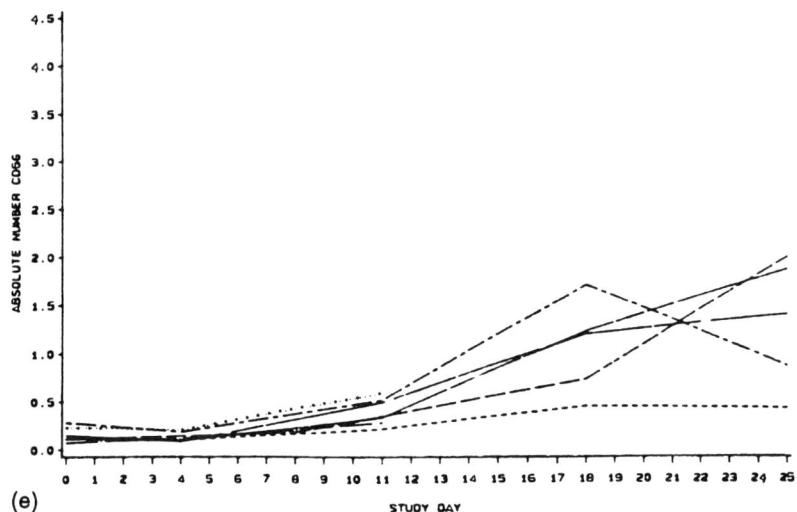

(e)

ABSOLUTE NUMBER OF CD56 BY STUDY DAY
RX_NO=1B

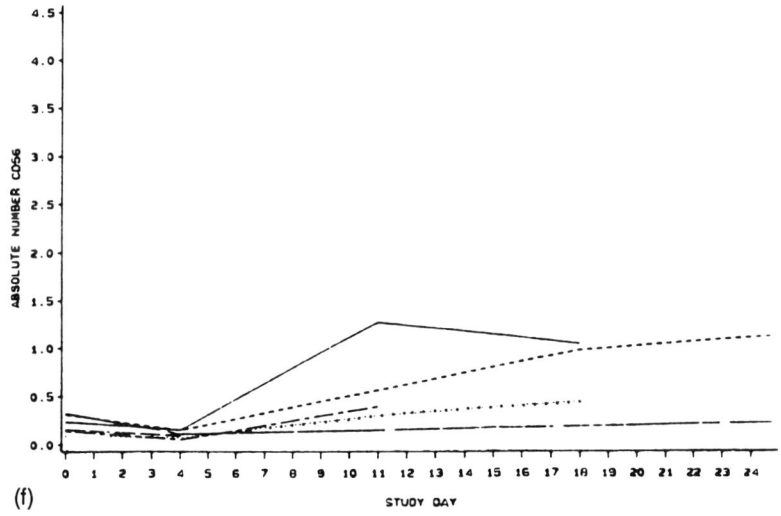

(f)

line for absolute numbers were examined and compared for the various dose levels and response groups in patients treated with rIL-2 given as CI and rhIFN-α_{2A} given IM. At day 5 the absolute number of lymphocytes decreased in most patients (data not shown). When the various subsets were examined, CD3[+] lymphocytes demonstrated the most consistent decrease (Fig. 2). No significant changes from baseline were seen, however, between dose levels or response groups. By day 12 of the study, CD3[+] lymphocytes had returned to but rarely exceeded baseline levels.

An analysis of the induction of activated T cell subsets in the peripheral blood during rIL-2 plus rhIFN-α_{2A} treatment revealed that after an initial decrease the number of activated T cells increased above baseline, with the peak response on day 12 (Fig. 2). The activated T cell population consisted of those cells expressing the IL-2α receptor (IL-2Rα; CD25) and HLA-DR, as well as some that expressed HLA-DR, but not CD25 (Fig. 2). Response categories were also examined for any correlation with changes in these lymphocyte subsets. No significant changes were noted; however, some low-level increases in the CD3[+]CD25[+]HLA-DR[+] population ($p = 0.11$) were present in responding patients ($n = 4$) compared with nonresponders ($n = 9$).

C. Immunohistologic Evaluation of Tumor Biopsies Before and During Therapy

Since changes in lymphocyte populations in peripheral blood may not mirror immune activity in the tumors themselves, the mononuclear infiltrate within primary and metastatic tumors were analyzed in patients administered rIL-2 plus rhIFN-α_{2A} therapy using immunohistologic examination of biopsies before and during treatment. Biopsy results obtained from patients with melanoma or renal cell carcinoma treated with either of two rIL-2 plus rhIFN-α_{2A} schedules are presented in Table 2. Because of patient status and disappearance of tumor, it was not possible to biopsy most of the regressing tumors. The results show that before treatment tumors displayed low to moderate infiltrates of CD3[+] cells comprised of both CD4 and CD8 subsets. Most tumors were devoid of NK and B cells but contained varying numbers of macrophages. In most patients few changes in the immunoregulatory cell types occurred. In some cases, treatment with rIL-2 and rhIFN-α_{2A} caused an increase in CD4[+] and CD8[+] T cells, with minimal changes in cells expressing the NK phenotype; however, the patterns were inconsistent (Table 2).

Serial biopsies of subcutaneous nodules were performed in one patient with metastatic malignant melanoma (patient 4) treated with the CI schedule.

ABSOLUTE NUMBER OF CD3 BY STUDY DAY
RX_NO=1A

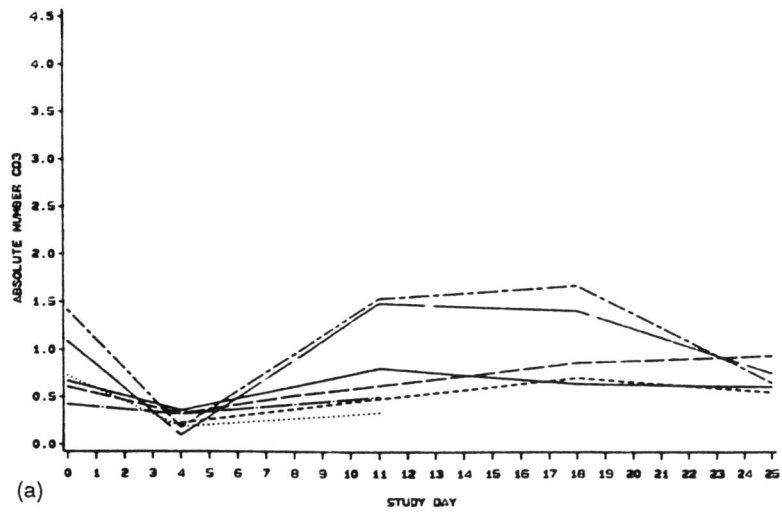

(a)

ABSOLUTE NUMBER OF CD3 BY STUDY DAY
RX_NO=1B

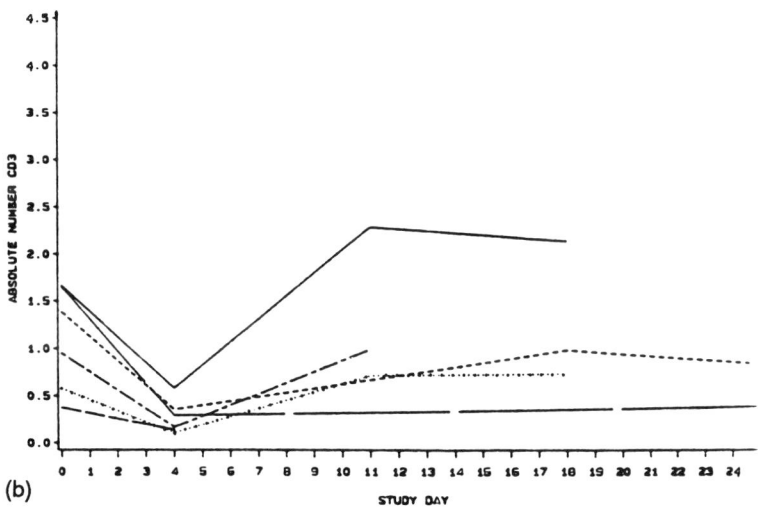

(b)

Figure 2 Analysis of total T cells and activated T cell subsets. Three-color flow analysis of PBL was performed on days indicated in Figure 1. (a, c, and e) patients in dose level a; (b, d, and f) patients in dose level b of protocol 2376 described in Figure 1. (a and b) Total CD3$^+$ cells; (c and d) CD3$^+$CD25$^-$HLA-DR$^+$ cells; and (e and f) CD3$^+$CD25$^+$HLA-DR$^+$ cells.

283

ABSOLUTE NUMBER OF CD3+CD25−HLADr+ BY STUDY DAY

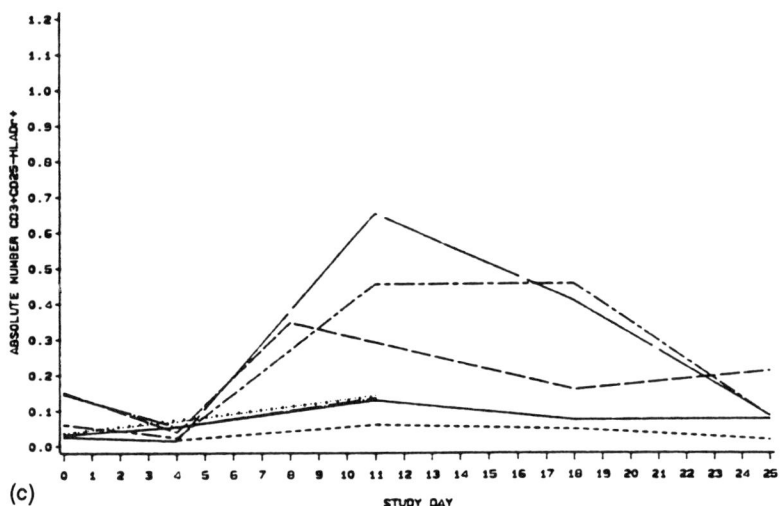

(c)

ABSOLUTE NUMBER OF CD3+CD25−HLADr+ BY STUDY DAY

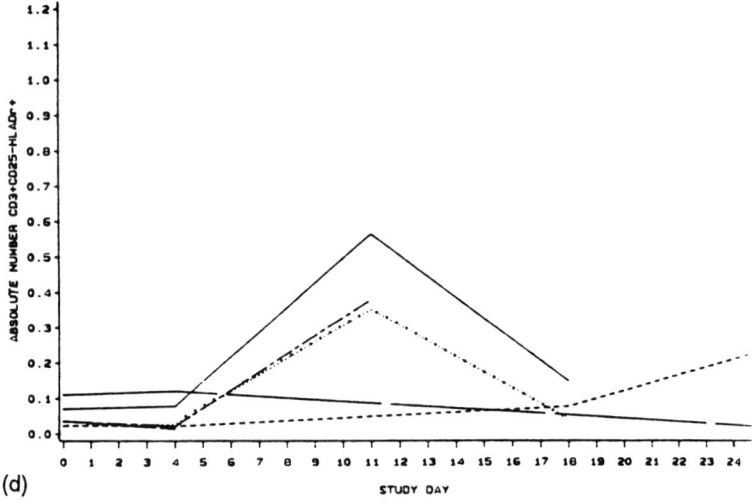

(d)

Figure 2 (Continued)

ABSOLUTE NUMBER OF CD3+CD25+HLADr+ BY STUDY DAY
RX_NO=1A

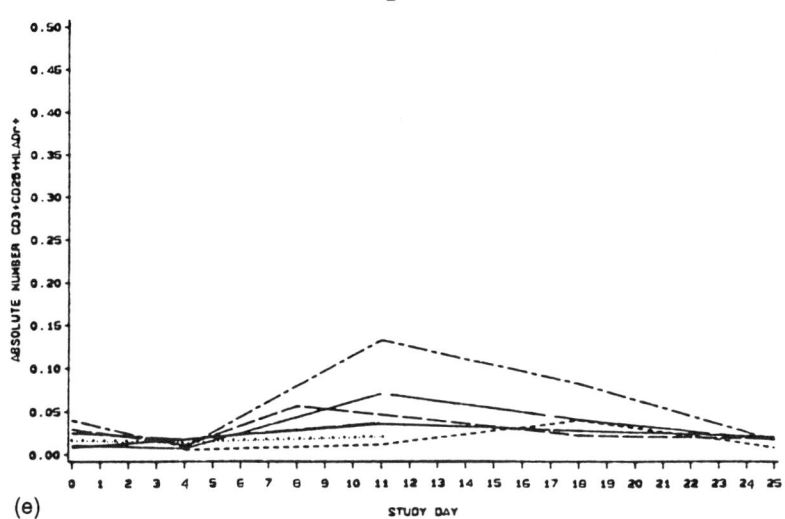

(e)

ABSOLUTE NUMBER OF CD3+CD25+HLADr+ BY STUDY DAY
RX_NO=1B

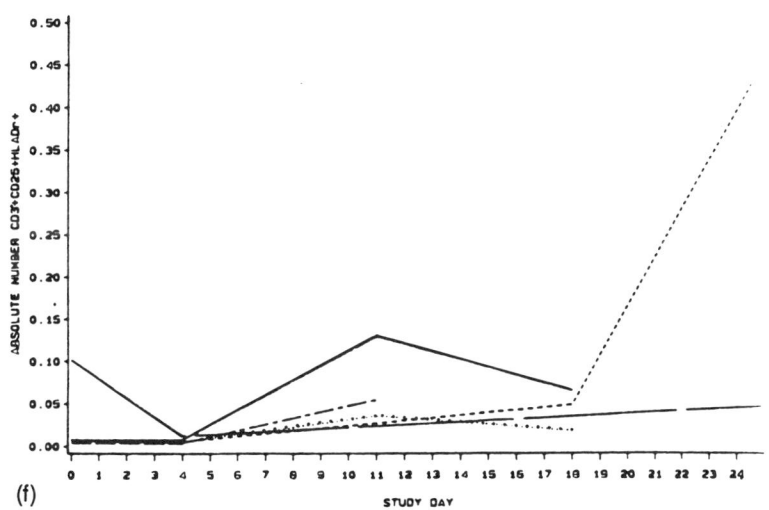

(f)

Table 2 Phenotype of Infiltrating Lymphocytes

Protocol	Protocol no.	Patient	Treatment day	Tumor	Immunohistologic results[a]								
					CD3	CD4	CD8	CD56	CD16	HLA-DR[b]	HLA-A, B, C[b]	CD22	CD14
CI IL-2 + IFN-α	2367	4	0	Melanoma	1$^+$	3$^+$	1$^+$	TP	—	—	ND	ND	2$^+$
			8		1$^+$	2$^+$	1$^+$	TP	—	2$^+$	ND	ND	2$^+$
			29		3$^+$	4$^+$	3$^+$	TP	TR	3$^+$	ND	ND	3$^+$
CI IL-2 + IFN-α	2681	1903	0	RCC	ND	ND	ND	ND	ND	ND	ND	ND	ND
			105		1$^+$	1$^+$	1$^+$	—	—	1$^+$	3$^+$	TR	—
CI IL-2 + IFN-α	2682	1804	16	Melanoma	3$^+$	4$^+$	3$^+$	1$^+$	1$^+$	1$^+$	ND	ND	3$^+$
			123		2$^+$	1$^+$	1$^+$	TP	1$^+$	1$^+$	1$^+$	—	1$^+$
	1808		0	Melanoma	2$^+$	3$^+$	TR	TR	—	—	1$^+$	—	2$^+$
			14		2$^+$	1$^+$	1$^+$	1$^+$	—	—	2$^+$	—	1$^+$
Bolus IL-2 + IFN-α	1964	071	0	Melanoma	2$^+$	3$^+$	1$^+$	TP	—	3$^+$	ND	ND	2$^+$
			15		1^{+b}	1$^+$	TR	TP	—	—	ND	1$^+$	1$^+$
	066		0	Melanoma	3$^+$	2$^+$	2$^+$	TR	TR	3$^+$	ND	ND	ND
			29		No viable cell: necrotic								

Case		Tumor									
081	0	Melanoma	TR	TR	TR	—	—	TR	4+	—	TR
	17		1+	1+	1+	TR	TR	—	1+	1+	TR
083	0	RCC	3+	2+	2+	TP	TR	4+	4+	—	2+
	13		3+	3+	3+	TP	—	3+	3+	—	2+
	19		4+	3+	3+	TP	—	4+	4+	—	2+
	26		4+	3+	4+	TP	—	4+	4+	—	3+
	33		4+	3+	3+	TP	—	4+	3+	TR	3+
086	0	Melanoma	2+	1+	1+	TP	—	1+	1+	—	1+
	12		4+	3+	3+	TP	—	4+	4+	TR	2+
	26		4+	3+	2+	TP	—	4+	4+	—	2+
091	0	RCC	4+	3+	1+	—	1+	4+	4+	—	2+
	16		4+	3+	3+	TR	TR	4+	4+	—	2+
90	0	Melanoma	TR	TR	—	TP	—	—	4+	—	4+
	93		1+	1+	TR	TP	—	—	4+	—	1+
076	0	RCC	ND	ND	ND	ND	ND	ND	ND	ND	ND
	54		1+	TR	TR	TP	—	—	—	—	TR

[a] Semiquantitative scale: TP, tumor cells positive; TR, trace, 5% of cells positive; 1+, 5–25% of cells positive; 2+, 25–50% of cells positive; 3+, 50–75% of cells positive; 4+, 75–100% of cells positive; ND, not determined. CD56 evaluated for both tumor cells and hematopoietic cells.
[b] HLA-DR and HLA-A, B, C evaluated selectively for tumor cells.

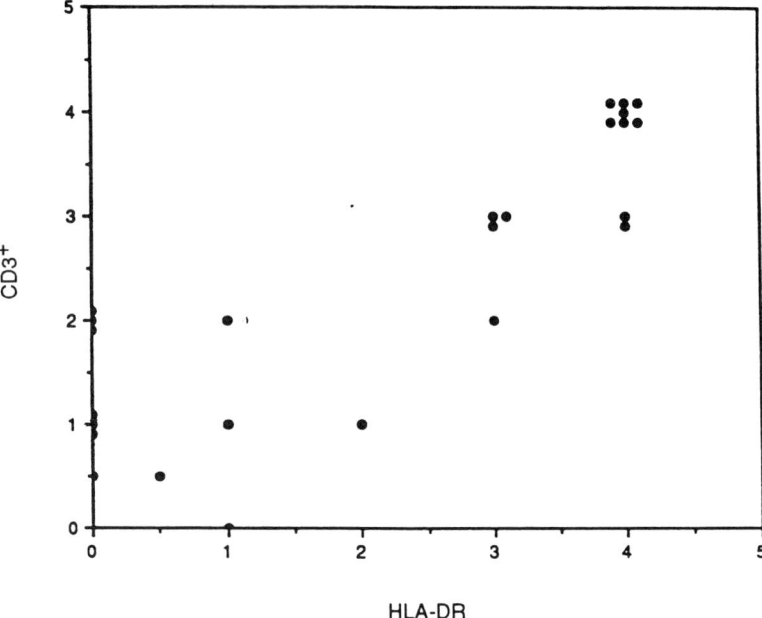

Figure 3 Relationship between CD3$^+$ infiltration and HLA-DR expression on tumor cells. Each dot represents an individual lesion evaluated by immunohistology. The degree of infiltration by CD3$^+$ lymphocytes was plotted against the number of tumor cells expressing HLA-DR. The same semiquantitative scale described in Table 3 was employed here.

Samples were obtained pretreatment and on days 8 and 28 of therapy. The results are summarized in Table 2. Tumor cells in the initial (pretreatment) sample did not express HLA-DR, and only scattered CD3$^+$ cells were identified in the tumor bed. Subsequent biopsies (days 8 and 28) demonstrated abundant expression of HLA-DR on tumor cells and marked T cell infiltration.

The relationship between the intensity of lymphocyte infiltrate and HLA-DR expression on tumor cells was examined further by analyzing the level of staining using anti-CD3 and anti-HLA-DR antibodies on 25 biopsies that included samples taken before and during treatment. As seen in Figure 3, the degree of infiltration by CD3$^+$ cells appeared to correlate with the level of HLA-DR expression on the tumor cells, as others have reported (18,19) for IL-2-based therapy.

D. Clonal Analysis of T Cells from the Tumor Biopsies

Preliminary studies were conducted to define the types of lymphocyte that could be expanded under limiting dilution condition from tumor biopsies and to determine if the clones had lytic activity for the autologous tumor. Cloning studies were conducted with three patients receiving rIL-2 and rhIFN-α_{2A} therapy, from samples taken at the times indicated in Table 3. Two samples were biopsies taken from metastatic lesions in the lung and liver, respectively, and the third was from the right kidney.

Collectively, 66 proliferating clones were detected, and of those, 38 were phenotyped. All expressed CD3, with approximately equal numbers expressing either CD4 or CD8 and one having the phenotype of a double-negative T cell. Most of the clones were negative for CD56. Cytolytic activity against the autologous tumor was examined using clones derived from two of the three patients (patients 1 and 3). In both cases, clones were detected that had lytic activity for the autologous tumor (Table 3). In addition, the clones derived from patient 3, which were lytic for the autologous tumor, did not lyse K562

Table 3 T Cell Clones Derived from Biopsy Specimens of Patients Treated with rIL-2 plus rhIFN-α_{2A}

| | | | | Tested clone | | | |
| | | | | Phenotype[c] | | Lytic activity[d] | |
Patient	Tumor site[a]	Initial TIL × 10^{5b}	Growing clones	CD4$^+$	CD8$^+$	CD4$^+$	CD8$^+$
1	Kidney	19.3	38	9	7	2/8	1/7
2	Liver metastasis	0.18	15	8	6	ND	ND
3	Lung metastasis	134.0	13	5	3	3/5	2/3

[a] Kidney tumor (patient 1) was obtained 6 days after completion of therapy. Biopsy was performed on day 17 of therapy from patient 2. Patient 3 had a surgical excision of a small lung nodule 9 days after stopping therapy. Patients 1 and 2 had cloning studies during the second cycle, and patient 3 had studies done after 2½ cycles of therapy. Patient status at time of biopsy or surgery: patient 1 (stable); patient 2 (stable); and patient 3 (responder).

[b] Number of lymphocytes obtained after a 2 h digest with collagenase (type III) and DNase (type I).

[c] When clones were of sufficient size they were phenotyped by staining cytospin using the immunoperoxidase method. All clones were CD3$^+$ and either CD4$^+$ or CD8$^+$.

[d] The ratio refers to the number of clones lytic for autologous tumor per total number of clones tested. Clones considered positive displayed greater than 10% lysis against the autologous tumor targets (effector-target ratio of 20:1). Short-term cultures of RCC were established from patients 1 and 3. Clones from patient 3 were also tested for lysis against K562, and all displayed less than 10% lysis.

target cells. These results demonstrate that $CD56^- CD4^+$ and $CD8^+$ T cell subsets are the predominant cell type expanded from tumor sites in patients on rIL-2 and rhIFN-α_{2A} therapy.

IV. DISCUSSION

We have examined the influence of rIL-2 and rhIFN-α_{2A} treatment on NK and T cell responses in cancer patients and attempted to relate these changes to clinical response. Although the data are preliminary, they suggest that the changes that occur during therapy in lymphocyte subpopulations observed within the tumor are distinct from those in the peripheral blood.

Increases in LAK cell number and activity were most pronounced in the peripheral blood. Treatment with rIL-2 and rhIFN-α_{2A} augmented NK activity and induced LAK activity on day 12 of the study. Budd et al. (1) demonstrated a relationship between the NK activity in the peripheral blood and the dose of rIL-2 administered: higher doses of rIL-2 were associated with greater NK activity. In addition, it was found that the NK response augmented by IL-2 and rhIFN-α_{2A} was inversely related to the dose of rhIFN-α_{2A}, with lower doses (0.1×10^6 U/m^2) inducing greatest activity. In the present study, much higher doses of rhIFN-α_{2A} were employed, and no differences were detected between patients receiving either 5.0 or 10×10^6 U/m^2 of rhIFN-α_{2A}.

Flow cytometry and cell-sorting studies demonstrated that the rise in NK and LAK activity paralleled an increase in the number of $CD56^+$ lymphocytes, including $CD3^- CD56^+ CD8^-$ cells. This latter population had significant LAK activity compared to the $CD56^-$ T cell population. Previous trials with CI rIL-2 also demonstrated that the majority of the LAK response was mediated by $CD56^+$ cells (17,20,21).

Whereas the total number of $CD3^+$ T cells in the peripheral blood did not rebound above baseline values during rIL-2 and rhIFN-α_{2A} treatment, the number of activated T cells appeared to increase above baseline levels. Interleukin-2 administered as immunotherapy has been shown to increase HLA-DR$^+$ cells and IL-2Rα cells in the peripheral blood (22). However, it was not clear from this report whether the increase in HLA-DR$^+$ and IL-2Rα ($CD25^+$) cells in the blood reflected changes in NK, T cells, or other populations. It was reported recently that NK cells activated in vivo by IL-2 administration respond to rIL-2 mainly through the p75 IL-2R protein and retain a p55-negative ($CD25^+$) phenotype (23). Our results show that rIL-2 and rhIFN-α_{2A} therapy caused an increase in activated T cells that express HLA-DR in the peripheral blood, some of which coexpress the CD25 protein

(α chain) of the IL-2 receptor. Whether these activated T cells represent part of the specific host immune response to tumor is not known. To date, changes in the number or activity of peripheral blood immune cells (lymphocyte subsets and NK and LAK activity) in patients treated with rIL-2 plus rhIFN-α_{2A} do not suggest an association between immune stimulation and subsequent clinical response. An increase in CD3$^+$CD25$^+$HLA-DR$^+$ lymphocytes was noted in responding patients, but this observation is preliminary, does not reach statistical significance, and requires additional study with larger numbers of patients. These analyses were all performed on peripheral blood, and the events in this compartment may not truly reflect changes occurring at the tumor site.

An analysis of the mononuclear cells infiltrating tumors before therapy revealed that T cells and macrophages represented the major immune populations. The number of cells expressing the NK markers CD16 and CD56 were either very low or not detectable, suggesting that NK cells constitute only a minor component of the local host immune response. These results are in general agreement with the results of others (18,19,24). We also noted from an analysis of 25 biopsies that the degree of CD3$^+$ T cell infiltration was directly proportional to the number of tumor cells expressing HLA-DR. In our study the correlation between HLA-DR expression and T cell infiltrate was irrespective of IL-2 therapy. However, Rubin et al. (19) reported that this correlation was associated with rIL-2-based therapy. This difference in our results and those of Rubin et al. may relate to differences in sample size, clinical trials employed, and variations in methodology of immunohistology between the two studies. Our finding that 87% of renal cell carcinoma (RCC) patients ($n = 8$) had HLA-DR expression on greater than 50% of the cells is slightly higher but in general agreement with the work of Rubin et al. (17), who reported that 58% RCC specimens expressed HLA-DR. The number of HLA-DR-positive melanomas (27%, $n = 17$) reported in our study is lower than that by Rubin et al., where they found that 53% of metastatic melanomas expressed HLA-DR. In most biopsy samples, tumor cells expressed class I major histocompatibility complex (MHC) antigens, although the level of expression on a per cell basis, as well as the percentage of cells positive for class I, varied considerably. It appears from animal studies that MHC class I and II expression on tumor cells is important to the development of an effective immune response to the tumor (25,26). T cells involved in antitumor immunity are composed of CD4$^+$ helper T cells that recognize antigen in concert with MHC class II molecules and CD8$^+$ cytotoxic cells that recognize antigen along with class I molecules (27–30). Recent transfection experiments with MHC genes suggest that MHC class I and II molecules expressed on tumors are involved in inducing CD8 and CD4 T cell antitumor responses, respectively (25,26). Weber et al. (25) reported that a class I-deficient murine melanoma, B16BL6, when transfected with K^b class I gene, made this tumor sensitive to immunotherapy with rIL-2. Lyt-2$^+$ (CD8$^+$) T cells appeared to be the predominant cell type responsible in vivo for eliminating the class I$^+$ B16BL6 cells. More recently it was shown that the transfection of MHC class II genes into a murine sarcoma allowed this tumorigenic line to be rejected when implanted into syngeneic mice (26). In addition, rejection of the MHC class II$^+$ tumor appeared to be due to the augmentation of helper T cell response (26). Although the role of MHC molecules in augmenting an immune response to human tumor is not well defined, it may be that the expression of MHC class II on tumors is important in stimulating a T cell infiltrate into the tumor. It is possible that the increase in the cellular infiltrate observed during therapy with rIL-2 plus rhIFN-α_{2A} is attributable to an increase in MHC class I and II expression on the tumors. Alternatively, the treatment with rIL-2 and IFN-α may induce TIL to produce cytokines (i.e., IFN-γ) that potentiate the expression of HLA-DR on tumor cells.

During the course of these studies we noted that some of the tumor cells themselves expressed CD56. CD56 (Leu-19) is expressed on many tumors, as well as various lymphocyte subsets (Tubbs et al., unpublished data). Neuroendocrine carcinomas, including undifferentiated small cell carcinoma, carcinoid tumors, and pancreatic islet cell tumors, express high levels of this antigen. In our experience, about 50% of renal cell carcinomas are also positive for CD56.

We were unable to obtain tissue in most responding patients because of patient status and disappearance of tumors and therefore were not able to determine if tumor regression was associated with the degree of cellular infiltrate. In some of the biopsies examined, treatment with rIL-2 and rhIFN-α_{2A} caused an increase in the infiltrate, with the most significant changes in the number of CD4$^+$ and CD8$^+$ cells. Increases were also noted in the macrophage population, whereas treatment induced only minimal changes in NK cells. There were multiple biopsies in one patient with melanoma who had a minor regression of his tumor, and immunohistochemical studies showed increases in CD3$^+$ cells. Rubin et al. (19) demonstrated that during rIL-2-based therapy all regressing metastatic lesion exhibited an increase in T cell infiltrate, suggesting an association between infiltrating T cells and clinical response. Clearly, additional studies are needed to determine if the clinical response observed with rIL-2 and rhIFN-α_{2A} therapy is correlated with T cell infiltrate.

Clonal analysis of TIL from small tumor biopsies and a primary lesion demonstrated that CD3$^+$CD4$^+$CD56$^-$ and CD3$^+$CD8$^+$CD56$^-$ are the predominant lymphocytes capable of responding under limiting dilution conditions. In one of the two biopsies, sufficient tumor cells were obtained for analysis of lytic activity. Although the number of clones tested was small, we found some CD4$^+$ and CD8$^+$ clones that were lytic for autologous tumor. In one case lytic clones were derived from a regressing lesion. However, it remains to be determined if the therapy causes a selective increase in specific cytotoxic T lymphocytes within the tumor, particularly in regressing lesions, and if this response differs from that observed in the peripheral blood. We also observed that a significant number of TIL were nonlytic, which may represent cells with helper function or cells that are not part of the host antitumor response. Additional studies to address these questions are underway.

In most studies the changes in immune cells as a consequence of cytokine therapy have been monitored in the peripheral blood, with only a few studies examining changes in the tumor bed (19). Here we have examined phenotypic and functional properties of immune cells in the blood and tumor of the same patients undergoing immunotherapy with rIL-2 and rhIFN-α_{2A}. This analysis, although preliminary, suggests that the changes in immune lymphocyte subsets in the blood and in the tumor are distinct. It appears that a greater emphasis should be placed on defining the phenotypic and functional characteristics of lymphoid cells infiltrating the tumor during therapy than in monitoring the peripheral blood.

V. SUMMARY

Presented here is a preliminary analysis of the immunomodulatory effects of rIL-2 administered as either a continuous infusion or intravenous bolus combined with rhIFN-α_{2A} to patients with advanced malignancies in a series of phase I or II trials. The influence of cytokine combination on NK and T cells in the peripheral blood and tumor were investigated. Treatment with CI IL-2 and rhIFN-α_{2A} resulted in an increase in peripheral blood LAK activity at all dose levels, which appeared greatest on day 12. The rise in lytic activity coincided with increases in the number of CD56$^+$ peripheral blood lymphocytes. The total number of CD3$^+$ peripheral blood lymphocytes decreased on day 4 and returned to prestudy values by day 10. Analysis of activated T cells demonstrated that both CD3$^+$CD25$^+$HLA-DR$^+$ and CD3$^+$CD25$^-$HLA-DR$^+$ cells increased by day 10 and declined by day 18. Immunohistologic studies were performed on tumor biopsies from patients on various rIL-2 plus rhIFN-α_{2A} protocols. Predominant infiltrates observed before and during therapy consisted of CD4$^+$ and CD8$^+$ T cells, with significant numbers of CD14$^+$ tissue macrophages and low numbers of CD56$^+$CD16$^+$ NK cells. Increases in T cells were sometimes observed during therapy, and the degree of infiltrate by CD3$^+$ cells correlated with the percentage of tumor cells expressing HLA-DR. Clonal analysis from biopsy specimens showed that all the IL-2-responsive cells were T cells (CD3$^+$CD56$^-$), with no detection of NK clones. The results suggest rIL-2 plus rhIFN-α_{2A} therapy augments NK and T cell responses in peripheral blood and T cell and macrophage response in tumor sites.

ACKNOWLEDGMENTS

We thank Matthew Owens and Michael McNealis for staining and analysis by three-color immunocytometry. Also, we are grateful to Lisa Gannon and Denise McLain for their assistance in coordinating the data and the nursing staff of M-70 for their devoted patient care. We also thank Diane Hall for typing this manuscript. This work was supported in part by a grant from Hoffmann-LaRoche.

REFERENCES

1. Budd GT, Osgood B, Barna B, et al. Phase I clinical trial of interleukin-2 and interferon-alpha: toxicity and immunologic effects. Cancer Res 1990; 49: 6432–6.
2. Lee KH, Talpaz M, Rothberg JM, et al. Concomitant administration of recombinant human interleukin-2 and recombinant interferon-a2a in cancer patients: a phase I study. J Clin Oncol 1989; 7:1726–32.
3. Rosenberg SA, Lotze MT, Yang JC, et al. Combination therapy with interleukin-2 and alpha interferon for the treatment of patients with advanced cancer. J Clin Oncol 1989; 7:1863–74.
4. Bukowski RM, Murthy S, Sergi JS, et al. Phase I trial of continuous infusion recombinant interleukin-2 and intermittent recombinant alpha-2A: toxicity and immunologic effect. J Biol Response Mod (in press).
5. Cameron RB, McIntosh JK, Rosenberg SA. Synergistic antitumor effects of combination immunotherapy with recombinant interleukin-2 and recombinant hybrid interferon in the treatment of established hepatic metastases. Cancer Res 1988; 48:5819–17.
6. Brunda MJ, Rosenbaum D, Stern L. Inhibition of experimentally-induced murine metastases by recombinant alpha interferon: correlation between the modulatory effect of interferon treatment on natural killer cell activity and inhibition of metastases. Int J Cancer 1984; 24:421–6.

7. Rosenberg SA, Schwarz SL, Spiess PJ. Combination immunotherapy for cancer: synergistic antitumor interactions of interleukin-2, alpha interferon and tumors infiltrating lymphocytes. J Natl Cancer Inst 1988; 80:1393–7.

8. Iigo M, Sukura M, Tamura T, Saijo N, Hoshi A. In vivo antitumor activity of multiple injections of recombinant interleukin-2, alone and in combination with three different types of recombinant interferon, on various syngeneic murine tumor models. Cancer Res 1988; 48:260–4.

9. Lanier LL, Loken MR. Human lymphocyte subpopulations identified by using three color immunofluorescence and flow cytometry analysis; correlation of Leu-2, Leu-3, Leu-7, Leu-8 and Leu-11 cell surface antigen expression. J Immunol 1982; 132:151–6.

10. Tubbs RR, Sheibani K. Immunohistology of lymphoproliferative disorders. Semin Diagn Pathol 1984; 1:272–84.

11. Herberman RB. Natural killer cell activity and antibody-dependent cell-mediated cytotoxicity. In: Rose NR, Friedman H, Fahey JL, eds. Manual of clinical immunology, 3rd ed. Washington, DC: American Society of Microbiology, 1986; 308–14.

12. Grimm EA, Muzumder A, Zhang HZ, Rosenberg SA. Lymphokine-activated killer cell phenomenon: lysis of natural killer-resistant fresh solid tumor cells by interleukin-2 activated autologous human peripheral blood lymphocytes. J Exp Med 1982; 155: 1823–41.

13. Finke JH, Rayman P, Alexander J, et al. Characterization of the cytolytic activity of CD4[+] and CD8[+] tumor-infiltrating lymphocytes in human renal cell carcinoma. Cancer Res 1990; 50:2363–70.

14. Moretta A, Pantaleo G, Moretta L, Cerottini JC, Mingur MC. Direct demonstration of the clonogenic potential of every human peripheral blood T cell. Clonal analysis of HLA-DR expression and cytolytic activity. J Exp Med 1983; 157:743–50.

15. Kruskal WH, Wallia WA. Use of ranks in one-criterion variance analysis. J Am Stat Assoc 1952; 47:583–621.

16. Wilcoxon F. Individual comparisons by ranking methods. Biometrics Bull 1945; 1:80–3.

17. Sosman JA, Kohler PC, Hank JA, et al. Repetitive weekly cycles of interleukin-2. II. Clinical and immunologic effects of dose, schedule, and addition of indomethacin. J Natl Cancer Inst 1988; 80:1451–61.

18. Cohen PJ, Lotze MT, Roberts JR, Rosenberg SA, Jaffee ES. The immunopathology of sequential tumor biopsies in patients treated with interleukin-2. Correlation of response with T-cell infiltration and HLA-DR expression. Am J Pathol 1987; 129:208–16.

19. Rubin JT, Elwood LJ, Rosenberg SA, Lotze MT. Immunohistochemical correlates of response to recombinant interleukin-2 based immunotherapy in humans. Cancer Res 1989; 49:7086–92.

20. McMannis JD, Fisher RJ, Creekmore SP, Braun DP, Harris JE, Ellis TM. In vivo effects of recombinant IL-2. I. Isolation of circulating Leu-19[+] lympho-

kines activated killer effector cells from cancer patients receiving recombinant IL-2. J Immunol 1988; 140:1335–40.

21. Ellis TM, Creekmore SP, McMannis JD, Braun DP, Harris JA, Fisher RI. Appearance and phenotypic characterizations of circulating Leu19$^+$ cells in cancer patients receiving recombinant interleukin-2. Cancer Res 1989; 48:6597.

22. Lotze MT, Matory YL, Ettinghausen SE, et al. In vivo administration of purified human interleukin-2. II. Half life, immunologic effects, and expansion of peripheral lymphoid cells in vivo with recombinant IL-2. J Immunol 1985; 135:2867–75.

23. Weil-Hillman F, Voss SD, Fisch P, et al. Natural killer cells activated by interleukin-2 treatment in vivo respond to interleukin 2 primarily through the P_{75} receptor and maintain the P_{55} (TAC) negative phenotype. Cancer Res 1990; 50:2683–91.

24. Banner BF, Burnham JA, Buhnson RR, Ernstoff MS, Auerbach HE. Immunophenotypic markers in renal cell carcinoma. Mod Pathol 1990; 3(2):129–34.

25. Weber JS, Jay G, Tanaka K, Rosenberg SA. Immunotherapy of a murine tumor with interleukin 2. Increased sensitivity after MHC class I gene trasfection. J Exp Med 1990; 166:1716–33.

26. Ostrand-Rosenberg S, Thakur A, Clements V. Rejection of mouse sarcoma cells after transfection of MHC class II genes. J Immunol 1990; 144:4068–71.

27. Swain SL. T cell subset and the recognition of MHC class. Immunol Rev 1983; 74:129.

28. Schwartz RH. T-lymphocytes recognition of antigen in association with gene products of the major histocompatibility complex. Annu Rev Immunol 1985; 3:237.

29. Towsend A, Bodmer H. Antigen recognition by class I restricted T lymphocytes. Annu Rev Immunol 1989; 7:601.

30. Germain R, Malissan B. Analysis of the expression and function of class II major histocompatibility complex encoded molecules. Annu Rev Immunol 1989; 4:251.

26

Treatment of Metastatic Renal Cell Carcinoma with High-Dose Interferon and Prednisone

Sophie D. Fosså, Ragnhild Gunderson, and Gustav Lehne

The Norwegian Radium Hospital, Oslo, Norway

Unni Hjelmaas

Roche Norge, Oslo, Norway

I. INTRODUCTION

Metastatic renal cell carcinoma (MRCC) is a malignancy that is highly resistant to available systemic treatment. The best response rates have been obtained with single-drug or combined immunotherapy.

Single-drug interferon (IFN) treatment has produced response rates of about 15%, displaying a weak dose-response relationship within certain dose limits (1). Clinical application of IFN is reduced by the drug's high subjective toxicity (flulike symptoms, fever, anorexia, and fatigue), however, leading to frequent and unwanted dose reductions and premature discontinuation.

In 1987 we made the observation that such subjective toxicity was considerably decreased when high-dose interferon treatment was combined with prednisone (P), without reduction in the response (2). This led to two consecutive phase II trials in our department using high-dose IFN + P.

II. PATIENTS AND METHODS

A. Patients

Patients fulfilling the following eligibility criteria were entered into the two subsequent trials: histologically confirmed renal cell carcinoma, progressive bidimensionally measurable disease manifestations, age $\leq$ 70 years, World Health Organization (WHO) performance status $\leq$ 2, no previous hormone treatment or chemotherapy, and informed consent.

In trial 18, 23 patients were treated with recombinant interferon-α (Roferon A and Roceron A, Hoffmann-LaRoche), 18×10^6 IU intermuscularly three times per week, together with oral prednisone (5 mg, four times per day for 4 weeks). Thereafter the prednisone dose was gradually reduced to the maintenance dose of 10 mg daily.

In trial 27, in 27 subsequent patients the interferon dose was increased to 27×10^6 IU three times per week given subcutaneously, whereas the prednisone doses were the same as in trial 18.

B. Follow-up

During treatment and at each of the monthly follow-up visits, the following parameters were determined: blood cell counts, serum creatinine, alkaline phosphatase, γ-GT, transaminases, and performance status. Hematologic and biochemical toxicity were scored according to WHO criteria (3). Subjective toxicity was arbitrarily graded as the presence or absence of flulike symptoms (none, mild, moderate, severe, or life threatening). The overall tolerability was evaluated as good (no dose modification necessary), poor (dose reduction or temporary treatment discontinuation necessary), or bad (permanent treatment discontinuation necessary).

Objective response was evaluated according to WHO criteria (3). Minimum treatment duration was 2 months, unless early progression was recorded before this period elapsed. Treatment was discontinued after 2 months for progression or after 3 months if the size reduction was <30% (4). All other patients continued until progression and/or the development of unacceptable toxicity. All treatment was discontinued after 1 year.

III. RESULTS

A total of 23 patients from trial 18 and 24 patients from trial 27 were finally evaluable for response (Table 1): 49 patients were evaluable for toxicity.

Table 1 Demographics

	Trial 18	Trial 27	Total
Number of patients	23	27	50
Ineligible	—	1	1
Unevaluable for response	—	2	2
Prior nephrectomy[a]	20	22	42
Performance status[a]			
0	8	15	23
1	12	10	22
2	3	1	4
Treatment duration,[a] months			
<2	6	6	12
2–4	10	15	25
>4	7	5	12
Site of indicator lesion[b]			
Lung	8	12	20
Soft tissue, locoregional	3	5	8
Liver	6	1	7
Lymph nodes	2	5	7
Bone[c]	2	1	3
Primary tumor	2	—	2

[a] All evaluable patients.
[b] Patients evaluable for response.
[c] With measurable surrounding soft tissue extension.

A. Response

An objective response was seen in five patients from trial 18 and four patients from trial 27 (Table 2; response rate, 19%; 95% confidence response rate, 9–33%). Of the nine responses two were complete, one in each trial. The median response duration was 8 months.

B. Toxicity

Hematologic, but not biochemical toxicity was more frequent and more pronounced in patients from trial 27 than those from trial 18 (Table 3). Subjective toxicity (flulike symptoms) contributed to the decision to discontinue the treatment with IFN + P after 3 months in two nonresponding patients from trial 18 and seven similar patients from trial 27. In an additional two patients from trial 27 treatment was discontinued before 4 weeks elapsed.

Table 2 Response[a]

	Trial 18 (23)	Trial 27 (24)	Total (47)
Overall response (%)	5 (22)	4 (17)	9 (19)
Complete response	1	1	2
Partial response	4	3	7
No change	6	14	20
Progression	12	6	18
Time to progression, months	8, 8, 21, 24, 30	4, 5, 8, 15[+]	4, 5, 8, 8, 8, 15[+], 21, 24, 30

[a] The 95% confidence intervals are 8–44% for trial 18, 5–37% for trial 27, and 9–33% for total.

C. Survival

The 1 year survival rate for all evaluable patients was 52%, without significant difference between the two different phase II studies (Fig. 1).

IV. DISCUSSION

The present study confirms that IFN has definite although limited activity in MRCC (5–12). IFN doses of 18×10^6 IU three times per week seem to be as effective as doses of 27×10^6 IU three times per week. Our overall response rate of 19% and our 1 year survival rate of 52% are in agreement with previous reports using similar doses of IFN in MRCC, either applied as monotherapy or in combination with vinblastine (1,5,12–14).

Most of these clinical investigators have reported significant and often dose-limiting flulike symptoms in 80–90% of the patients treated with IFN doses similar to those used in the present study. In contrast to these reports, dose-limiting toxicity was observed in only 11 of our 49 evaluable patients receiving IFN together with prednisone. IFN doses of 27×10^6 IU three times per week led to significant flulike symptoms in one-third of the patients, whereas only two of 23 of the patients from trial 18 developed dose-limiting IFN toxicity. Prednisone itself may cause toxicity, however, particularly in patients with a history of peptic ulcer.

Responses of MRCC to high-dose IFN are partly induced by the direct cytotoxic effects of the drug (15). IFN may in addition have an immuno-stimulating effect that can be monitored by natural killer (NK) cell activity (1). Our results suggest that low-dose prednisone treatment does not interfere with any immunostimulating effect of high-dose IFN, as far as the response

Table 3 Toxicity

	Trial 18	Trial 27	Total
Evaluable patients	23	26	49
Leukocytes[a]			
0	22	19	41
1	1	6	7
2			
3		1	1
Thrombocytes			
0	22	23	45
1	1	3	4
γ-GT[a]			
0	9	12	21
1	7	8	15
2	5	5	10
3	2	1	3
Creatinine[a]			
0	17	25	42
1	6	1	7
Tolerability[b]			
Good	19	17	36
Poor, bad	4	9	13
Flulike symptoms[b]			
None or mild	21	20	41
Moderate	2	4	6
Severe	—	2	2
Toxicity-associated treatment discontinuation	2	9	11

[a] WHO toxicity grading.
[b] For grading, see text.

rate in MRCC is considered. However, in future studies combining IFN and Prednisone, the NK activity should be monitored together with other parameters of treatment-induced immune response.

V. CONCLUSION

The present study confirms previous observations (2,16) that the combination of interferon and prednisone is as effective in MRCC as interferon monotherapy, with a response rate of 19%. The addition of low-dose prednisone leads to considerably reduced subjective toxicity during interferon treatment without reduction in the response rate.

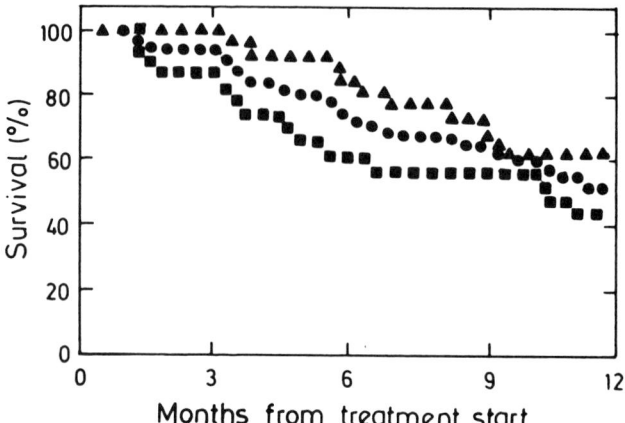

Figure 1   One year survival in 49 patients with MRCC treated with IFN + prednisone. All evaluable patients (49, circles): trial 18 (23, squares); and trial 27 (26, triangles).

REFERENCES

1. Porzsolt F, Digel W, Jacobsen H, Mittnacht S, Kirchner H, Heimpel H. Different antitumor mechanisms of interferon-alpha in the treatment of hairy cell leukemia and renal cell cancer. Cancer 1988; 61:288–93.
2. Fosså SD. Improved subjective tolerability of interferon by combination with prednisolone. Eur J Cancer Clin Oncol 1987; 23:875–6.
3. Miller AB, Hoogstraten B, Staquet M, Winkler A. Reporting results of cancer treatment. Cancer 1981; 47:207–14.
4. Fosså SD, Nesland JM, Melvik JE, Jacobsen AB, Moe AB. Prediction of objective response to recombinant interferon-alpha with or without vinblastine in metastatic renal cell carcinoma. Acta Oncol 1990; 29:303–6.
5. Bergerat J–P, Herbrecht R, Dufour P, et al. Combination of recombinant interferon alfa-2A and vinblastine in advanced renal cell cancer. Cancer 1988; 62:2320–4.
6. Muss HB, Costanzi JJ, Leavitt R, et al. Recombinant alfa interferon in renal cell carcinoma: a randomized trial of two routes of administration. J Clin Oncol 1987; 5:286–91.
7. Schornagel JH, Verweij J, Ten Bokkel Huinink WW, et al. Phase II study of recombinant interferon alpha-2-A and vinblastine in advanced renal cell carcinoma. J Urol 1989; 142:253–6.
8. Figlin RA, deKernion JB, Mukamel E, Palleroni AV, Itri LM, Sarna GP. Recombinant interferon alfa-2a in metastatic renal cell carcinoma: assessment of

antitumor activity and anti-interferon antibody formation. J Clin Oncol 1988; 6:1604–10.

9. Quesada JR, Rios A, Swanson D, Trown P, Gutterman JU. Antitumor activity of recombinant-derived interferon alpha in metastatic renal cell carcinoma. J Clin Oncol 1985; 3:1522–8.

10. Creagan ET, Buckner JC, Hahn RG, Richardson RR, Schaid DJ, Kovach JS. An evaluation of recombinant leucocyte A interferon with aspirin in patients with metastatic renal cell cancer. Cancer 1988; 61:1787–91.

11. Krown SE. Therapeutic options. Semin Oncol 1985; 12:13–7.

12. Trump DL, Elson PJ, Borden EC, et al. High-dose lymphoblastoid Interferon in advanced renal cell carcinoma: an Eastern Cooperative Oncology Group Study. Cancer Treat Rep 1987; 71:165–9.

13. Fosså SD, Raabe N, Moe B. Recombinant interferon-alpha with or without vinblastine in metastatic renal cell carcinoma: results of a randomized phase-II study. Br J Urol 1989; 64:468–71.

14. Neidhart JA, Anderson SA, Harris JE, et al. Vinblastine fails to improve response of renal cancer to interferon alfa-n1: high response rate in patients with pulmonary metastases. J Clin Oncol 1991; 9:832–7.

15. Welander CE. Overview of preclinical and clinical studies of interferon alfa-2b in combination with cytotoxic drugs. Invest New Drugs 1987; 5:47–59.

16. Fosså SD, Gunderson R, Moe B. Recombinant Interferon-alpha combined with prednisone in metastatic renal cell carcinoma. Reduced toxicity without reduction of the response rate—a phase II study. Cancer 1990; 65:2451–4.

27

Interleukin-2 and Interferon-α in Renal Cell Carcinoma

Europe

Jens Atzpodien, Alfred Körfer, Axel Schomburg, Thomas Menzel, Werner De Riese, Hubert Poliwoda, and Hartmut Kirchner

Medizinische Hochschule Hannover, Hannover, Germany

I. INTRODUCTION

Metastatic renal cell carcinoma continues to present a therapeutic challenge. Spontaneous regression of metastatic disease has been observed in a small proportion of patients, but prognosis remains poor, with 1- and 3-year survival rates of 26 and 4%, respectively, in patients with recurrent or metastatic disease (1,2).

Given the lack of effective hormonal or chemotherapeutic agents in metastatic renal carcinoma, immunomodulatory treatment approaches are warranted.

Clinical trials employing recombinant interferon-α (rIFN-α) at doses of three or more megaunits daily three to five times per week have yielded objective remissions in 5–27% of patients treated, with an overall response rate of approximately 16% (3,4).

In initial studies, the systemic administration of high-dose intravenous (IV) recombinant interleukin-2 (rIL-2) in conjunction with lymphokine-activated killer cells has produced a response rate of 33%, including complete remissions in patients with metastatic renal cell carcinoma (5).

In this and subsequent clinical trials, however, the severity of adverse reactions (life-threatening fluid retention, hypotension, and pulmonary edema) has limited the IV use of rIL-2 to the inpatient and/or intensive care setting, depending on the schedule employed (5–10).

More recently, the use of rIL-2 has provided evidence for a nonlinear dose-response curve, resulting in biologic and therapeutic responses at dosages up to 10-fold below the maximum tolerated dose. In the European Immunotherapy Trials Program conducted at our institution, low-dose rIL-2 has been self-administered as a subcutaneous (SC) bolus (11). This novel mode of application has been employed as home therapy; when compared to intravenous rIL-2 regimens it reduced systemic toxicity while preserving therapeutic efficacy in patients with metastatic renal cell carcinoma (11).

Recent studies at our institution have also demonstrated a synergism between rIL-2 and rIFN-α in the preclinical and clinical settings (12,13).

Here, we report our cumulative experience using SC rIL-2 and rIFN-α as home therapy in patients with metastatic renal cell carcinoma. In addition to objective tumor regressions, we evaluated systemic toxicity and long-term survival of patients as parameters of palliative tumor therapy.

II. PATIENTS AND METHODS

A. Patients

A group of 50 patients with progressive metastatic renal cell cancer were treated with this protocol and received SC rIL-2 and SC rIFN-α (Table 1). All patients had histologically confirmed tumors and clinically evaluable progressive disease. Most patients (90%) entered in the study had an Eastern Cooperative Oncology group performance status of zero or one. In all patients, tumor nephrectomy was always performed before systemic therapy.

B. Treatment Plan and Patient Evaluation

All patients were treated as outpatients. Upon rIL-2/rIFN-α combination therapy, patients received a 2 day rIL-2 (EuroCetus, Amsterdam) pulse at 14.4–18.0 million IU/m^2/day, followed by 3.6–4.8 million IU/m^2/day, 5 days/week, over 6 consecutive weeks, and rIFN-α_{2B} (Essex Pharma, München) at 3.0–6.0 million U/m^2 administered two to three times weekly for 6 weeks. Treatment courses were repeated unless progression of disease occurred.

Reevaluation of the patient's tumor status was performed at regular 2 month intervals. A complete remission was defined as the disappearance of all

Table 1 Patient Characteristics

Evaluable patients	50
Sex	
Male	36
Female	14
Age (years)	
Median	55
Range	23–69
Pretreatment	
Surgery	50
Chemotherapy	6
Radiotherapy	15
Hormones	10
Immunotherapy	14

signs of disease for a minimum of 4 weeks, a partial remission as a minimum of 50% reduction in the sum of the products of the greatest perpendicular diameters of measurable lesions without an increase in size of any lesion, or the appearance of new lesions, stable disease as less than a partial response in the absence of disease progression for at least 8 weeks, and progression as an increase of at least 25% in the sum of the products of the longest perpendicular diameters of measurable lesions, or the development of new lesions.

C. Evaluation of Patient Sera

To quantitate serum levels of anti-IL-2 and anti-IFN-α IgG antibodies, an indirect enzyme-linked immunosorbent assay was used as reported previously (14). For the detection of neutralizing activity against rIL-2, patient sera were heat inactivated (52°C for 30 minutes) and tested for inhibition of mouse cytotoxic T lymphocytes, employing a [3H]thymidine proliferation assay. A neutralizing titer > 100, defined as fold reduction in IL-2-induced proliferation times the final serum dilution, was considered positive (15).

D. Hematologic Studies

The hematologic effects of rIL-2 were evaluated using differential blood counts obtained from all patients at weekly intervals.

E. Statistical Analyses

Statistical significance was assessed using the *t*-test, the paired *t*-test, and the Wilcoxon and Cox multivariate analyses wherever applicable.

III. RESULTS

In this clinical trial, 50 evaluable patients were treated (Table 1).

A. Treatment Response

Of the 50 evaluable patients who received SC rIL-2 and SC rIFN-α, four had a complete response and 10 a partial remission. Objective tumor regressions occurred in lungs ($n = 13$), liver ($n = 1$), lymph nodes ($n = 4$), bone ($n = 2$), and other tumor sites ($n = 2$), including a pleural metastasis (Table 2). All objective tumor remissions were observed during the first treatment cycle. The median response duration was 23^+ months in patients with complete tumor regression. An additional 20 patients presented with stable disease upon therapy.

B. Survival

Overall median survival from start of therapy was calculated at 20^+ months in all patients irrespective of the tumor response. Size of metastatic lesions was identified as an independent prognostic parameter (Cox analysis); thus, 1 and 2 year survival rates of 71% were calculated in patients with small lesions (≤ 20 mm ϕ), as opposed to 35 and 23% in patients with larger metastases (i.e., >20 mm ϕ). Long-term survival rates from time of diagnosis of metastatic disease were 78, 65, and 31% at 1, 2, and 5 years, respectively, in all patients treated.

Table 2 Clinical Response and Tumor Site[a]

	Evaluable	Complete response	Partial response	Stable disease	Progressive disease
rIL-2/rIFN-α	50	4	10	20	16
Tumor site					
Lung	40	4	9	16	11
Liver	8	—	1	4	3
Lymph nodes	25	2	2	8	13
Bone	14	—	2	7	5
Local relapse	6	—	—	5	1
Other	15	1	1	9	4

[a] All patients evaluable completed at least one cycle of treatment.

C. Toxicity

Recombinant IL-2 and rIFN-α produced World Health Organization grade I or II fevers, chills, and malaise in 85, 64, and 85% of treatment cycles. Anorexia (grade I/II) was seen in 89% of cycles and was often accompanied by nausea and vomiting (82% of treatment courses) and/or diarrhea (36% of treatment courses). Transient elevations in serum alkaline phosphatase or serum transaminases occurred in 44% of treatment cycles. Hypotension was seen in 25% of courses and was usually mild. Respiratory distress was noted in 36% of cycles but was never associated with pulmonary fluid retention. In all patients, rIL-2/rIFN-α-related systemic toxicity resolved after cessation of treatment. Capillary leak-induced fluid retention and weight gain did not occur. No toxic deaths occurred.

The subcutaneous administration of rIL-2 resulted in transient inflammation and local induration at the injection sites, which persisted for up to 2 weeks following treatment.

D. Neutralizing Antibodies Against rIL-2 or rIFN-α

Tumor response was never abrogated by neutralizing serum activity to rIL-2 ($n = 3$) or rIFN-α ($n = 0$). None of the patients exhibited neutralizing antibodies during the first 2 months of therapy.

E. Hematologic Effects

Systemic administration of rIL-2 resulted in a mean 1.7-fold increase in circulating lymphocytes. Subset analyses revealed a significant expansion of natural killer cells as a statistical correlate to treatment response (data not shown).

IV. DISCUSSION

As part of the European Immunotherapy Trials Program, in the present clinical study we evaluated the outpatient combination of rIFN-α and rIL-2 in patients with advanced progressive renal cell carcinoma. All patients received immunotherapy at home.

The mechanisms by which interleukin-2 and interferon-α mediate tumor regression have been extensively studied but are not yet fully understood. It has been hypothesized that IFN-α may augment IL-2-induced killing through activation of cytotoxic lymphocytes and via enhanced expression of major histocompatibility complex class I antigens on tumor cells (13,16,17).

In this clinical study, tumor regressions occurred in 28% of patients receiving rIL-2 and rIFN-α combination therapy for progressive metastatic renal cell carcinoma. Response rates appeared to exceed those observed with hormonal therapy (less than 5%) (18) and chemotherapy alone (less than 10% for vinblastine and other cytoxic agents) (3). Remission rates between 0% and 18% have been reported with rIL-2 alone (5,19,20).

In the present study, low-dose subcutaneous rIL-2 was used with a standard dose of rIFN-α. The overall toxicity of the combination was low, compared to that with the intravenous administration of single-agent rIL-2 (5–10). The clinical efficacy in our patients (8% complete and 20% partial responses) has been comparable to the most aggressive rIL-2 regimen available (5).

In addition, with this home therapy, the survival of metastatic progressive renal cell carcinoma patients has been significantly extended beyond the survival of historic controls (1,2,21–23). Although no cure is available in this disease, it appears that long-term systemic administration low-dose immunotherapy may prolong patient survival while limiting systemic toxicity and preserving overall quality of life.

Randomized prospective clinical trials are needed to establish the risk-benefit advantage and therapeutic efficacy of recombinant subcutaneous interleukin-2 and interferon-α at systemic outpatient doses far below the maximum tolerated dose.

REFERENCES

1. Buzaid AC, Todd MB. Therapeutic options in renal cell carcinoma. Semin Oncol 1989; 16:12–9.
2. Patel NP, Lavengood RW. Renal cell cancer: neutral history and results of treatment. J Urol 1977; 119:722–6.
3. Krown SE. Therapeutic options in renal cell carcinoma. Semin Oncol 1985; 12:13–7.
4. Muss HB. Interferon therapy for renal cell carcinoma. Semin Oncol 1987; 14:36–42.
5. Rosenberg SA, Lotze MT, Muul LM, et al. A progress report on the treatment of 157 patients with advanced cancer using lymphokine-activated killer cells and interleukin-2 or high-dose interleukin-2 alone. N Engl J Med 1987; 316:889–97.
6. West WH, Tauer KW, Yannelli JR, et al. Constant-infusion recombinant interleukin-2 in adoptive immunotherapy of advanced cancer. N Engl J Med 1987; 316:898–905.
7. Fisher RI, Coltman CA, Doroshow JH, et al. Metastatic renal cancer treated with interleukin-2 and lymphokine-activated killer cells. Ann Intern Med 1988; 108:518–23.

8. Rosenberg SA, Packard BS, Aebersold PM, et al. Use of tumor-infiltrating lymphocytes and interleukin-2 in the immunotherapy of patients with metastatic melanoma. N Engl J Med 319:1676–80.

9. Rosenstein M, Ettinghausen SE, Rosenberg SA. Extravasation of intravascular fluid mediated by the systemic administration of recombinant interleukin-2. J Immunol 1986; 137:1735–42.

10. Lee RE, Lotze MT, Skibber JM, et al. Cardiorespiratory effects of immunotherapy with interleukin-2. J Clin Oncol 1989; 7:7–20.

11. Atzpodien J, Körfer A, Evers P, et al. Low dose subcutaneous recombinant interleukin-2 in advanced human malignancy: a phase II outpatient study. Mol Biother 1990; 2:18–26.

12. Atzpodien J, Shimazaki C, Wisniewski D, et al. Interleukin-2 und interferon-α in der adoptiven Immuntherapie des Plasmozytoms: Ein experimentelles Modell. In: Lutz D, Heinz R, Nowotny H, Stacher A, eds. Leukämien und Lymphome. München: Urban & Schwarzenberg, 1988; 211–2.

13. Atzpodien J, Körfer A, Franks CR, Poliwoda H, Kirchner H. Home therapy with recombinant interleukin-2 and interferon-α2b in advanced human malignancies. Lancet 1990; 335:1509–12.

14. Engvall E, Perlman P. Enzyme-linked immunosorbent assay (ELISA). Quantitative assay of immunoglobulin G. Immunochemistry 1971; 8:871–4.

15. Gillis S, Ferm MM, Ou W. T cell growth factor: parameters of production and a quantitative microassay for activity. J Immunol 1978; 120:2027–32.

16. Spiegel RE. The alpha interferons: clinical overview. Semin Oncol 1986; 13:207–17.

17. Brunda MJ, LBellantoni D, Sulich V. In vivo anti-tumor activity of combinations of interferon alpha and interleukin-2 in a murine model. Correlation of efficacy with the induction of cells resembling natural killer cells. Int J Cancer 1987; 40:3948–53.

18. Harris DT. Hormonal therapy and chemotherapy of renal cell carcinoma. Semin Oncol 1983; 10:422–30.

19. Whitehead RP, Ward DL, Hemingway LL. Effect of subcutaneous recombinant interleukin 2 in patients with disseminated renal cell carcinoma. Proc Am Soc Clin Oncol 1987; 6:241.

20. Sosman JA, Kohler PC, Hank J. Repetitive weekly cycles of recombinant human interleukin-2: responses of renal carcinoma with acceptable toxicity. J Natl Cancer Inst 1988; 80:60–3.

21. Elson PJ, Witte RS, Trump DL. Prognostic factors for survival in patients with recurrent or metastatic renal cell carcinoma. Cancer Res 1988; 48:7310–3.

22. Onishi T, Machida T, Masuda F, et al. Nephrectomy in renal carcinoma with distant metastasis. Br J Urol 1989; 63:600–4.

23. Maldazys JD, deKernion JB. Prognostic factors in metastatic renal carcinoma. J Urol 1986; 136:376–9.

VII

Chemotherapy and Chemoimmunotherapy

28

Interleukin-2 and Vinblastine for Renal Cell Carcinoma

Frederick R. Aronson

University of California, San Francisco, San Francisco, California

I. INTRODUCTION

Renal cell carcinoma accounts for approximately 2% of all malignancies and approximately 2% of all cancer deaths. The prognosis for patients with recurrent or metastatic renal cancer is poor, with mortality rates of 74 and 96% at 1 and 3 years, respectively (1). Treatment of advanced disease with hormonal or chemotherapy has generally been of limited benefit. Recent enthusiasm for infusional floxuridine treatment, with generally tolerable toxicity and an objective response rate of nearly 20%, must be tempered by the limited duration of objective responses (median 10.8 months, range 1–18 months) (2). Interferons α, β, and γ are active alone or in combination, but most responses are partial, of limited duration, and occur in patients with lung as the only site of metastatic disease (3–7).

High-dose interleukin-2 (IL-2)-based therapy induces objective responses in approximately 20% and durable complete responses in 5–10% of patients but is associated with significant acute toxicity that limits its use to carefully selected patients (8,9). To date, results have not improved by combining IL-2 with other biologic agents (10). IL-2 and vinblastine (11) are both active against renal cell carcinoma and have distinct toxicities and mechanisms of action. In an effort to improve the efficacy and reduce the toxicity of IL-2 therapy for renal cell carcinoma, we conducted a phase II trial of moderate-dose IL-2 given by continuous infusion alternating with vinblastine. Despite accruing a relatively poor risk group of patients, 3 of 20 patients entered have achieved responses that are ongoing at greater than 2 years off treatment.

II. METHODS

A. Patients

All patients had histologically confirmed, bidimensionally measurable stage III or IV renal cell carcinoma. Other eligibility criteria included age > 18 years, Eastern Cooperative Oncology Group (ECOG) performance status of 0 (asymptomatic) or 1 (symptomatic but fully functional), anticipated survival of at least 4 months, and adequate organ function defined by leukocyte count greater than 3500 μl^{-1}, platelet count greater than 100,000 μl^{-1}, serum creatinine less than 2.0 mg/dl, normal serum bilirubin, SGOT less than twice the upper limit of normal, forced expiratory volume in one second greater than 2.0 liters, or ≥75% of predicted, and no evidence of congestive heart failure, prior myocardial infarction, serious arrhythmias, or signs of ischemia on electrocardiography and exercise stress test. A negative pregnancy test was required for women of child-bearing potential. Patients were excluded if hepatitis B surface antigen or antibodies to human immunodeficiency virus were detected in serum, if the use of pressors was contraindicated, if corticosteroid use was likely to be required, or if active infection was present. Furthermore, subjects with prior malignancy other than basal cell carcinoma, with brain metastases, organ allografts, or significant comorbid illness were ineligible. Prior hormonal therapy, radiotherapy, or immunotherapy was permitted if completed at least 3 weeks before IL-2 therapy was begun. However, patients previously treated with IL-2 or vinca alkaloids were excluded. Investigational review board (IRB) approval was obtained, and all patients gave written informed consent.

B. Treatment

The treatment scheme is described in Table 1. IL-2 therapy was administered on the regular oncology wards of the University of California, San Francisco (UCSF) Medical Center and the San Francisco Veterans Administration (VA) Hospital. Recombinant human IL-2 [specific activity 18 million international units (MIU) per mg protein] was provided by Cetus Corporation (Emeryville, CA). Patients received IL-2 (18 MIU/m^2 per 24 h) by continuous intravenous (IV) infusion for up to 96 h on days 1–5 and 12–16. The dose was reduced by

Table 1 Interleukin-2 and Vinblastine Treatment Scheme

Days 1–5 and 12–16: interleukin-2, inpatient oncology ward, continuous
  intravenous infusion for up to 96 h; dose, 18 million IU/m^2 per 24 h[a]
Days 24 and 26: vinblastine, outpatient oncology clinic, rapid intravenous
  injection; dose,[a] 4 mg/m^2
Next cycle begins on day 36

---

[a] Dose reductions required for significant toxicity (see text).

50% for grade III toxicity (hypotension unresponsive to fluids, dyspnea at
rest, symptoms or signs of myocardial ischemia, life-threatening arrhythmias,
change in mental status, or other severe toxicity). A second dose reduction, to
25% of the full dose, was permitted for persistent grade III toxicity. At any
point, treatment was discontinued rather than reduced if persistence of the
toxicity was considered potentially life-threatening. Treatment was resumed
when toxicity abated to grade I or better. Patients whose dose was reduced by
50% began subsequent infusions at full dose; those whose dose was reduced
by 50% on two occasions for the same toxicity and those whose dose was
reduced to 25% or less began subsequent infusions at 75% of the original
dose. Treatment was discontinued in patients who developed grade IV (life-
threatening) toxicity. Acetaminophen, indomethacin, and ranitidine were
given on a regular basis during IL-2 therapy. In addition, IV merepidine was
given for rigors, antihistamines were given for pruritius, and antiemetics and
antidiarrheal agents were given as needed. Furosemide was given for several
days after each IL-2 treatment to eliminate fluids retained during therapy.
Corticosteroids were administered only for life-threatening toxicity. Vinblastine (4 mg/m^2 per dose) was given in the outpatient clinic by IV bolus on
days 24 and 26 of each 35 day cycle. The vinblastine dose was reduced by
50% for white blood count (WBC) < 3500 μl^{-1}, platelets $< 100,000$ μl^{-1},
or bilirubin at 1.5–3.0 mg/dl or by 75% for bilirubin > 3.0 mg/dl and was
omitted for WBC < 3000 μl^{-1} or platelets $< 75,000$ μl^{-1} as measured on
day 24.

Patients were evaluated for response after completing two cycles of treatment. Those without evidence of tumor progression could receive two additional cycles of treatment. Patients with stable disease after four cycles were
removed from the study. Responding patients were eligible to continue
therapy; therapy was discontinued when patients had no further response to
treatment or had disease progression or severe toxicity. Patients who achieved
a complete response were eligible to receive two additional cycles of treat-

ment. Responding patients and those with stable disease were followed until disease progression; patients with progressive disease were removed from the study.

C. Response Evaluation

Complete responses were defined as the total disappearance of all tumor for at least 4 weeks at all sites on physical examination, computed tomographic scans, and, in patients with bone lesions, plain radiographs. Partial responses were defined as $\geq 50\%$ reduction in the sum of the products of the longest perpendicular diameters of all measurable lesions for at least 4 weeks without the appearance of new lesions. Patients with less than 50% tumor regression or less than 25% tumor growth and no new lesions were considered to have stable disease. Patients with a $\geq 25\%$ increase in tumor bulk or with new lesions were considered to have progressive disease. Response durations were calculated from the date patients completed therapy.

III. RESULTS

A. Patients

A total of 20 patients with advanced renal cell carcinoma were enrolled in this study between August 1988 and June 1991. It is important to note that all patients enrolled on this study either declined or were ineligible to be enrolled on the National Cancer Institute-sponsored high-dose IL-2-based therapy protocols that were active at UCSF during this time. All patients had evidence of progressive disease at the time of entry in the study, and all patients were considered evaluable for response and toxicity; their characteristics are listed in Table 2.

B. Treatment

The 20 patients have thus far received a total of 55 courses of IL-2 and vinblastine. One patient with stable disease after 2 cycles of therapy is continuing treatment at this time. Both patients who were accrued at the San Francisco VA Hospital elected to discontinue therapy before completing 1 cycle of treatment. All the remaining patients completed between 2 and 6 complete cycles of therapy. At least one IL-2 dose reduction was required during 36 of the 55 cycles, and only two patients completed all of the planned treatment without IL-2 dose reduction. Nonetheless, patients received a median of 86% of the planned IL-2 dose (range 44–100%), and 16 of the 20 patients received at least 75% of the planned IL-2 dose. Aside from the 2 VA

Table 2 Patient Characteristics ($N = 20$)

Sex	
Male	15
Female	5
Age, years	
Median	64.5
Range	41–81
ECOG performance status	
Asymptomatic, 0	7
Symptomatic but fully functional, 1	13
Previous treatment	
Nephrectomy	15
Radiation	4
Hormonal	1
No prior systemic therapy	19
Tumor bulk, cm^2	
Median	40.4
Range	5–234
Tumor sites	
Lung	16
Nodes	10
Liver	9
Bone	6
Renal primary	5
Renal bed	3
Mesentery	2
Spleen	1
Adrenal	1
Lung only	1
Lung and nodes only	4

Hospital patients, seven patients required vinblastine dose reductions; however, the average dose received was 89% of the planned dose among the 18 patients who received vinblastine. Thus, although most patients required some dose reductions, the majority of patients received at least 75% of the maximum possible dose of IL-2 and vinblastine.

C. Response

Of the 20 patients treated, there were two complete responses and one partial response. These responses are all ongoing at 29^+, 29^+, and 27^+ months. The patient who achieved a partial response had complete regression of all lung and liver metastases, clinical evidence of response in multiple bone metastases, and partial regression of a 7 cm primary renal lesion after completing four cycles of therapy. After completing a total of six cycles, she underwent partial nephrectomy and has subsequently been free of disease, aside from a residual abnormality on bone scan at the site of a previously irradiated lesion. One of the complete responders developed life-threatening gastrointestinal bleeding from the small bowel 6 days after completing the first 4 day IL-2 infusion. Despite extensive subsequent evaluation, no structural abnormality was identified at the site of bleeding. Response evaluation, however, revealed obvious regression of the multiple lung, lymph node, and renal bed masses and, with the permission of the IRB and the study sponsor and with the patient's informed consent, treatment was resumed without recurrence of bleeding. The other complete responder presented with a subcutaneous lesion and underwent nephrectomy and resection of the subcutaneous lesion and an ileal lesion found at laparotomy but developed multiple lung and liver lesions 2 months later. He achieved a complete response after four cycles and has remained free of disease since completing six cycles. No patient's pretreatment characteristics suggested an increased likelihood of response.

An additional three patients have achieved minor responses: two of these patients recently discontinued treatment because of toxicity (peripheral neuropathy in one patient with a remote history of severe alcohol abuse and life-threatening *staphylococcal* infection in the other) and continue to be followed for evidence of additional response. The other patient was a 41-year-old man with von Hippel-Lindau disease who presented with bilateral bulky renal primary tumors, lung, nodal, and liver lesions, and hypercalcemia. He had no evidence of central nervous system or ocular abnormalities and tolerated therapy with minimal toxicity. He rapidly achieved a complete response, aside from his renal lesions, which showed minimal regression despite six cycles of therapy. After six months off therapy without evidence of extrarenal recurrence, he underwent attempted ex vivo partial nephrectomy and then bilateral nephrectomy; within 2 months of beginning hemodialysis he developed new lung lesions and died 4 months later. One patient had a mixed response, with regression of multiple lung lesions in the face of progressive bone disease. As noted earlier, one patient with stable disease remains on treatment. All the other 12 patients had progressive disease, and 10 of these have died of disease.

D. Toxicity

Overall, the toxicity of this regimen was similar to that reported for other moderate-dose IL-2 regimens (Table 3). Multiple toxic side effects were common, but these were generally mild to moderate in severity. Essentially all patients had some nausea, vomiting, diarrhea, skin rash, hypotension, fluid retention, and elevation in blood creatinine levels; fever, stomatitis, neurologic toxicity, and mild granulocytopenia occurred frequently. Toxicities resolved rapidly in all but one patient with a remote history of alcohol abuse who developed persistent peripheral neuropathy attributed temporally to vinblastine administration. A total of 18 patients required one or more IL-2 dose reductions during treatment. Hypotension unresponsive to IV fluids was the most common dose-limiting toxicity and occurred in 12 patients. Other dose-limiting toxicities included pulmonary toxicity (five patients), neurologic toxicity (four patients), and gastrointestinal toxicity (three patients); five patients had nadir neutrophil counts of less than 1000 μl^{-1}, but none of these patients developed infections. Of 14 patients tested three developed hypothyroidism, including the patient who achieved a partial response and two minor responders. Another three patients had grade IV (life-threatening) toxicities, including hypotension requiring pressors (two patients), pulmonary edema requiring intubation (one patient), gastrointestinal bleeding (one patient), and infection (one patient). There were no treatment-related deaths. In summary, although mild to moderate toxicity was common, treatment was readily managed on the regular oncology ward in most cases, with only 3 of the 55 courses delivered resulting in transfers to the intensive care unit.

Table 3 Toxicity $(N = 20)$[a]

Toxicity	Number of patients	
	Grade I or II	Grade III or IV
Hypotension	8	12
Pulmonary	8	5
Neurologic	6	4
Infection	1	1
Fever	15	0
Cutaneous	17	1
Diarrhea	18	2
Nausea or vomiting	18	1
Bilirubin	4	0
SGOT	8	0
Creatinine	13	4
Granulocytopenia	6	5
Thrombocytopenia	2	0

[a] There were no patient deaths or episodes of myocardial toxicity.

IV. DISCUSSION

This study demonstrates the activity of moderate-dose IL-2 and vinblastine therapy in a group of relatively poor risk patients with advanced renal cell carcinoma. Patients accrued to this study tended to be older, with worse performance status and less favorable sites of disease than patients accrued to other recently reported phase II trials of biologic agents for renal cell carcinoma. This can be accounted for primarily because patients were only accrued to this study if they were not eligible for, or declined to participate in, high-dose IL-2-based trials. In view of the strong effect of these characteristics on response rate, the observation of three objective and durable responses among 20 poor-risk patients is remarkable. Although all three responders had lung lesions, two also had liver metastases and the other had involved lymph nodes and a renal bed recurrence. It is of course not clear that this regimen is superior to high-dose IL-2-based regimens. Further study of this regimen in selected patients is needed before its utility can be confirmed and better defined. To this end, accrual to this trial was extended to investigators at the University of California–Davis and McGill University during late 1990; an additional 12 patients have since been accrued, but an analysis of the final results of the study is not yet possible.

Whether vinblastine contributed significantly to the efficacy of the regimen is unknown. Recent studies using similar doses of IL-2 alone or in combination with other biologics have also shown activity against renal carcinoma (10,12). In addition, at least one patient responded to treatment before receiving vinblastine. Additional data regarding the efficacy of the regimen are required to better address this question. Further study of the combination is not inappropriate since it appears that vinblastine did not add appreciably to toxicity.

Even in this relatively poor risk group of patients, toxicity was almost always manageable on a regular oncology ward. The daily dose used in this regimen is comparable to that of high-dose continuous-infusion regimens, but each infusion was limited to 96 h and the dose was reduced at a lower threshold of toxicity than that used with high-dose regimens given in the intensive care unit. The lower intensity of treatment was particularly beneficial in responders who underwent repeated cycles of treatment in the hospital.

In summary, moderate-dose IL-2 alternating with vinblastine is active against renal cell carcinoma and can induce durable remissions in patients with visceral metastatic disease. Toxicity is similar to that seen with moderate doses of IL-2 alone and was managed on a regular oncology ward almost exclusively. Further study in more selected patients is needed to better define the objective and durable response rates of this regimen and to determine whether vinblastine contributes to efficacy.

V. SUMMARY

Interleukin-2 and vinblastine are active in renal cell carcinoma, have mainly nonoverlapping toxicities, and have distinct mechanisms of action. Between August 1988 and June 1991, 20 patients with advanced renal cell carcinoma were treated in a phase II study with moderate-dose IL-2 (18 million international units per m^2/day, days 1–4 and 12–16) and intravenous injections of vinblastine (4 mg/m^2) on days 24 and 26 of each 35 day cycle. All patients received IL-2 on a regular oncology ward. Toxicity was typical of moderate-dose IL-2 therapy, with frequent but mild nausea, emesis, diarrhea, stomatitis, fever, hypotension, and fluid retention. A total of 18 patients required IL-2 dose reductions, but 80% of patients received at least 75% of the planned doses. Hypotension (12 patients) and pulmonary toxicity (five patients) were the most common dose-limiting side effects. Although three patients had grade IV toxicity (hypotension requiring pressors, pulmonary edema, gastrointestinal bleeding, and infection), there were no treatment-related deaths. Of 14 patients tested three developed hypothyroidism: all three showed evidence of tumor regression. Complete responses were seen in two patients, and one patient had a partial response with subsequent resection of the residual primary renal lesion; all three responses are ongoing at 29^+, 29^+, and 27^+ months off therapy. Another three patients had minor responses, and two of these have not yet been reevaluated after completing therapy. One patient with stable disease after two cycles is still receiving treatment. Moderate-dose IL-2 and vinblastine can be given on a regular oncology ward and appear to have activity comparable to that of high-dose IL-2-based treatment, with some patients achieving durable remissions.

ACKNOWLEDGMENTS

I am grateful to Drs. Frank Valone, Michael Bar, and Kenneth Fink, as well as to the many UCSF fellows and house staff; and to the staff of the Cancer Research Institute ward of UCSF Medical Center for their help in selecting and caring for the patients; and to Mary Lou Ernest, Brigid Hobbs, Yuke Hong, and Michael Tasch for their help with data management and patient care. This study was supported in part by the Cetus Corporation and by NIH Contract NO1-CM73702.

REFERENCES

1. Patel NP, Lavengood RW. Renal cell cancer: natural history and results of treatment. J Urol 1977; 119:722.
2. Hrushesky WJM, von Roemeling R, Lanning RM, Rabatin JT. Cicadian-shaped infusions of floxuridine for progressive metastatic renal cell carcinoma. J Clin Oncol 1990; 8:1504.
3. Quesada JR. Biologic response modifiers in the therapy of metastatic renal cell carcinoma. Semin Oncol. 1988; 15:396.
4. Figlin RA, deKernion JB, Mukamel E, Palleroni AV, Itri LM, Sarna GP. Recombinant interferon alfa-2a in metastatic renal cell carcinoma: assessment of antitumor activity and anti-interferon antibody formation. J Clin Oncol 1988; 6:1604.
5. Kinney P, Triozzi P, Young D, et al. Preliminary report of a phase II trial of interferon-beta serine in metastatic renal cell carcinoma. Proc Am Soc Clin Oncol 1988; 7:162.
6. Aulitzky W, Gastl G, Aulitzky WE, et al. Successful treatment of metastatic renal cell carcinoma with a biologically active dose of recombinant interferon-gamma. J Clin Oncol 1989, 7:1875.
7. Ernstoff MS, Nair S, Bahnson RR, et al. A phase IA trial of sequential administration recombinant DNA-produced interferons: combination recombinant interferon gamma and recombinant interferon alfa in patients with metastatic renal cell carcinoma. J Clin Oncol 1990; 8:1637.
8. Weiss GR, Margolin KA, Aronson FR, et al. A randomized comparison of bolus versus continuous infusion interleukin-2 and lymphokine-activated killer cells in advanced renal cell carcinoma. J Clin Oncol 1992; 10:275.
9. Atkins MB, Sparano J, Fisher RI, et al. Randomized phase II trial of high dose IL-2 either alone or in combination with interferon alpha 2B in advanced renal cell carcinoma. J Clin Oncol 1993, in press.
10. Sznol M, Thurn A, Aronson FR. Treatment with interleukin-2 in combination with other biologic agents. In: Atkins MB, Mier JW, eds. Clinical biology of interleukin-2. New York: Dekker, in press. 1992.
11. Linehan WM, Shipley WU, Longo DL. Cancer of the kidney and ureter. In: DeVita VT Jr, Hellman S, Rosenberg, SA, eds. Cancer: principles and practice of oncology. Philadelphia: Lippincott, 1989; 992.
12. Sossman JA, Kohler PC, Hank J, et al. Repetitive weekly cycles of recombinant human interleukin-2: responses of renal carcinoma with acceptable toxicity. J Natl Cancer Inst 1988; 80:60.

29

Kidney Cancer

Chronochemotherapy

William J. M. Hrushesky

Albany Medical College and Stratton Veterans Administration Medical Center, Albany, New York

I. INTRODUCTION

In 1972, a paper appeared in *Science* that reported that the arrangement within the day of doses every 3 h of cytosine arabinoside (cytarabine, Ara-C) had a pronounced effect on the survival rate of mice inoculated with L1210 leukemia cells (1). This study was built on extensive prior work demonstrating that all Ara-C toxicities are markedly dependent on the time during the day-night cycle at which the drug is administered (2). Together the experiments showed unequivocally that, in mice, the timing of Ara-C administration predictably modulates its therapeutic index (Fig. 1).

Surprisingly, nearly 20 years later, this simple hypothesis has still not been extended to clinical trials for human leukemia, even though the mainstay treatment for the most common deadly acute leukemias has remained Ara-C, used at higher and higher dose intensities with greater and greater toxicity (3). In the meantime, it has been shown that all anthracyclines, which are generally coupled with Ara-C to treat the nonlymphocytic leukemias, also exhibit a pronounced circadian time dependence in their pharmacology, toxicology, and efficacy in mice and in humans (4–6). Furthermore, many combination chemotherapy studies, done in follow-up to the initial Ara-C study, have demonstrated that the addition of a second or third drug to the regimen seldom

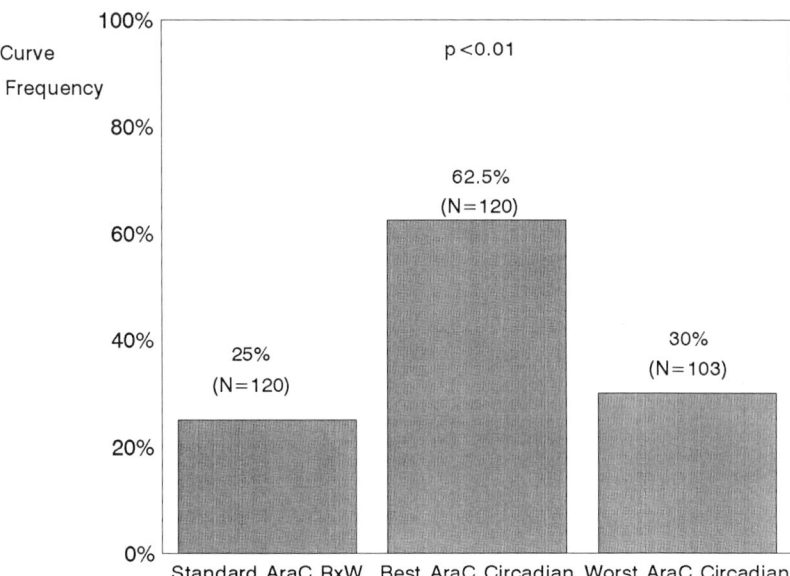

Figure 1   The best Ara-C schedule, peaking 2–6 h before daily awakening, cures over 60% of mice with L1210 leukemia compared to 25% treated by standard non–time-modified administration. The worst circadian schedule, peaking daily, cures 30% of the animals. (From Haus et al. Science 1972; 177:80–82.)

interferes with the enhancement in therapeutic index resulting from circadian optimization of each drug (Fig. 2).

In Minnesota, we began a series of studies in rodents that led to the circadian optimization of the doxorubicin-cisplatin combination (Fig. 3) (8). National Cancer Institute-sponsored randomized clinical studies then revealed that every occurrence of doxorubicin and cisplatin toxicity is largely dependent upon the circadian timing of these agents in human beings (Fig. 4) (4,9). In patients with widespread ovarian cancer, optimal circadian drug timing resulted in safer administration of higher doses of drug and, in turn, an improvement in the 5-year survival rate of women with advanced ovarian cancer. (10).

II. RECENT METHODS AND RESULTS

More recently, a shift in patient accrual and the availability of programmable, implantable drug delivery devices have pointed us toward studies of the time

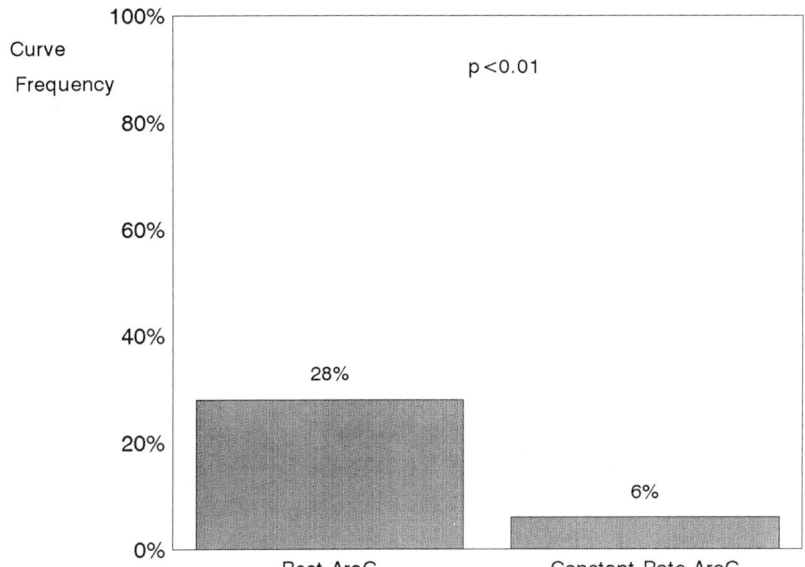

Figure 2 In this study, Ara-C and cyclophosphamide were given to mice after an overwhelming dose of intraperitoneal L1210 leukemia cells. When the best circadian pattern of Ara-C was employed and when cytoxan was given at its daily optima, 28% of mice were cured. When a human nonchronobiologic constant-rate pattern of Ara-C was given and cyclophosphamide was given at either its best or worst time of the mouse day, the average cure rate was 6%. (From Ref. 7.)

dependence of fluoropyrimidine pharmacology, toxicology, and efficacy. As with cytosine arabinoside, doxorubicin-cisplatin, and other anticancer agents, the fluoropyrimidine story began with rodent experimentation. Studies with mice in the early 1980s revealed that the LD_{50} of 5-fluorouracil (5-FU), a mainstay of solid tumor treatment, is markedly and reproducibly higher when given in the sleep span (11,12). Peters et al. confirmed this early work and extended it to show that both nonspecific 5-FU toxicity and toxicity toward a murine colon carcinoma are each dependent on circadian timing (13).

The programmable automatic delivery systems initially available for clinical cancer treatment were small in volume and thus required highly concentrated drug. In anticipation of new clinical trials of chronobiologic chemotherapy studies, fluorodeoxyuridine (FUDR), a more highly concentratable fluoropyrimidine, was studied in mice and rats. Chronotoxicology studies of intravenous and intraperitoneal bolus FUDR administration in mice revealed

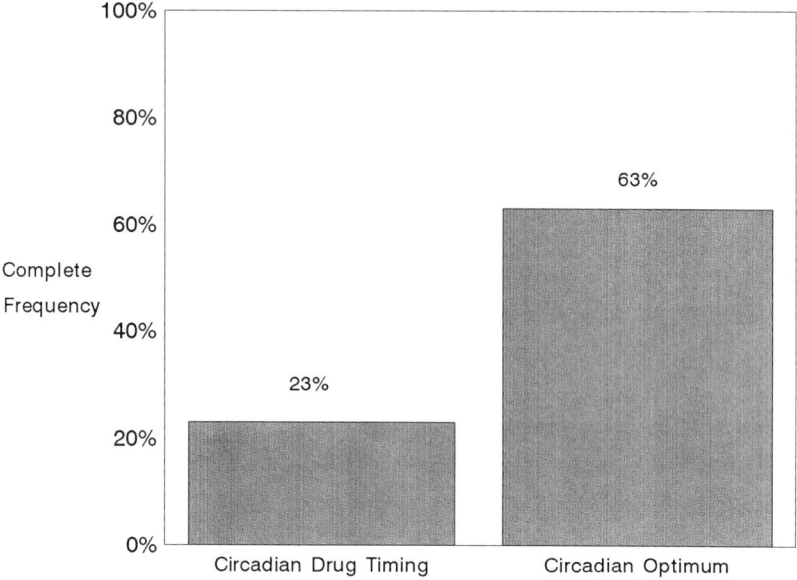

Figure 3 After establishment of a transplanted solid tumor mass, therapy was begun and complete remission frequency was contrasted as a function of circadian drug timing. Doxorubicin was given to all rats just before usual awakening (circadian optimum). When cisplatin was given in daily activity, 23% of rats had complete disappearance of the tumor. When cisplatin was given late in daily activity, approximately three times as many rats had total tumor disappearance. This was the case no matter which agent was given first and whether there were 0–24 or 72–96 h between the drugs. [From Sothern et al. J Natl Cancer Inst 1989; 81 (2).]

that the safest time for this drug was several hours earlier in the day than for 5-FU (14). The highest LD_{50} (lowest toxicity) occurred reproducibly late in the daily activity span. FUDR has an extremely short half-life and hence must be administered by constant infusion. Extensive continuous-infusion studies performed upon Fisher 344 rats afflicted with the fluoropyrimidine-sensitive 13762MT adenocarcinoma revealed that continuous infusions weighted in the late activity and usual sleep span are reproducibly less toxic and more effective than constant-rate infusions or infusions that delivered peak levels of the drug at other times during the day (Fig. 5) (15).

With this preclinical information, we initiated a series of randomized clinical studies to investigate whether the systemic or intrahepatic toxicities of FUDR can be lessened and the dose intensity safely increased by administer-

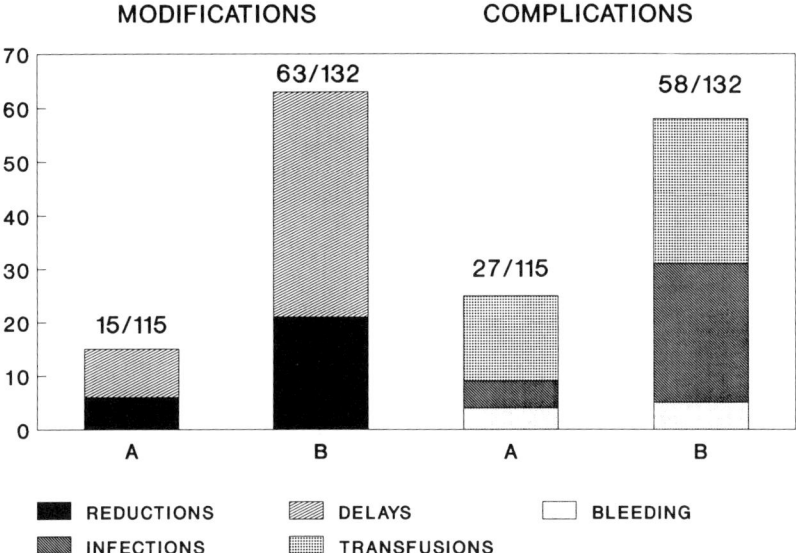

Figure 4 When doxorubicin was given in the morning and cisplatin in the evening (A), fewer dose reductions or treatment delays were required ($p<0.01$) than when doxorubicin was given in the evening and cisplatin was given in the morning (B). Even though less drug was given less often, there was a higher complication frequency with B.

ing the drug late in the cancer patient's usual daily activity span (16). So far we have shown that optimal drug timing offers a clinical advantage for systemic FUDR infusion in patients with metastatic renal cell cancer (17) and for intrahepatic FUDR infusion in colorectal cancer patients with liver metastases (Wesen et al., unpublished). Moreover, Levi et al. (18) demonstrated a clinical advantage to shaping 5-FU infusion (to peak at 4 a.m.) in patients with widespread colorectal cancer.

III. KIDNEY CANCER RESULTS

Continuous long-term 5-fluoro-2'-deoxyuridine (floxuridine) infusion frequently causes severe and dose-limiting gastrointestinal toxicity when administered at a constant rate at commonly prescribed dose levels. In preclinical studies, a circadian infusion pattern peaking late in the daily activity phase was better tolerated and had superior antitumor activity against a transplanted tumor than a constant infusion. Based upon these data and upon other

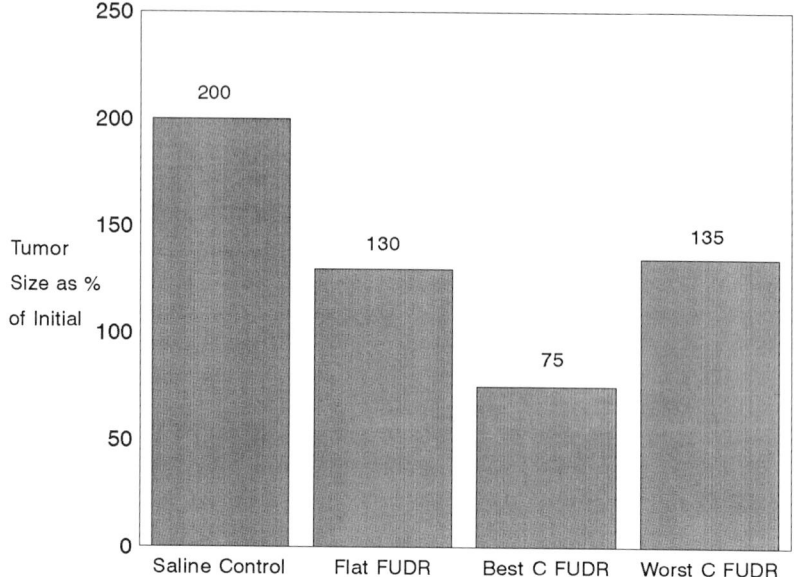

Figure 5 Continuous-infusion FUDR at a constant rate diminished tumor growth compared to saline control. The best circadian regimen, peaking during sleep, resulted in halving tumor size compared to flat infusion. A circadian infusion (C) peaking during wakefulness was equivalent to the flat infusion.

chronobiologic cytokinetic and pharmacologic considerations, we compared a circadian-patterned variable-rate infusion with a maximal flow rate in the late afternoon or early evening and minimum flow rate during the early morning hours to a constant-rate infusion in 54 patients with widespread cancer (Fig. 6). All FUDR infusions were administered using implanted drug pumps. In a pilot crossover study and a second randomized trial, patients with metastatic malignancies treated with equal dose intensities experienced less frequent and less severe diarrhea, nausea, and vomiting following variable-rate infusion (Tables 1 and 2). In a third study, the dose intensity of variable-rate infusion was escalated stepwise to determine the maximum tolerated dose. Patients receiving time-modified FUDR infusion tolerated an average of 1.45-fold more drug per unit time while evincing minimal toxicity (Fig. 7). FUDR infusion was found to have activity against progressive metastatic renal cell cancer (RCC). The increased dose intensity achieved by optimal circadian shaping may improve the therapeutic index of infusional FUDR and may help control malignancies that are refractory to conventional chemotherapy (Fig. 8).

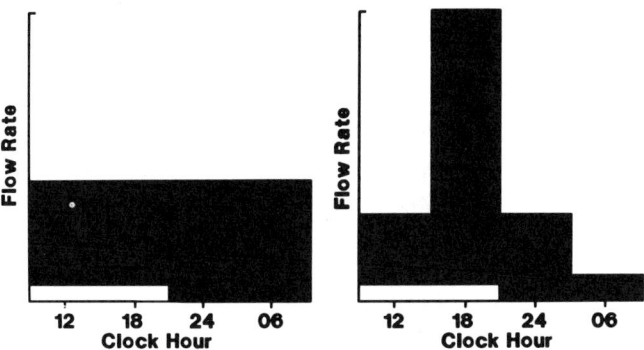

Figure 6 Schedules of FUDR infusions. Area under the curve for each pattern is equivalent.

Table 1 Toxicity of FUDR Infusions: Results of Pilot Study

Type FUDR infusion[a]	Patient	Courses	Dose intensity (mg/kg/week)	Nausea, vomiting (%)	Diarrhea (%)	Hospitalization (%)
Flat	5	12	0.45	60[b]	80[b]	20
Time modified	5	26	0.46	40	20	0

[a] Patients were started on continuous FUDR and crossed over to time-modified infusion.
[b] $p < 0.05$.

Table 2 Randomized Trial of FUDR Infusion in Patients with Metastatic Malignancies

Type FUDR infusion	Patient	Course	Dose intensity (mg/kg/week)	Nausea, vomiting (%)	Diarrhea (%)	Hospitalization (%)
Flat	14	29	0.45	50[a]	43[a]	21
Time modified	16	57	0.48	19	6	0

[a] $p < 0.05$.

A total of 68 unselected consecutive patients with progressive metastatic renal cell carcinoma were treated between March 1985 and November 1988 with continuous-infusion floxuridine. Of these patients, 37% had previously received and failed systemic treatment. Using implantable pumps for automatic drug delivery, FUDR was continuously infused for 14 days at monthly intervals. The starting dose was 0.15 mg/kg/day (intravenous, IV; $n = 61$) or

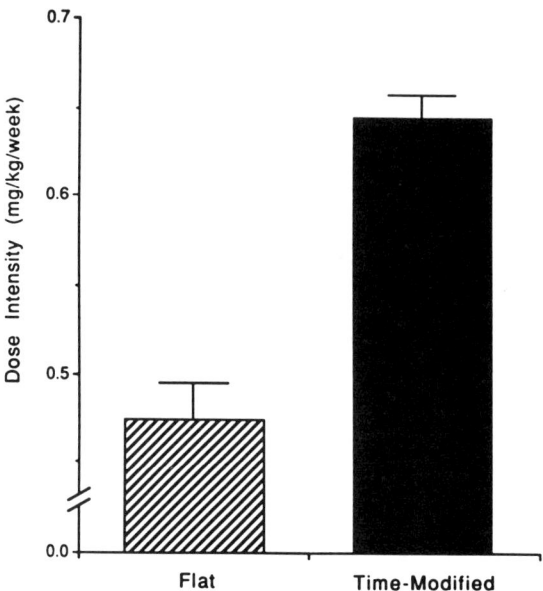

Figure 7   Dose intensity of FUDR administered by flat or time-modified infusions of FUDR.

0.25 mg/kg/day (intraarterial, IA; $n = 7$); IV doses were increased or decreased in increments of 0.025 mg/kg/day as permitted by toxicity. Diarrhea (with or without mild abdominal cramping) and nausea or vomiting limited the FUDR IV infusion, and hepatic function abnormalities limited FUDR IA infusion. The use of a circadian-modified infusion schedule permitted high FUDR doses to be safely given compared with a constant-rate infusion schedule. Of 63 patients assessable for response, 56 received systemic FUDR infusion: four complete responses (CR, 7.1%) and seven partial responses (PR, 12.5%) were observed (objective response rate, CR plus PR, 19.6 ± 5.1%, 95% confidence limits). The median objective response duration was 10.8 months (range 1–18 months; mean 9.4 ± 1.6). An additional four patients had minor tumor responses (MR, 7.1%). In a subgroup of seven assessable patients receiving hepatic arterial FUDR, we observed one CR and three PR (57.2 ± 42.8%). Overall, objective response (CR plus PR) was seen in a quarter of assessable patients treated, 15 of 63, but only 15 of the 63 assessable patients (25.4%) have had objective tumor progression. The median follow-up time for all 68 patients is 28 months (range 1–42), and their

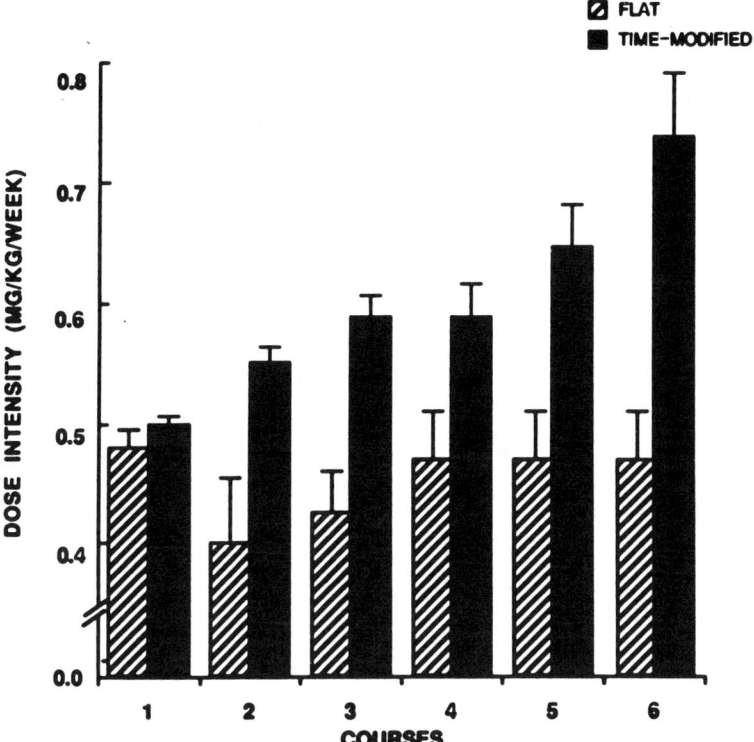

Figure 8 Increases in dose intensity of time-modified FUDR infusion in patients with metastatic renal cell carcinoma compared with a flat infusion schedule.

median survival duration is 15 months (range 3–37 months) (Fig. 9). Continuous-infusion FUDR is an effective outpatient treatment for progressive metastatic RCC, producing durable tumor response and causing little toxicity. In summary, the circadian timing of anticancer drugs markedly affects their pharmacology, toxicology, and efficacy. When giving cytotoxic cancer therapy without regard to its circadian timing, as in continuous infusions, the timing of the peak drug infusion rate results in apparently variable and poorly reproducible therapeutic results and unnecessary drug toxicity.

We and other investigators have begun to attempt to define the mechanisms that underlie the circadian time dependence of fluoropyrimidine toxicity and anticancer activity. Of potential importance is the way drugs are handled by the organs primarily responsible for catabolism or excretion (drug pharmacol-

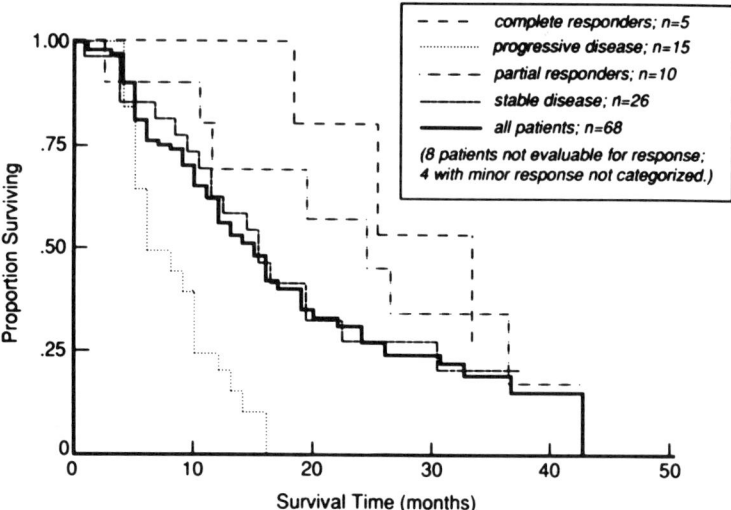

Figure 9 Survival of 68 patients with metastatic renal cell carcinoma receiving time-modified FUDR infusion.

ogy), the way drugs are handled by the targets of toxicity (biochemical pharmacology), and, correlatively, the cell cycle phase of the target cells at the time of drug exposure (circadian cytokinetics) (19–23).

IV. MECHANISMS OF FLUOROPYRIMIDINE CIRCADIAN PHARMACODYNAMICS

The circadian-dependent pharmacology of continuous, constant-rate 5-FU infusion, as measured by rhythmic fluctuations in plasma levels of the drug throughout the day, was first demonstrated by Petit et al. (24) and later by Harris et al. (25). Each group noted marked variations in pharmacokinetics at different times of the day, although the timing of peak FU levels differed between the two groups of patients. The difference may be related to the fact that the patients in the first study received cisplatin at a fixed time of day before each 5-day 5-FU infusion, whereas the patients in the second study received only 5-FU and for much longer spans. Nonetheless, both papers clearly demonstrate that there are large, reproducible differences within studies and across subjects in plasma levels of 5-FU at different times of the day during a continuous, constant-rate drug infusion.

Work by Tuchman (26, 28) and, later, by Diasio et al. (27) demonstrated the importance of dihydropyrimidine dehydrogenase (DPD) as the rate-limiting enzyme involved in the breakdown of 5-FU to nontoxic metabolites. When human peripheral blood mononuclear cells were isolated around the clock in seven subjects, we found that DPD levels were much higher just after usual sleep onset than at other times of the day (Fig. 10) (28). In their recent elegant ex vivo rat liver perfusion study, Harris et al. demonstrate unequivocally that 5-FU clearance and metabolism by the liver are critically circadian stage dependent. Eight times as much 5-FU was extracted per unit time from perfused rat livers removed in mid- to late sleep compared to those removed in midactivity (29). Tuchman's data showing that the levels of human mononuclear DPD (28) peak during sleep are consistent with the results of the perfusion experiments in rodents. In aggregate, these data suggest that a prominent circadian rhythm in DPD activity exhibited by both organs of

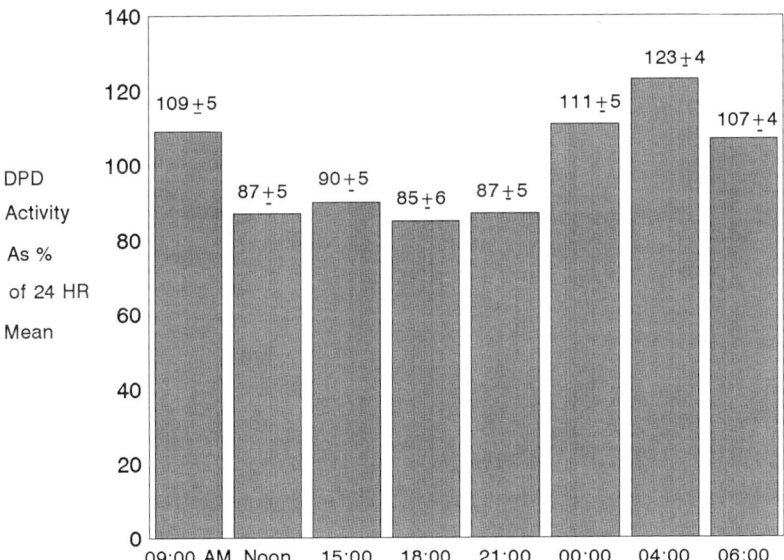

Figure 10 Dihydropyridine dehydrogenase activity in the circulating lymphocytes of seven normal subjects was found to vary throughout the day, with clearly higher levels during the middle of the night sleep span ($F = 7.29$, $p < 0.001$).

metabolism, as well as by cells more peripheral to 5-FU catabolism, may be responsible, at least in part, for the circadian dependence of 5-FU toxicity in rodents and humans and perhaps also for the circadian dependence of its anticancer efficacy documented in rodent models and, more recently, suggested by work with cancer patients.

The circadian pharmacology and biochemical pharmacology of FUDR are less clearly established than those of 5-FU, in part because the former drug is administered in much lower milligram amounts and requires much more sensitive analytic methods. This picture is also complicated by the fact that these two fluoropyrimidines are interconvertible. In preliminary experiments, von Roemeling et al. observed a twofold circadian difference in the convertibility of FUDR to 5-FU, indicating that FUDR pharmacodynamics may depend upon the circadian DPD rhythms at some times of the day but not others (30). The activities of other enzymes important in the activation of FUDR to FdUMP (i.e., dihydrouracil dehydrogenase, uridine phosphorylase, and thymidine phosphorylase) have each been shown to be subject to circadian rhythms in mouse liver (31); however, assessment of the exact contribution of these enzymes to the crisp, high-amplitude circadian rhythm in FUDR toxicity and efficacy requires further work in murine and human systems. Together, these preclinical and clinical results with fluoropyrimidine indicate that circadian time structure in the organs of catabolism and excretion and the biochemical enzyme activity rhythms in normal or malignant target cells may independently be critically important in determining the optimal time of day for bolus drug administration or the optimal circadian shape of continuous-infusion fluoropyrimidine therapy. Because the metabolic processes necessary to catabolize these two closely related drugs are different yet related and the intracellular targets are overlapping but to some extent distinct, the two agents have distinct optimal circadian timings that are nearly a third of a day apart (14).

In addition to the circadian patterns of crucial enzyme activities, circadian patterns of cytokinetic activity in malignant and nonmalignant tissues damaged by fluoropyrimidines may be of equal importance in explaining the circadian pharmacodynamics. Both 5-FU and FUDR are most active against dividing cells undergoing DNA synthesis in all tissues studied throughout the circadian cycle is nonrandomly distributed throughout the day (32). Depending on dose and duration of infusion, the gut, skin, and bone marrow are the primary targets of fluoropyrimidine toxicity. Human skin (33), bone marrow (34,35), colorectal mucosa have been found to exhibit marked circadian rhythms in DNA synthesis (36). When FUDR is infused such that lower levels are delivered during the early morning hours, the clinical toxicity is markedly diminished and the dose intensity can be safely elevated. In humans, the dose-limiting target of FUDR infusional toxicity is the colorectal mucosa. Serial biopsies of rectal mucosa every 3 h for 24 h from 24 human volunteers in both the fed and fasted states revealed that there is much greater in vitro uptake of [^{3}H]thymidine (presumably reflecting DNA synthesis) in colonic epithelial cells removed during the early morning hours than later in the day or evening (Buchi et al., unpublished). This circadian stage coincidence of minimal [^{3}H]thymidine uptake and minimal FUDR toxicity in colon epithelial cells is intriguing and warrants further study.

Few data are available to evaluate whether spontaneous human malignancies are cytokinetically coordinated on the circadian time scale. The most thorough evaluation of this difficult question was accomplished in patients with ovarian cancer. Klevecz et al. sampled cells washed from the peritoneal cavities of a large number of women every 2–4 h for up to 4 days. Using sophisticated cytofluorometric techniques, these investigators found circadian coordination of the proportion of malignant epithelial and nonmalignant mesothelial cells synthesizing DNA: that is, a higher proportion of malignant cells were engaged in DNA synthesis in the evening hours (37). In another study, a smaller number of patients with non-Hodgkin's lymphoma underwent thin-needle aspiration of tumor masses every 4 h for a minimum of 24 h. Some individuals and the group as a whole were found to exhibit large time-dependent differences, with peak activities clustering in the early morning hours (38). Serial biopsies of tumor and normal skin in one of our patients with widespread cutaneous epidermoid carcinoma revealed high-amplitude circadian rhythms in mitotic index of the tumor cell population with the same phase as in the patient's normal skin. Mitotic indices of tumor and normal tissues were identical at the times of lowest daily values, whereas tumor cell mitoses were manyfold more frequent at times during the day associated with the usual highest daily mitotic activity (Hrushesky et al., unpublished). These limited data suggest that the cytokinetic activity of tumor tissues is likely to be coordinated in circadian time and that there may well be windows in circadian time when cell cycle stage-specific attacks on these cells may be more or less effective.

V. CONCLUSION

Taken together, the preclinical and clinical data defining optimum timings of 5-FU and FUDR are compelling. The time-dependent differences in toxic-therapeutic ratios of these drugs are substantial, and we are now beginning to understand the biochemical and cellular mechanisms that contribute to these differences.

A complete understanding of circadian control mechanisms should not be a prerequisite for incorporation of these ideas into clinical trials. It is clear that many advances in the chemotherapeutic control of human malignancy have been gained without a sophisticated understanding of the mechanisms of action of each drug in effective chemotherapy regimens. In my view, our present knowledge of circadian pharmacology is sufficient to enable us not only to optimize the effectiveness of the chemotherapeutic agents currently in use but perhaps also to expand the repertoire of effective anticancer agents. It is daunting to realize that the scores of anticancer drugs discovered in murine screens and subsequently rejected in phase I trials because of unacceptably high toxicity were recommended for clinical study on the basis of murine toxicology and efficacy studies performed during the animals' usual sleep span and were later rejected clinically on the basis of studies routinely performed during the activity span of cancer patients.

As newer therapeutic approaches are developed with growth factors and other genetically engineered proteins, temporal questions become ever more important. We have already found, for example, that the LD_{50} for tumor necrosis factor varies by 1 log and its curative efficacy varies some sevenfold, depending on the time of day it is administered (39), that recombinant human erythropoietin increases reticulocyte response sevenfold if it is given at an optimal circadian stage (Wood et al., submitted), and that recombinant human interleukin-2 either doubles splenocyte (putative) natural killer cell number or fails to increase it, depending on whether it is given during the rest or activity phase of the murine circadian cycle (von Roemeling et al., submitted). A wide variety and rapidly growing number of programmable drug delivery strategies are being perfected and applied to the practical challenges of circadian-optimized treatment (40). We can no longer afford to deny either the existence or the importance of the circadian time structure of living organisms if we are to optimally apply both established and new technologies to effective cancer therapy.

VI. SUMMARY

For decades oncologists have been frustrated by the relentless biology of metastatic kidney cancer, which has resulted in an expected 3–6 month survival for its 12,000–15,000 annual victims. Although the disease's behavior, in aggregate, has been highly predictable and uniformly dismal, rare exceptions of prolonged survival or spontaneous regression indicate to the open minded that the overall balance between cancer and host can make a critical difference in determination of the ultimate outcome of this fascinating disease. This hopelessness associated with the diagnosis of metastatic renal cell carcinoma has been cracking during the last 5 years. Immunomodulation with interferons or interleukin-2 has clearly been shown to favorably modulate the host-tumor balance in a real minority of treated patients. Our approach of carefully examining a novel way of administering an antimetabolite shown previously not to have been useful in this disease has also yielded interesting results. FUDR is a pyrimidine nucleotide analog that damages cells (following conversion to FdUMP) only during the process of DNA synthesis by binding to thymidylate synthase. RCC is usually a very low growth fraction in tumor, and therefore we employed long-term continuous infusion for 14 of every 21–28 days. Normal gut and bone marrow cells synthesize DNA most actively in the later half of the night and first half of the morning: we therefore modulated the FUDR infusion so that most of each day's continuous daily dose is given in the early evening and first half of the night. With this approach, we have been able to increase the average safe dose intensity by 50%, diminish toxicity, and control progressive RCC in the majority of patients treated. Objective responses have occurred in 29% of patients, 40% of whom failed prior therapy. This therapy is accomplished entirely in an outpatient setting with a single visit every 2 weeks and minimal toxicity of life-style disruption. Recent results indicate that interleukin and interferon circadian timing are far more critical than the timing of FUDR. In fact, in our hands using a mouse tumor model system, improper IL-2 timing is as likely to result in tumor growth stimulation as proper timing is to result in tumor growth control. This chapter has briefly reviewed both the concepts and some recent results of circadian chronopharmacodynamics.

REFERENCES

1. Haus E, Halberg F, Scheving LE, et al. Increased tolerance of leukemic mice to arabinolsylcytosine with schedule adjusted to circadian system. Science 1972; 177:80–82.
2. Scheving LE, Haus E, Kuhl JFW, et al. Close reproduction by different laboratories of characteristics of circadian rhythm in 1-β-D-arabino-furanosylcytosine. Cancer Res 1976; 36:1133–7.
3. Freireich E. Ara-C: a twenty year update. J Clin Oncol 1987; 5(4):523–4.
4. Hrushesky WJM. Circadian timing of cancer chemotherapy. Science 1985; 228:73–5.
5. Levi F, Mechkouri M, Roulon A, et al. Circadian rhythm in tolerance of mice

for the new anthracycline analog 4'-O-tetrahydropyranyl adriamycin (THP). Eur J Cancer Clin Oncol 1985; 21:1245–51.

6. Mormont MC, von Roemeling R, Sothern RB, Berestka JS, Langevin TR, Hrushesky WJM. Circadian rhythm and seasonal dependence in tolerance of mice to 4'-epi-doxorubicin. Invest New Drugs 1988; 6:273–83.

7. Scheving LE, Burns ER, Pauly JE, et al. Survival and care of lukemic mice after circadian optimization of treatment with cyclophosphamide and 1-β-D-arabinofuranosylcytosine. Cancer Res 1977; 37:3648–55.

8. Sothern RB, Levi F, Haus E, Halberg F, Hrushesky WJM. Doxorubicin-cisplatin control of a murine plasmacytoma depends upon circadian stage of treatment. J Natl Cancer Inst 1988; 80:1232–7.

9. Hrushesky WJM. The clinical application of chronobiology to oncology. Am J Anat 1983; 168:519–42.

10. Hrushesky WJM, von Roemeling R, Sothern RB. Circadian chronotherapy: from animal experiments to human cancer chemotherapy. In: Lemmer B, ed. Chronopharmacology: cellular and biochemical interactions. New York: Dekker, 1989; 439–73.

11. Popovic P, Popovic V, Baughman J. Circadian rhythm and 5-fluorouracil toxicity in C3H mice. Biomed Therm 1982; 25:185–7.

12. Burns ER, Beland SS. Effect of biological time on the determination of the LD50 of 5-fluorouracil in mice. Pharmacology 1984; 28(2):96–300.

13. Peters GJ, Van Dijk J, Nadal JC, Van Groeningen CJ, Lankelma J, Pinedo HM. Diurnal variation in the therapeutic efficacy of 5-fluorouracil against murine colon cancer. In Vivo 1987; 1:113–8.

14. Gonzalez JL, Sothern RB, Thatcher G, Nguyen N, Hrushesky WJM. Substantial difference in timing of murine circadian susceptibility to 5-fluorouracil and FUDR. Proc AACR 1989; Abstract 2452.

15. Von Roemeling R, Hrushesky WJM. Circadian FUDR infusion pattern determines its therapeutic index. J Natl Cancer Inst 1990; In press.

16. Van Roemeling R, Hrushesky WJM. The advantage of circadian shaping of fluoropyrimidine infusions. In: Lokich JL, ed. Cancer chemotherapy by infusion, Vol. 2. Chicago: Precept Press, 1990; In press.

17. Hrushesky WJM, von Roemeling R, Lanning RM, Rabatin JT. Circadian shaped infusions of FUDR for progressive metastatic renal cell carcinoma. J Clin Oncol 1990; In press.

18. Levi F, Soussan A, Adam R, et al. Programmable-in-time pumps for chronotherapy of patients with colorectal cancer with 5-day circadian-modulated venous infusion of 5-fluorouracil (CVI-5FUra). Proc ASCO 1989; Abstract 429.

19. Sothern RB, Levi F, Haus E, Halberg F, Hrushesky WJM. Control of a murine plasmacytoma with doxorubicin-displatin: dependence in circadian stage of treatment. J Natl Cancer Inst 1989; 81:135–45.

20. Hrushesky WJM. Circadian timing of cancer chemotherapy. Science 1985; 228:73–5.

21. Von Roemeling R, Hrushesky WJM. Circadian patterning of continuous flox-uridine infusion reduces toxicity and allows higher dose intensity in patients with widespread cancer. 1989; 7:1710–9.

22. Hrushesky WJM, von Roemeling R, Lanning RM, Rabatin JT. Circadian-shaped infusions of floxuridine for progressive metastatic renal cell carcinoma. J Clin Onol 1990; 8:1504–13.

23. Hrushesky WJM, Bluming AZ, Gruber SA, Sothern RB. Menstral influence on surgical cure of breast cancer. Lancet 1989; 2:949–52.

24. Petit E, Milano G, Levi F, Thyss A, Bailleul F, Schneider M. Circadian rhythm-varying plasma concentration of 5-fluorouracil during a five-day continuous venous infusion at a constant rate in cancer patients. Cancer Res 1988; 48: 1676–9.

25. Harris BE, Song R, Soong SJ, Diasio RB. Relationship between dihy-dropyrimidine dehydrogenase activity and plasma 5-fluorouracil levels with evidence for circadian variation of enzyme activity and plasma drug levels in cancer patients receiving 5-fluorouracil by protracted continuous infusion. Cancer Res 1990; 50:197–201.

26. Tuchman M, Stoeckeler JS, Kiang DT, O'Dea RF, Ramnaraine ML, Mirkin BL. Familial pyrimidinemia and pyrimidinuria associated with severe fluorouracil toxicity. N Engl J Med 313:2445–9.

27. Diasio RB, Beavers TL, Carpenter JT. Familial deficiency of dihydropyrimidine dehydrogenase biochemical basis for familial pyrimidinemia and severe 5-fluorouracil-induced toxicity. J Clin Invest 1988; 81:47–51.

28. Tuchman M, von Roemeling R, Lanning R, Sothern RB, Hrushesky, WJM. Sources of variability of dihydropyrimidine dehydrogenase (DPD) activity in human blood mononuclear cells. Chronopharmacol 1988; 5:399–402.

29. Harris BE, Song R, Soong SJ, Diasio RB. Circadian variation of 5-fluorouracil catabolism in isolated perfused rat liver. Cancer Res 1989; 49:6610–4.

30. Von Roemeling R, Fukuda E, Rudin J, Mormont MC, Sothern R, Hrushesky WJM. Are FUDR pharmacokinetics circadian stage dependent? Proc AACR 1989; Abstract, 2345.

31. El Kouni MH, Naguib FMN, Cha S. Circadian rhythm of dihydrouracil dehy-drogenase (DHUDase), uridine phosphorylase (UrdPase), and thymidine phos-phorylase (dThdPase) in mouse liver. FASEB J 1989; 3:A397.

32. Scheving LE, Tsai TH, Feuers RJ, Scheving LA. Cellular mechanisms involved in the action of anticancer drugs. In: Lemmer B, ed. Chronopharmacology: cellular and biochemical interactions. New York: Dekker, 1989; 317–69.

33. Scheving LE. Mitotic activity in the human epidermis. Anat Rec 1959; 135: 7–19.

34. Mauer AM. Diurnal variation of proliferative activity in the human bone mar-row. Blood 1965; 26:1–7.

35. Smaaland R, Sletvold O, Bjerknes R, Lote K, Laerum OD. Circadian variations of cell cycle distribution in human bone marrow. Chronobiologia 1987; 14:239.

36. Buchi KN, Rubin NJ, Moore JG. Circadian cellular proliferation in human rectal mucosa. Annu Rev Chronopharmacol 1989; 5:355.
37. Klevecz RR, Shymko RM, Blumenfeld D, Braly PS. Circadian gating of S phase in human ovarian cancer. Cancer Res 1987; 47:6267–71.
38. Smaaland R, Lote K, Laerum OD, Vokac Z. A circadian study of cell cycle distribution in non-Hodgkin lymphomas. Annu Rev Chronopharmacol 1989; 5:383.
39. Langevin T, Young J, Walker K, von Roemeling R, Nygaard S, Hrushesky WJM. The toxicity of tumor necrosis factor (TNF) is reproducibly different at specific times of the day. Proc AACR 1987; 28:Abstract 281.
40. Hrushesky WJM. The rationale for non-zero-order drug delivery using automatic, computer-based drug delivery systems (chronotherapy). J Biol Response Mod 1988; 6:587–98.

Index

Adjuvant nephrectomy survival
  (*see also* Surgical
  treatment), 19
Adoptive immunotherapy:
  with bispecific monoclonal
    antibodies, 75
  with interferons, 6
  with LAK cells and IL-2, 6
  with tumor necrosis factor, 6
Adriamycin, 5

Bispecific monoclonal antibodies
  (*see* Monoclonal
  antibodies, bispecific)
Bone metastases as prognostic
  factor, 13, 14
Brain metastases as prognostic
  factor, 13–14

CD3 complex, 68
  T cell activation and, 68
Cell lines:
  expression of gp160 by, 87–88
  genetic changes in, 38, 57
  growth inhibition by IFN-α, 86
  oncogene transformation of,
    58–62
  properties of, 54
  viral transformation of, 56
Chromosome 3 (*see* Genetic
  changes, chromosome 3
  abnormalities)
Chromosome 7 (*see* Genetic
  changes, chromosome 7
  abnormalities)
Chronochemotherapy:
  definition of, 325–327
  with FUDR, 327–329

About the Editors

ERIC A. KLEIN is Head, Section of Urologic Oncology in the Department of Urology at The Cleveland Clinic Foundation, Ohio. The author or coauthor of more than 60 book chapters and professional papers, he is a Fellow of the American College of Surgeons and a member of the Society of Urologic Oncology, the American Urological Association, the Society for Basic Urological Research, and the American Association for Cancer Research, among other organizations. Dr. Klein received the M.D. degree (1981) from the University of Pittsburgh School of Medicine, Pennsylvania. He is a diplomate of the American Board of Urology.

RONALD M. BUKOWSKI is Director of the Experimental Therapeutics Program of the Cleveland Clinic Cancer Center at The Cleveland Clinic Foundation, and serves as a Professor of Medicine, Ohio State Medical School, Columbus, Ohio. A Fellow of the American College of Physicians and a member of the American Urological Association, the American Society of Clinical Oncology, and the American Society for Clinical Pharmacology and Therapeutics, among other organizations, he is the author of one book, the coeditor of two books, and the author or co author of over 130 professional papers and book chapters. Dr. Bukowski received the M.D. degree (1967) from Northwestern University, Evanston, Illinois, and is board certified in medical oncology and hematology.

JAMES H. FINKE is a Staff Scientist in the Department of Immunology at The Cleveland Clinic Foundation, Ohio. He is the author or coauthor of over 40 professional papers and a member of the American Association of Immunologists, the International Society for Interferon Research, and the American Association for Cancer Research, among other organizations. His research interests include particular attention to tumor immunology lymphokines/monokines, the generation of cytotoxic T lymphocytes, and immunotherapy. Dr. Finke received the Ph.D. degree (1973) in immunology from the University of Missouri, Columbia, and completed a postdoctoral Fellowship at the Albert Einstein College of Medicine, Bronx, New York.